W9-CPH-147

AIDS

AIDS

Cultural Analysis
Cultural Activism

edited by Douglas Crimp

contributions by Leo Bersani, Gregg Bordowitz, John Borneman, Douglas Crimp, Martha Gever, Sander L. Gilman, Jan Zita Grover, Amber Hollibaugh, Mitchell Karp, Carol Leigh, Max Navarre, PWA Coalition, Suki Ports, Katy Taylor, Paula A. Treichler, and Simon Watney

An OCTOBER Book

The MIT Press
Cambridge, Massachusetts
London, England

Third printing, 1991

First MIT Press edition, 1988

©1987 Massachusetts Institute of Technology and
October Magazine, Ltd. Originally published as
"Aids: Cultural Analysis/Cultural Activism,"
October 43, Winter 1987.

Printed and bound in the United States of America.

Library of Congress Cataloging-in-Publication Data

AIDS: cultural analysis/cultural activism.

   Bibliography: p.
   1. AIDS (Disease) — Social aspects. I. Crimp,
Douglas
RA644.A25A357 1988 362.1′9697′92 88-11148
ISBN 0-262-03140-X
ISBN 0-262-53079-1 (pbk.)

AIDS: Cultural Analysis/
Cultural Activism

DOUGLAS CRIMP

"I assert, to begin with, that 'disease' does not exist. It is therefore illusory to think that one can 'develop beliefs' about it to 'respond' to it. What does exist is not disease but practices." Thus begins François Delaporte's investigation of the 1832 cholera epidemic in Paris.[1] It is a statement we may find difficult to swallow, as we witness the ravages of AIDS in the bodies of our friends, our lovers, and ourselves. But it is nevertheless crucial to our understanding of AIDS, because it shatters the myth so central to liberal views of the epidemic: that there are, on the one hand, the scientific facts about AIDS and, on the other hand, ignorance or misrepresentation of those facts standing in the way of a rational response. I will therefore follow Delaporte's assertion: AIDS does not exist apart from the practices that conceptualize it, represent it, and respond to it. We know AIDS only in and through those practices. This assertion does not contest the existence of viruses, antibodies, infections, or transmission routes. Least of all does it contest the reality of illness, suffering, and death. What it *does* contest is the notion that there is an underlying reality of AIDS, upon which are con-structed the representations, or the culture, or the politics of AIDS. If we recognize that AIDS exists only in and through these constructions, then hope-fully we can also recognize the imperative to know them, analyze them, and wrest control of them.

Within the arts, the scientific explanation and management of AIDS is largely taken for granted, and it is therefore assumed that cultural producers can respond to the epidemic in only two ways: by raising money for scientific research and service organizations or by creating works that express the human suffering and loss. In an article for *Horizon* entitled "AIDS: The Creative Response," David Kaufman outlined examples of both, including benefits such as "Music for Life," "Dancing for Life," and "Art against AIDS," together with descriptions

---

1.   François Delaporte, *Disease and Civilization: The Cholera in Paris, 1832*, trans. Arthur Gold-hammer, Cambridge, Massachusetts, and London, England, MIT Press, 1986, p. 6.

of plays, literature, and paintings that take AIDS as their subject.[2] Regarding these latter "creative responses," Kaufman rehearses the clichés about art's "expressing feelings that are not easily articulated," "shar[ing] experiences and values through catharsis and metaphor," "demonstrating the indomitability of the human spirit," "consciousness raising." Art is what survives, endures, transcends; art constitutes our legacy. In this regard, AIDS is even seen to have a positive value: Kaufman quotes Michael Denneny of St. Martin's Press as saying, "We're on the verge of getting a literature out of this that will be a renaissance."[3]

In July 1987, PBS's *McNeil/Lehrer Newshour* devoted a portion of its program to "AIDS in the Arts." The segment opened with the shibboleth about "homosexuals" being "the lifeblood of show business and the arts," and went on to note the AIDS-related deaths of a number of famous artists. Such a pretext for a special report on AIDS is highly problematic, and on a number of counts: First, it reinforces the equation of AIDS and homosexuality, neglecting even to mention the possibility that an artist, like anyone else, might acquire AIDS heterosexually or through shared needles when shooting drugs. Secondly, it suggests that gay people have a *natural* inclination toward the arts, the homophobic flip side of which is the notion that "homosexuals control the arts" (ideas perfectly parallel with anti-Semitic attitudes that see Jews as, on the one hand, "making special contributions to culture," and, on the other, "controlling capital"). But most pernicious of all, it implies that gay people "redeem" themselves by being artists, and therefore that the deaths of other gay people are less tragic.[4] The message is that art, because it is timeless and universal, transcends individual lives, which are time-bound and contingent.

Entirely absent from the news report (and the *Horizon* article) was any mention of *activist* responses to AIDS by cultural producers. The focus was instead on the dramatic effect of the epidemic upon the art world, the coping with illness and death. Extended interviews with choreographers Bill T. Jones and his lover Arnie Zane, who has been diagnosed with AIDS, emphasized the "human face" of the disease in a way that was far more palatable than is usual in broadcast television, simply because it allowed the positive self-representations of both a person with AIDS and a gay relationship. Asked whether he thought "the

2.   David Kaufman, "AIDS: The Creative Response," *Horizon*, vol. 30, no. 9 (November 1987), pp. 13–20.
3.   Denneny is the editor of Randy Shilts's *And the Band Played On*, a discussion of which appears in my essay "How to Have Promiscuity in an Epidemic," pp. 237–271.
4.   Redemption, of course, necessitates a prior sin — the sin of homosexuality, of promiscuity, of drug use — and thus a program such as "AIDS in the Arts" contributes to the media's distribution of innocence and guilt according to who you are and how you acquired AIDS. Promiscuous gay men and IV drug users are unquestionably guilty in this construction, but so are all people from poor minority populations. The special attention paid to artists and other celebrities with AIDS is nevertheless contradictory. While a TV program such as "Aids in the Arts" virtually beatifies the stricken artist, for personalities such as Rock Hudson and Liberace the scandal of being found guilty of homosexuality tarnishes the halo of their celebrity status.

arts are particularly hit by AIDS," Zane replied, "That's the controversial question this month, right?" but then went on to say, "Of course I do. I am in the center of this world, the art world. . . . I am losing my colleagues." Colleen Dewhurst, president of Actors Equity, suggested rather that "AIDS-related deaths are not more common among artists, only more visible," and continued, "Artists are supposed to represent the human condition . . ." (a condition that is, of course, assumed to be universal).

"Art lives on forever"—this idealist platitude came from Elizabeth Taylor, National Chairman of the American Foundation for AIDS Research, shown addressing the star-studded crowd at the gala to kick off "Art against AIDS." But strangely it was Richard Goldstein, writer for the *Village Voice* and a committed activist on the subject of AIDS, who contributed the broadcast's most unabashed statement of faith in art's transcendence of life: "In an ironic sense, I think that AIDS is good for art. I think it will produce great works that will outlast and transcend the epidemic."

It would appear from such a statement that what is at stake is not the survival of people with AIDS and those who might now be or eventually become infected with HIV, but rather the survival, even the flourishing, of art. For Goldstein, this is surely less a question of hopelessly confused priorities, however, than of a failure to recognize the alternatives to this desire for transcendence—a failure determined by the intractability of the traditional idealist conception of art, which entirely divorces art from engagement in lived social life.

Writing in the catalogue of "Art against AIDS," Robert Rosenblum affirms this limited and limiting view of art and the passivity it entails:

> By now, in the 1980s, we are all disenchanted enough to know that no work of art, however much it may fortify the spirit or nourish the eye and mind, has the slightest power to save a life. Only science can do that. But we also know that art does not exist in an ivory tower, that it is made and valued by human beings who live and die, and that it can generate a passionate abundance of solidarity, love, intelligence, and most important, money.[5]

There could hardly be a clearer declaration of the contradictions inherent in aesthetic idealism than one which blandly accepts art's inability to intervene in the social and simultaneously praises its commodity value. To recognize this as contradictory is not, however, to object to exploiting that commodity value for the purpose of fundraising for AIDS research and service. Given the failure of government at every level to provide the funding necessary to combat the epidemic, such efforts as "Art against AIDS" have been necessary, even crucial to our survival. I want, nevertheless, to make three caveats.

5.   Robert Rosenblum, "Life Versus Death: The Art World in Crisis," in *Art against AIDS*, New York, American Foundation for AIDS Research, 1987, p. 32.

1. Scientific research, health care, and education are the *responsibility and purpose* of government and not of so-called "private initiative," an ideological term that excuses and perpetuates the state's irresponsibility. Therefore, every venture of this nature should make clear that it is necessitated strictly because of criminal negligence on the part of government. What we find, however, is the very opposite:

> Confronting a man-made evil like the war in Vietnam, we could assail a government and the people in charge. But how do we confront a diabolically protean virus that has been killing first those pariahs of grass-roots America, homosexuals and drug addicts, and has then gone on to kill, with far less moral discrimination, even women, children, and heterosexual men? We have recourse only to love and to science, which is what *Art against AIDS* is all about.[6]

2. Blind faith in science, as if it were entirely neutral and uncontaminated by politics, is naive and dangerous. It must be the responsibility of everyone contributing to fundraisers to know enough about AIDS to determine whether the beneficiary will put the money to the best possible use. How many artists and dealers contributing to "Art against AIDS," for example, know precisely what kinds of scientific research are supported by the American Foundation for AIDS Research? How many know the alternatives to AmFAR's research agenda, alternatives such as the Community Research Initiative, an effort at testing AIDS treatments initiated at the community level by PWAs themselves? As anyone involved in the struggle against AIDS knows from horrendous experience, we cannot afford to leave anything up to the "experts." We must become our own experts.[7]

3. Raising money is the most passive response of cultural practitioners to social crisis, a response that perpetuates the idea that art itself has no social function (aside from being a commodity), that there is no such thing as an engaged, activist aesthetic practice. It is this third point that I want to underscore

---

6.   *Ibid.*, p. 28. I hope we can assume that Rosenblum intends his remarks about "pariahs" and "moral discrimination" ironically, although this is hardly what I would call politically sensitive writing. It could easily be read without irony, since it so faithfully reproduces what is written in the press virtually every day. And the implication of the "even women" in the category distinct from "homosexuals" is, once again, that there's no such thing as a lesbian. But can we expect political sensitivity from someone who cannot see that AIDS is political? that *science* is political? It was science, after all, that conceptualized AIDS as a gay disease — and wasted precious time scrutinizing our sex lives, theorizing about killer sperm, and giving megadoses of poppers to mice at the CDC — all the while taking little notice of the others who were dying of AIDS, and thus allowing HIV to be injected into the veins of vast numbers of IV drug users, as well as of hemophiliacs and other people requiring blood transfusions.

7.   I do not wish to cast suspicion on AmFAR, but rather to suggest that no organization can be seen as neutral or objective. See, in this regard, the exchange of letters on AmFAR's rejection of the Community Research Initiative's funding applications in the *PWA Coalition Newsline*, no. 30 (January 1988), pp. 3–7.

by insisting, against Rosenblum, that art *does* have the power to save lives, and it is this very power that must be recognized, fostered, and supported in every way possible. But if we are to do this, we will have to abandon the idealist conception of art. We don't need a cultural renaissance; we need cultural practices actively participating in the struggle against AIDS. We don't need to transcend the epidemic; we need to end it.

What might such a cultural practice be? One example appeared in November 1987 in the window on Broadway of New York's New Museum of Contemporary Art. Entitled *Let the Record Show* . . . , it is the collective work of ACT UP (the AIDS Coalition to Unleash Power), which is — I repeat what is stated at the beginning of every Monday night meeting — "a nonpartisan group of diverse individuals united in anger and committed to direct action to end the AIDS crisis." More precisely, *Let the Record Show* . . . is the work of an ad hoc committee within ACT UP that responded to the New Museum's offer to do the window installation. The offer was tendered by Curator Bill Olander, himself a participant in ACT UP.

> I first became aware of ACT UP, like many other New Yorkers, when I saw a poster appear on lower Broadway with the equation: SILENCE=DEATH. Accompanying these words, sited on a black background, was a pink triangle — the symbol of homosexual persecution during the Nazi period and, since the 1960s, the emblem of gay liberation. For anyone conversant with this iconography, there was no question that this was a poster designed to provoke and heighten awareness of the AIDS crisis. To me, it was more than that: it was among the most significant works of art that had yet been done which was inspired and produced within the arms of the crisis.[8]

That symbol, made of neon, occupied the curved portion of the New Museum's arched window. Below it, in the background, and bathed in soft, even light, was a photomural of the Nuremberg Trials (in addition to prosecuting Nazi war criminals, those trials established our present-day code of medical ethics, involving such things as informed consent to experimental medical procedures). In front of this giant photo are six life-size, silhouetted photographs of "AIDS criminals" in separate, boxed-in spaces, and below each one the words by which he or she may be judged by history, cast — literally — in concrete. As the light goes on in each of these separate boxed spaces, we can see the face and read the words:

8.   Bill Olander, "The Window on Broadway by ACT UP," in *On View* (handout), New York, New Museum of Contemporary Art, 1987, p. 1. The logo that Olander describes is not the work of ACT UP, but of a design collective called the SILENCE=DEATH Project, which has lent the logo to ACT UP.

The logical outcome of testing is a quarantine of those infected.
— Jesse Helms, US Senator

It is patriotic to have the AIDS test and be negative.
— Cory Servaas, Presidential AIDS Commission

We used to hate faggots on an emotional basis. Now we have a good reason.

— anonymous surgeon

AIDS is God's judgment of a society that does not live by His rules.
— Jerry Falwell, televangelist

Everyone detected with AIDS should be tattooed in the upper forearm, to protect common needle users, and on the buttocks to prevent the victimization of other homosexuals.
— William F. Buckley, columnist

And finally, there is a blank slab of concrete, above which is the silhouetted photograph of President Reagan. We look up from this blank slab and see, once again, the neon sign: SILENCE=DEATH.

But there is more. Suspended above this rogues' gallery is an electronic information display programmed with a running text, portions of which read as follows:

Let the record show . . . William F. Buckley deflects criticism of the government's slow response to the epidemic through calculations: "At most three years were lost . . . Those three years have killed approximately 15,000 people; if we are talking 50 million dead, then the cost of delay is not heavy . . .

Let the record show . . . The Pentagon spends in one day more than the government spent in the last five years for AIDS research and education . . .

Let the record show . . . In June 1986, $47 million was allocated for new drug trials to include 10,000 people with AIDS. One year later only 1,000 people are currently enrolled. In that time, over 9,000 Americans have died of AIDS.

Let the record show . . . In 1986, Dr. Cory Servaas, editor of the *Saturday Evening Post*, announced that after working closely with the National Institutes of Health, she had found a cure for AIDS. At the time, the National Institutes of Health officials said that they had never heard of Dr. Cory Servaas. In 1987, President Reagan appointed Dr. Cory Servaas to the Presidential AIDS Commission.

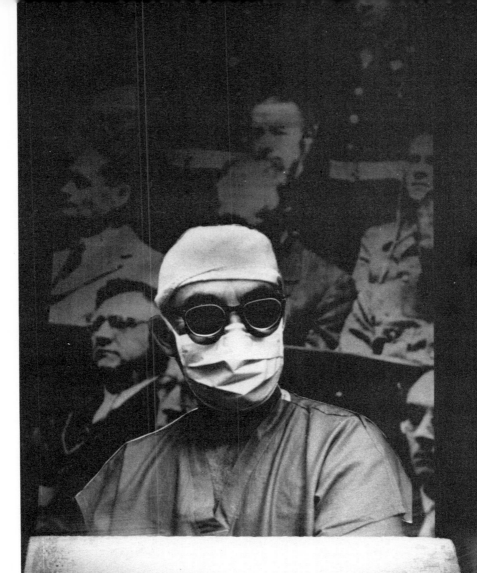

"WE USED TO HATE FAGGOTS
ON AN EMOTIONAL BASIS.
NOW WE HAVE GOOD REASON."

ANONYMOUS SURGEON

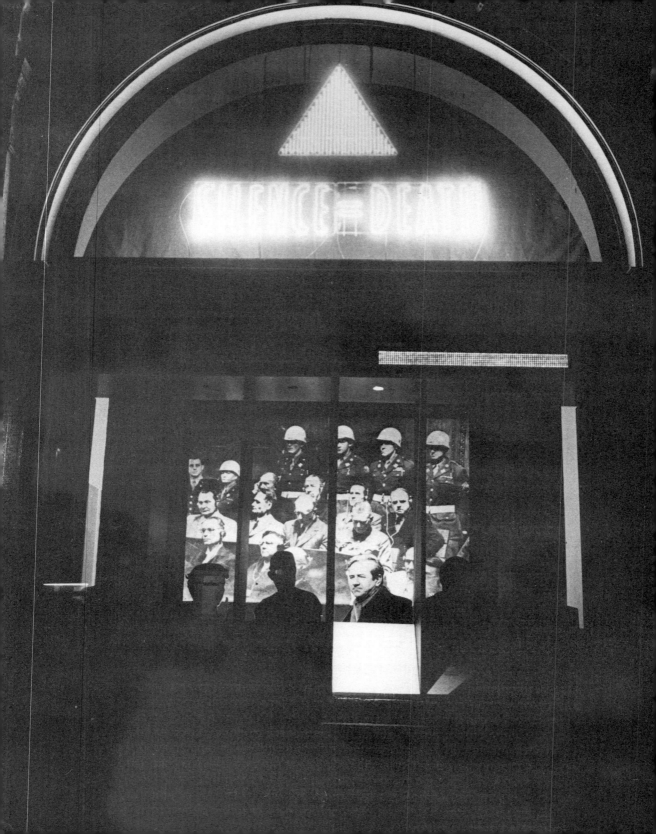

Let the record show . . . In October of 1986, $80 million was allocated for public education about AIDS. 13 months later there is still no national education program. In that time, over 15,000 new cases have been reported.

Let the record show . . . 54% of the people with AIDS in New York City are black and Hispanic. The incidence of heterosexually transmitted AIDS is 17 times higher among blacks than whites, 15 times higher among Hispanics than whites. 88% of babies with AIDS are black and Hispanic. 6% of the US AIDS education budget has been targeted for the minority community.

And finally:

By Thanksgiving 1981, 244 known dead . . . AIDS . . . no word from the President.

By Thanksgiving 1982, 1,123 known dead . . . AIDS . . . no word from the President.

The text continues like this, always with no word from the President, until finally:

By Thanksgiving 1987, 25,644 known dead . . . AIDS . . . President Reagan: "I have asked the Department of Health and Human Services to determine as soon as possible the extent to which the AIDS virus has penetrated our society."

After each of these bits of information, the sign flashes, "Act Up, Fight Back, Fight AIDS," a standard slogan at ACT UP demonstrations. Documentary footage from some of these demonstrations could be seen in the videotape *Testing the Limits: New York*, programmed at the New Museum simultaneously with the window display. The video about AIDS activism in New York City is the work of a collective (also called Testing the Limits) "formed to document emerging forms of activism arising out of people's responses to government inaction in the global AIDS epidemic."

The SILENCE=DEATH Project, the group from ACT UP who made *Let the Record Show* . . . , and Testing the Limits share important premises that can teach us much about engaged art practices. First, they are *collective* endeavors. Second, these practices are employed by the collectives' members as an essential part of their AIDS activism. This is not to say that the individuals involved are not artists in the more conventional sense of the word; many of these people work within the precincts of the traditional art world and its institutions. But involvement in the AIDS crisis has not left their relation to that world unaltered. After making *Let the Record Show* . . . for the New Museum, for example, the group from ACT UP reconvened and decided to continue their work. Among the general principles discussed at their first meeting, one was unanimously voiced: "We have to get out of Soho, get out of the art world."

The New Museum has been more hospitable than most art institutions to socially and politically committed art practices, and it was very courageous of the museum to offer space to an activist organization rather than to an artist. It is also very useful that the museum has a window on lower Broadway that is passed by many people who would never set foot in an art museum. But if we think about art in relation to the AIDS epidemic—in relation, that is, to the communities most drastically affected by AIDS, especially the poor and minority communities where AIDS is spreading much faster than elsewhere—we will realize that no work made within the confines of the art world as it is currently constituted will reach these people. Activist art therefore involves questions not only of the nature of cultural production, but also of the location, or the means of distribution, of that production. *Let the Record Show . . .* was made for an art-world location, and it appears to have been made largely for an art-world audience. By providing information about government inaction and repressive intentions in the context of shocking statistics, its purpose is to inform—and thereby to mobilize—its presumably sophisticated audience (an audience presumed, for example, to be able to recognize a photograph of the Nuremberg Trials).[9] Such information and mobilization *can* (contra Rosenblum) save lives; indeed, until a cure for AIDS is developed, *only* information and mobilization can save lives.

In New York City, virtually every official campaign of highly visible public information about AIDS—whether AIDS education in schools, public service announcements on TV, or posters in the subways—must meet with the approval of, among others, the immensely powerful and reactionary Cardinal John J. O'Connor. This has resulted in a murderous regime of silence and disinformation that virtually guarantees the mounting deaths of sexually active young people—gay and straight—and of IV drug users, their sex partners, and their children, most of them from poor, minority populations. Recognizing this, small coalitions of cultural workers, including a group calling itself the Metropolitan Health Association and the ACT UP committee that created *Let the Record Show . . .* , have taken to the streets and subways to mount education campaigns of their own. Employing sophisticated graphics and explicit information, printed in English and Spanish, these artists and activists are attempting to get the unambiguous word out about how safe sex and clean works can protect people from contracting HIV. Even apart from the possibility of arrest, the difficulties faced by these people are daunting. Their work demands a total reevaluation of the nature and purpose of cultural practices in conjunction with an understand-

9.   Whether or not the audience was also presumed to be able to see a connection between *Let the Record Show . . .* and the procedures and devices of artists such as Hans Haacke, Jenny Holzer, and Barbara Kruger is an open question.

*Metropolitan Health Association. Clean works
information for New York City subways. 1988.
(Photo: Diane Neumaier.)*

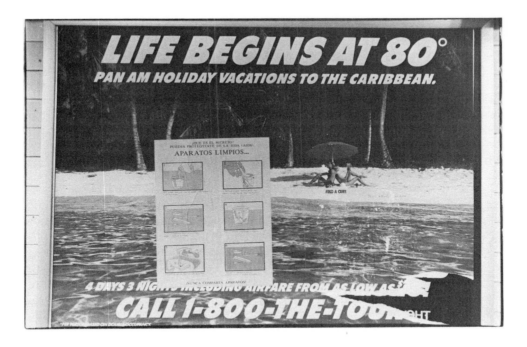

ing of the political goals of AIDS activism. It requires, in addition, a comprehensive knowledge of routes of HIV transmission and means of prevention, as well as a sensitivity to cultural specificity — to, say, the street language of Puerto Ricans as opposed to that of Spanish-speaking immigrants from Central or South America.

Even having adopted new priorities and accumulated new forms of knowledge, the task of cultural producers working within the struggle against AIDS will be difficult. The ignorance and confusion enforced by government and the dominant media; the disenfranchisement and immiseration of many of the people thus far hardest hit by AIDS; and the psychic resistence to confronting sex, disease, and death in a society where those subjects are largely taboo — all of these conditions must be faced by anyone doing work on AIDS. Cultural activism is only now beginning; also just beginning is the recognition and support of this work by art-world institutions.

Among those institutions, apart from the New Museum, I want to mention and credit two. Due to momentum gathering among students and faculty at the California Institute of the Arts in the previous year, the school developed a program of AIDS-related activities for 1987–88. These included a course entitled "Media(ted) AIDS" given by Jan Zita Grover and open to the entire student body; an agreement by the faculty to spend one-tenth of the overall budget for visiting artists and lecturers on presentations about AIDS-related work; a commitment by the library to spend one-quarter of its video acquisition budget on tapes about AIDS; and the inclusion of AIDS information in the monthly student newsletter (this information was also regularly silkscreened onto the school's walls). The value of such a coordinated program is that students can both receive (but also generate) information that can help them personally *and* begin to reconsider their roles as artists working in a moment of social crisis.

To date, a majority of cultural producers working in the struggle against AIDS have used the video medium. There are a number of explanations for this: Much of the dominant discourse on AIDS has been conveyed through television, and this discourse has generated a critical counter-practice in the same medium; video can sustain a fairly complex array of information; and cable access and the widespread use of VCRs provide the potential of a large audience for this work.[10] In October 1987, the American Film Institute Video Festival included a series entitled "Only Human: Sex, Gender, and Other Misrepresentations," organized by Bill Horrigan and B. Ruby Rich. Of eight programs in the series, three were devoted to videotapes on AIDS. Among the more than twenty videos, a full range of independent work was represented, including tapes made for broadcast TV (*AIDS in the Arts*), AIDS education tapes (*Sex, Drugs, and AIDS*, made for the New York City school system), and "art" tapes (*News from Home*, by Tom Kalin and Stathis Lagoudakis); music videos (*The ADS Epidemic*, by John Greyson), documentaries (*Testing the Limits*), and critiques of the media (*A Plague on You*, by the Lesbian and Gay Media Group). The intention of the program was not to select work on the basis of aesthetic merit, but rather to show something of the range of representations and counter-representations of AIDS. As B. Ruby Rich stated it in the catalogue:

> To speak of sexuality and the body, and not also speak of AIDS, would be, well, obscene. At the same time, the peculiarly key role being played by the media in this scenario makes it urgent that counter-images and counter-rhetoric be created and articulated. To this end, we have grouped the AIDS tapes together in three special programs to allow the dynamic of their interaction to produce its own discourse — and to allow the inveterate viewer to begin making the aesthetic diagnosis that is quickly becoming every bit as urgent as (particularly in the absence of) the medical one.[11]

10.   For a good overview of both commercial television and independent video productions about AIDS, see Timothy Landers, "Bodies and Anti-Bodies: A Crisis in Representation," *The Independent*, vol. 11, no. 1 (January–February 1988), pp. 18–24.
11.   B. Ruby Rich, "Only Human: Sex, Gender, and Other Misrepresentations," in *1987 American Film Institute Video Festival*, Los Angeles, 1987, p. 42.

*

The preparation of this OCTOBER publication on AIDS stemmed initially from my encounters with several works both in and about the media: Simon Watney's book *Policing Desire: AIDS, Pornography, and the Media*; Stuart Marshall's video *Bright Eyes*, made for Britain's Channel 4; and the documentary about AIDS activism in New York, *Testing the Limits*. In addition, I learned that Amber Hollibaugh, of the AIDS Discrimination Unit of the New York City Commission on Human Rights, was at work on *The Second Epidemic*, a documentary about AIDS-related discrimination. From the beginning my intention was to show, through discussion of these works, that there was a critical, theoretical, activist alternative to the personal, elegiac expressions that appeared to dominate the art-world response to AIDS. What seemed to me essential was a vastly expanded view of culture in relation to crisis. But the full extent to which this view would have to be expanded only became clear through further engagement with the issues. AIDS intersects with and requires a critical rethinking of all of culture: of language and representation, of science and medicine, of health and illness, of sex and death, of the public and private realms. AIDS is a central issue for gay men, of course, but also for lesbians. AIDS is an issue for women generally, but especially for poor and minority women, for child-bearing women, for women working in the health care system. AIDS is an issue for drug users, for prisoners, for sex workers. At some point, even "ordinary" heterosexual men will have to learn that AIDS is an issue for them, and not simply because they might be susceptible to "contagion."

The unevenness with which these questions are addressed in this publication, the priority given to gay issues (and to gay writers), reflects, in part, the history of organized response to AIDS in the US. Gay men and lesbians joined the struggle first and are still on its front lines. The unevenness is compensated, however, by the involvement of these people (and, increasingly, of straight women) in *all* the issues raised by AIDS, a development that is reflected in the work published here. (A gay friend about to embark on a poster campaign— using the recently released statistic that one in sixty-one babies born in New York City are HIV positive—spoke of the irony of a bunch of faggots trying to educate heterosexuals about safe sex practices.)[12] But there are lacunae that I regret, the most important of which is attention to the cataclysmic problem of AIDS in the Third World, a problem about which one hears only a deafening silence in the dominant media in the US.

---

12. An even more profound irony is the fact that often only gay people are willing to act as foster parents for HIV-positive children, and at a time when gay parenting is increasingly coming under attack by both federal and state governments. A special commission of the Reagan Administration has recommended against lesbians and gay men as potential foster parents, and several states have passed laws explicitly forbidding gay people to adopt children. In addition, gay parents are often refused custody of their natural children solely on the grounds of sexual orientation.

*

It has taken the work of many people to make this publication what it is. I want to thank all of the contributors, both those who turned their attentions from usual concerns to think and write about AIDS and those activists who found the extra time and energy to write for an academic publication. The People with AIDS Coalition in New York generously put the full run of their *Newsline* at my disposal and granted me a free hand in making selections from it. Information, leads, and illustrational materials were provided by the Gay Men's Health Crisis, Jan Zita Grover, Isaac Julien, Tom Kalin, Diane Neumaier, Jim Steakley, Frank Wagner, and Michael Wessmann; and Terri Cafaro, Joan Copjec, and Cathy Scott helped with various aspects of production.

My own education about AIDS was made considerably easier by the agreement of members of my reading group to spend several months discussing the subject and looking at videotapes, and I therefore want to acknowledge the participation of Terri Cafaro, Carlos Espinosa, Martha Gever, Timothy Landers, Eileen O'Neill, and our short-term guests Lee Quinby and Jane Rubin. Attendance at the regular Monday night meetings of ACT UP provided me with up-to-the-minute information and helped clarify many issues. Finally, I want to acknowledge the sustained involvement of Gregg Bordowitz, who has helped in countless ways.

AIDS: Keywords

JAN ZITA GROVER

In 1956 Raymond Williams delivered to his publisher the manuscript of *Culture and Society*, which contained a lengthy appendix tracing the shifting meanings of sixty words Williams considered central to explorations of culture. The publisher demanded a shorter text, and Williams's "keywords" were sacrificed. But twenty years and many entries later, *Keywords: A Vocabulary of Culture and Society* was published; its aim was "to show that some important social and historical processes occur *within* language, in ways which indicate how integral the problems of meanings and relationships really are."[1]

The kinds of words that Williams traced were invented or reimagined at the straining points where old social relationships were giving way to new ones. These words were neologisms (*capitalism*), adaptations or alterations of existing terms (*society* and *individual*), extensions (*interest*) or transfers (*exploitation*) of earlier meanings. Williams read such changes in commonly held meanings as barometers of more widespread shifts in society and culture, as indicators of "very interesting periods of confusion and contradiction of outcome, latencies in decision, and other processes of a real social history, which can be located rather precisely in this other [i.e., linguistic] way, and put alongside more familiar kinds of evidence."[2]

The advent of AIDS as a socially meaningful fact in the West has generated an enormous outpouring of words. Across journalistic, political, and medical discourses, a number of terms recur with such regularity that we might be tempted to conclude that AIDS has brought the worlds of the scientist and the humanist closer together. But we might also—and with greater plausibility— explain this phenomenon as an indication that certain shared assumptions are already embedded in these discourses.

1. Raymond Williams, "Introduction" to *Keywords*, revised edition, New York, Oxford University Press, 1983, p. 22 (the first edition was published by Fontana, London, in 1976). Williams's account of the history of *Keywords* can be found in this introduction, pp. 11–15, and in *Raymond Williams: Politics and Letters*, London, Verso, 1981, pp. 175–177.
2. Williams, *Politics and Letters*, p. 177.

It was Williams's hope that his *Keywords* might open up critical public scrutiny of "a crucial area of social and historical discussion" so that the language used to describe our world could be adapted or changed to fit that reality, rather than passively accepted as an already authorized tradition. Such a critical attention to language is essential to our understanding of and response to AIDS as the cultural construction that it is. AIDS is not simply a physical malady; it is also an artifact of social and sexual transgression, violated taboo, fractured identity — political and personal projections. Its keywords, like those isolated by Williams, are primarily the property of the powerful. "AIDS: Keywords" is my attempt to identify and contest some of the assumptions underlying our current knowledge. In this I am joined by many AIDS activists, including people living with AIDS.

It is my hope, as it was Williams's, that identification of some of these terms might contribute "not resolution but perhaps, at times, just that extra edge of consciousness. In a social history in which many crucial meanings have been shaped by a dominant class, and by particular professions operating to a large extent within its terms, the sense of edge is accurate. This is not a neutral review of meanings."[3]

*

acquired immune deficiency syndrome (AIDS) Jacques Leibowitch asks in *A Strange Virus of Unknown Origin* (1985): How do we know when we are faced with a new sickness, something that has not existed before, that cannot be understood and treated under an already existing rubric?

What is now called AIDS was first pieced together in 1981, when physicians in New York, Los Angeles, and San Francisco, some of whom had noted long-term enlarged lymph nodes (persistent generalized lymphadenopathy) in many of their gay clients as early as 1979, began seeing gay men with cases of *Pneumocystis carinii* pneumonia (PCP) and Kaposi's sarcoma (KS), a cancer of the blood vessels that usually follows a slow and relatively benign course and had most often been found among Central Africans and elderly men of Mediterranean origin.

The virulency of PCP and KS in these young men pointed to an underlying immune deficiency, since adults with intact immune systems are not normally prey to either disease, although both had been seen before in organ-transplant patients with deliberate, drug-induced immunosuppression and cancer patients whose immunosuppression was due to chemotherapy. Initially the complex of KS/PCP was termed GRID (gay-related immunodeficiency) or AID (acquired immune deficiency). As more symptoms, diseases, and invading organisms were identified, the complex was further qualified by the medical term *syndrome*, "a set of symptoms which occur together; the sum of signs of any morbid state; a

---

3.   Williams, *Keywords*, p. 24.

symptom complex.''[4] The term *AIDS,* for acquired immune deficiency syndrome, was officially adopted by the Centers for Disease Control (CDC) in 1982.

There is a significant distinction to be made between a syndrome and a disease (see below), a distinction that is *not* commonly made in the case of AIDS: a syndrome is a pattern of symptoms pointing to a ''morbid state,'' which may or may not be caused by infectious agents; a disease, on the other hand, is ''any deviation from or interruption of the normal structure or function of any part, organ, or system (or combination thereof) of the body that is manifested by a characteristic set of symptoms or signs and whose etiology, pathology, and prognosis may be known or unknown.''[5] In other words, a syndrome points to or signifies the underlying disease process(es), while a disease is constituted in and by those processes.

This is not merely a semantic distinction. Diseases can be communicable, syndromes cannot. What constitutes AIDS is an immune deficiency produced by the Human Immunodeficiency Virus (HIV). In the US, a severe immune deficiency results in a fairly invariable set of symptoms—in this case *diseases as symptoms*: PCP, KS, severe cytomegolovirus and herpes infections, and so on. In poor, tropical countries, the frequency of particular infections is different. In Central Africa, for example, tuberculosis and toxoplasmosis are more common than they are in the US. In Haiti, PCP is hardly seen at all, but the incidence of cryptosporidiosis and isospora infections is much higher. These differences point to the fact that immune suppression evincing itself as AIDS works with whatever is already present, though generally quiescent, in an HIV-infected population.

Unlike most infectious diseases, those that commonly afflict people with AIDS are usually incapable of causing overt illness in people with intact immune systems; because they are seizers of the opportunity provided by immune suppression, these diseases are called opportunistic infections. Thus, the syndrome AIDS cannot itself be contracted, nor can the opportunistic infections that constitute the syndrome be readily communicated to those with healthy immune systems. What *can* be contracted is the Human Immunodeficiency Virus.

AIDS . . . the disease The popular press, politicians, and physicians regularly move from ''acquired immune deficiency syndrome . . . AIDS'' to ''AIDS . . . the disease.'' What are the consequences of this shift?

Diseases, we are taught, are often communicable, the general term applied to both infectious and contagious diseases. In discussions of AIDS, because of distinctions *not* made—between syndrome and disease, between infectious and contagious—there is often a casual slippage from *communicable* to *contagious.*

4.   *Dorland's Medical Dictionary,* 26th edition, Philadelphia, W. B. Saunders, 1985.
5.   *Ibid.*

From this semantic error flow many consequences, not the least of which is widespread public terror about "catching" AIDS through casual contact.

Public health reports on the cause of AIDS initially and repeatedly compared it to the hepatitis B virus (HBV), since both appeared to be blood-borne and sexually transmitted, and both were found with great frequency among urban gay men. But in significant ways, HIV and HBV are not similar at all: HBV is far more infectious and far smaller, making it more difficult to control (for example, HBV can pass through natural-membrane condoms whereas HIV cannot). Nevertheless, the similarities — sexual and intravenous transmission — are such socially charged ones that they have masked the more important differences between HIV and HBV. The result is that AIDS, a terminal phase of HIV infection, is firmly fixed in people's minds as an HBV-like "disease" — highly infectious, easily spread to the unsuspecting drinker or diner.

AIDS test In 1983–84, French and American researchers managed to isolate and culture HIV-infected human T-cell lines, which led to the identification of HIV as the principal causative agent of AIDS. Once HIV could be grown in quantity, it became possible to use protein extracted from inactivated virus as a basis for an HIV antibody test. The enzyme-linked immunosorbent assay (ELISA) was rapidly developed and placed on the commercial market in March 1985 to be used as a screening test for donor blood in US blood banking.

The ELISA reacts to the presence of antibodies to HIV in a subject's serum; antibodies indicate that the subject's immune system is fighting a foreign protein or sugar molecule (in this case, HIV) that has signaled its presence. There is no consensus among scientists and physicians on the significance of HIV antibody positivity. It may signal either active infection or the body's successful fight against infection. Practically, however, HIV antibody positivity is taken as an indicator of infection with the virus, and the antibody positive person is *assumed* to be infectious (i.e., the person's blood, semen, breast milk, and organs and tissues for transplant are assumed to be capable of infecting another).

Like the term *AIDS virus* (see below), use of the term *AIDS test* implies that the invariable outcome of HIV antibody positivity is AIDS, that HIV positivity *is* AIDS. The phrase is employed regularly in the *New York Times* and *Los Angeles Times, Time* and *Newsweek*, the tabloids and television commentary. Among the consequences of this causal and *casual* linkage between antibody positive status and the end-drome, AIDS, are statutes such as the Illinois state law mandating "the AIDS test" as a condition for taking out a marriage license, and John Doolittle's California Senate Bill 1001, which the *Los Angeles Times* dutifully reported as "requir[ing] that the AIDS test be offered . . . to all applicants for marriage licenses." State bills mandating "the AIDS test" for convicted prostitutes, prisoners, and inmates of state mental institutions are under consideration nationwide; the federal government is already implementing "routine AIDS testing" of immigrants, the military, job corps personnel, some State Department personnel, and federal prisoners.

AIDS virus A seemingly ineradicable term, *AIDS virus* is almost universally employed by the popular press and is increasingly used by physicians, scientists, and public health planners. The effect of this usage, which conflates HIV with a terminal phase of HIV infection—AIDS—is to equate infection with death. It also supposes that the invariable outcome of HIV infection is death, whereas every other known virus's natural history suggests that a spectrum of outcomes is possible, ranging from quiescent, asymptomatic infection to symptomatic but subacute, to, in the case of HIV infection, immune exhaustion and subsequent infection by opportunistic infections and neoplasms; only the latter is clinically defined as AIDS.

AIDS virus, then, is a term more projective than descriptive. It imposes a mortal sentence on anyone infected with HIV, a projection of hostility and fear that bespeaks another's death in order to quell one's own anxieties.

bisexual Popular faith in the balkanization of sexual desire being what it is, how can we explain the "spread" (see below) of HIV infection into "the general population" (see below)? Enter the epidemic's new bête noire, the bisexual. Only *he* (in AIDS discussions, bisexuals are always male) can account for and absolve the heterosexual majority of any taint of unlawful desire.

The bisexual is seen as a creature of uncontrollable impulses—"their internal desire may make them more dangerous"—whose activities are invariably covert—"because of their double lives, they may be the most difficult group to reach and counsel" (Chris Norwood, *Advice for Life: A Woman's Guide to AIDS Risks*, 1987). Dr. Art Ulene, the *Today Show*'s resident "family physician," fingers the bisexual as the furtive source of spread: "It also takes only one bisexual to introduce the AIDS virus [*sic*] into the heterosexual community [see below]. . . . The risk is easily hidden when they are having sex with women" (*Safe Sex in a Dangerous World*, 1987). In these scapegoating accounts, the bisexual is characterized as demonically *active*, the carrier, the source of spread, the sexually insatiable. At the same time, sexual desire is parceled into two exclusive realms, the homosexual and heterosexual "communities," with the bisexual— understood as a homosexual *posing* as a heterosexual—acting as the secret conveyor of the diseases of the former to the healthy bodies of the latter. Such a characterization is necessary to preserve the virtue of heterosexual "victims" (see below).

carrier *Webster's Third* defines the medical meaning of *carrier* as "a person, animal, or plant that harbors and disseminates the specific microorganism or other agent causing an infectious disease from which it has recovered or to which it is immune and that may therefore become a spreader of disease." The term, as used in media discussions of AIDS, is accompanied by a faint suggestion of covertness, as if a "carrier" had indeed recovered or become immune to that now-invariable accompaniment of *carrier*: "the AIDS virus." The unspoken model is Typhoid Mary, who—asymptomatically infected with the typhoid bacillus—in popular fancy *willfully* continued to work as a food handler after her infectious state was made known to her (the fact that Mary Mallon was untrained for any other kind of work does not enter the fable).

Randy Shilts's "Patient Zero," a French Canadian airline steward, plays this role in the recently published *And the Band Played On* (1987). Being openly gay did not prevent Shilts from devising this highly marketable narrative pivoting on the treachery of a single (now dead) man infected with HIV. Shilts's treatment of Gaetan Dugas collapses the young man's entire life into his sexual habits with an avidity and prurience tailor-made for the mass media. The media, in turn, dutifully reported the "Patient Zero" story as if its discovery of this single early "carrier" resolved the problem of blame, so central to the construction of AIDS as a moral issue.

condone In the distinctive public discussion of AIDS, the verb *condone* is used most frequently by conservative commentators to obscure and stigmatize practices of which they disapprove: "To instruct teenagers about condom use is to *condone* teenage sex." "To provide condoms to prison inmates is to *condone* homosexual practices in prison." "To give IV drug users clean works is to *condone* illegal drug use." "To print an account of the economic effects of AIDS on a gay couple"—as *Money* did in June 1987—is "to condone homosexuality"—as a California doctor wrote the magazine in complaint. Simple acknowledgment of empirical fact is deliberately confused with endorsement of controversial practices.

The mass media have not challenged this specious reasoning. To do so would be to open themselves to the same charges leveled by right-wing critics against public health workers—that by raising unpopular issues, they *condone* unpopular practices such as intravenous drug use and teenage sexuality.

The nearly universal slippage, in discussions of prevention, from transmission modes (e.g., shared needles, penetrative sex) to traditionally stigmatized social categories (e.g., non-middle-class drug users, urban gay men) produces the desired effect: condemnation of social categories and silencing of the opposition (those who are said to *condone* their practices). Like Nancy Reagan's "Just say no" strategy for keeping kids off drugs, those at risk are treated not as historical subjects functioning within already existing historical and social formations, but as tabulae rasae upon which the powerful may write their own cultural scripts.

family When California state Senator John Doolittle sponsored a Senate bill on AIDS and the family in the 1986 legislative session, it passed without a single opposition vote. The bill legalized the creation of designated-donor pools to keep donated blood *within families* so as to prevent transmission of HIV from anonymous donors to "the general population." Who, after all, would oppose such a bill? It would be like voting against your mother.

Implicit in the bill, however, is the notion that the family has already cast out its HIV "carriers," if indeed it had any. And implicit in this is the belief that those infected with HIV are readily identifiable. Nowhere in Doolittle's bill is there any acknowledgment that families often contain and accept openly gay and lesbian children—and parents—as well as IV drug users. Doolittle's law is written around an idealized notion of the family as a locus of certainty, of moral and social purity, a zone exempt from conflicts and contagion, or one that has expelled such problems from its midst.

general population *Heterosexual* is not a polite word. It is commonly used only in gay circles or in those liberal settings where there are a large number of professed *non*heterosexuals present, in which case it functions as a self-conscious preface: "Well, I'm heterosexual, but . . . ." In gatherings where lesbians and gays are not visibly present, the term is seldom used, because the presumed identity of everyone *is* heterosexual. The term thus plays its differentiating role only in the presence of its implicit or explicit opposite. Even then, it smacks of distaste. To employ it around other heterosexuals suggests that heterosexuality is not a given, but something to be accounted for, a cultural rather than a natural construction.

Because such troubling associations accompany the word, how much more diplomatic to employ a term that doesn't raise the specter of sexual practices or identities at all. Hence, *general population*. As a term, it bespeaks neither sex nor revolution. Its very amorphousness guarantees widespread identification. Who, after all, would not regard him- or herself as part of the general population?

The answer, of course, is that no self-respecting queer can or should. James Hurley, a person with AIDS (PWA; see below), noted in the August 10, 1987, issue of *Newsweek*, "It hurts me very deeply to read that I'm not part of the general population." Well, think again. The asexuality, the vagueness of the term stands in opposition to the descriptive terms applied to most PWAs—homosexuals, gays, junkies, IV drug users. According to the term's users—the media, public health officials, politicians—"the general population" is virtuously going about its business, which is not pleasure-seeking (as drugs and gay life are uniformly imagined to be), so AIDS hits *its* members as an assault from diseased hedonists upon hard-working innocents.

Gary Bauer, President Reagan's assistant, told *Face the Nation* that the reason Reagan had not even uttered the word *AIDS* publicly before a press conference held late in 1985 was that the Administration did not until then perceive AIDS as a problem: "It hadn't spread into the general population yet."

Like the Nixon/Agnew "silent majority," the "general population" is the repository of everything you wish to claim for yourself and deny to others.

gay/homosexual community Whether used by spokespersons for said community or by its enemies, the people characterized as the *gay/homosexual community* are too diverse politically, economically, demographically to be described meaningfully by such a term. (One only has to attempt its opposite, *the heterosexual community*—a few right-wing politicians have—for the full absurdity of the term to become clear; see below.) Yet its expedience is undeniable: the great diversity of humankind is reduced by means of the term to a single stereotype. It fastens upon that which is most frightening and alluring in the other—for example, gay men's fantasized freedom from sexual and family constraints—and projectively makes it the sole marker of identity. Like the disembodied "they" of the childhood plaint ("All the other kids get to"), the vague "they" of the *homosexual community* get everything we're denied—both extreme pleasure and extreme pain. Just don't ask who *they* are: *they* are those who have already been defined as victims of their own excesses, those-who-have-AIDS.

heterosexual community Embattled conservatives have discovered another discriminated-against community—their own. Though the unquestioned primacy of heterosexuality in our nation's laws, education, politics, medicine, and culture would seem sufficiently to guarantee the security of male-female units, making it unnecessary to distinguish its identity from the minority's, the compulsion to define oneself in opposition to an other operates with clear extravagance here. Williams notes in *Keywords* that, from the mid-nineteenth century,

> the sense of immediacy or locality was strongly developed in the context of larger and more complex industrial societies. *Community* was the word normally chosen for experiments in an alternative kind of group-living. . . . [The term *community* implies] on the one hand the sense of direct common concern; on the other hand the materialization of various forms of common organization. . . . What is most important, perhaps, is that unlike all other terms of social organization . . . it seems never to be used unfavorably, and never to be given any positive opposing or distinguishing term.[6]

Particularly since the mid-1960s in the US, the term *community* has been most frequently invoked in oppositional terms to identify a local, ethnic, racial, or political variant to the mainstream. To find the mainstream defining itself as a variant is therefore surprising. The political conservative battling for the rights of the *heterosexual community* clearly does not struggle against social and cultural

6.   Williams, *Keywords*, pp. 75–76.

forces that have shut him out. But the *opposing term*, as Williams stresses—that is, the hypothesized *homosexual community*—must be seen here as the powerful and, crucially, the *active* community. Viewed from within as a site of unique privilege, heterosexuality becomes the mirror of the victimized minority community, besieged from without.

lesbian Since sexual desire is one of the chief determinants of modern identity, the woman whose desire turns toward members of her own sex has been marked out as essentially and socially different from "the general population." She shares this status with, among others, gay men, blacks, intravenous drug users. Since these latter are members of known "risk groups" (see below) for AIDS, lesbians must also be at high risk for AIDS. How is that for logic? It's played just fine with the blood banks. In 1982–83, the American Red Cross advised lesbians to defer donating blood, as gay men were urged to do. In Britain the debate still occupied space in the pages of the *Lancet*, the country's most prestigious medical journal, as late as 1986 ("Should Lesbians Give Blood?" in the issues of August 16 and 30, 1986). In the summer of 1987, the Sonoma County (California) Red Cross turned down a proposal by a group of women's motorcycle clubs to turn a weekend run to the Russian River into a blood drive. Sonoma County didn't want lesbian blood.

It probably restates the obvious to note that there is a lower reported incidence of HIV infection among lesbians than any other population group. So the scare about "lesbian blood" has less to do with rational fears about transmission of HIV than with fears of sexual and social taint (the kind of taint that obsessively appears in the guise of lesbian vampire fantasies in such films as *Daughters of Darkness* and *The Hunger*).

prostitute Prostitutes have been blamed for breaches of national security,[7] the fall of principalities and mighty men, the desecration of hearth and home. Now they are being blamed in many quarters for the "spread" (see below) of AIDS. HIV-infected prostitutes in Florida, Texas, and California have received a great deal of media attention, including that given to a convicted prostitute in Florida whose sentence included wearing an electronic collar that alerted police whenever she left her house. The media's—and medical, public health, and political officials'—focus on prostitutes as a source of infection functions primarily as a scapegoating device. In most epidemiological studies no distinction is made between prostitutes who are needle-sharing IV drug users and those who are not. Thus the category *prostitute* is taken as an undifferentiated "risk group" rather than as an occupational category whose members should, for epidemiological purposes, be divided into IV drug users and nonusers—with significantly differ-

7.   See Alan Brandt, *No Magic Bullets*, New York, Oxford University Press, 1985, for an account of the scapegoating of prostitutes during World Wars I and II.

ent rates of HIV infection—as other groups are (e.g., homosexual/bisexual non-IV drug users).

In the long-term study of women who are sexually active (professionally and nonprofessionally) conducted by Project AWARE at San Francisco General Hospital, the incidence of HIV infection among non-IV-drug-using sex-industry workers was found to be slightly *lower* than it was among nonprofessional, non-IV-drug-using women. The difference is accounted for by the widespread use of condoms by prostitutes' clients, something that sex workers demand while most other sexually active women do not. Other US and European studies that distinguish between prostitutes who use IV drugs and those who do not have produced similar results.

As is the case for lesbians, then, prostitutes are taken as embodiments of infectiousness less for their actual risks and rates of infection than for their symbolic and historical status. This is even more sensationally the case when the prostitutes in question are *male* prostitutes. Dr. Art Ulene, in his *Safe Sex in a Dangerous World*, reserves his deepest contempt (and fear) for male prostitutes, who "still *dot* the streets of my city [like the plague? like Kaposi's sarcoma?]—men so lacking in self-respect and restraint that they are lost to all appeals to decency." That male prostitution, like its female counterpart, is primarily an *economic* formation remains, of course, unutterable.

We might well wonder about science's claims to objectivity when public health and medical investigators can overlook the differences in degree of risk involved in protected sex, on the one hand, and needle sharing, on the other, in favor of the more socially resonant category of *prostitution*.

PWA (Person with AIDS) At the second AIDS Forum, held in Denver in 1983, a group of men and women with AIDS and ARC (AIDS-Related Complex) met to form an organization that would speak their own needs—in their own words. The Advisory Committee of People with AIDS, forerunner of today's National Association of People with AIDS, issued the following statement: "We condemn attempts to label us as 'victims,' which implies defeat, and we are only occasionally 'patients,' which implies passivity, helplessness, and dependence on the care of others. We are 'people with AIDS.'"

At the October 1987 March on Washington for Lesbian and Gay Rights, PWAs from all over the US took the naming of their condition one step further, announcing that they are "people *living* with AIDS." It is a measure of the need of the press—left, center, and right—to distance itself from AIDS that few of its journalists have chosen to employ either term. The most common usage by far is *AIDS victim* (see below). Nor is *PWA* widely used by physicians, for whom the PWA is first and foremost a patient. Politicians, particularly on the right, rarely use *any* term to describe people with AIDS; their manifest concern is with those who remain uninfected. This is perhaps a prudent move on their parts: calling attention to the need to *protect* the healthy majority from the *AIDS-victim* minority would make its absurdity clear.

The PWA's insistence upon naming as a key to identity, though partially aimed at the press, the public, the government, and the medical profession, is primarily an act of self-acclaim:

> We do not see ourselves as victims. We will not be victimized. We have the right to be treated with respect, dignity, compassion, and understanding. We have the right to live fulfilling, productive lives — to live and die with dignity and compassion. . . . We are born of and inextricably bound to the historical struggle for rights — civil, feminist, disability, lesbian and gay, and human. We will not be denied our rights![8]

risk group The concept of *risk group* is an epidemiological one; its function is to isolate identifiable characteristics that are predictive of where a disease or condition is likely to appear so as to contain and prevent it. In the case of AIDS, the syndrome was first identified in gay men, leading the Centers for Disease Control and others to speculate on the possibility that something they termed "the gay life-style" might itself be responsible for the condition (among factors considered were amyl nitrate "poppers," rogue genes, repeated bouts of common sexually transmitted diseases, too much sex ["excessive assaults on the immune system"], fast-lane living). The discovery in late 1981 that Haitians and IV drug users were also affected by the syndrome did not square with this theory, and a virus became the prime suspect, though it was not identified until the spring of 1983.

Still, the *risk group* concept was useful for public health, preventive purposes in the early years of the epidemic. It roughly identified people whose membership in a group practicing certain risk behaviors was likely to bring them into contact with the virus. What should have followed from this, however, did not. Before 1986, public health officials in the US did not make a nationwide, visible effort to inform people about how the virus was transmitted. Even now, what few efforts at nationwide preventive education do exist are hedged with euphemisms ("avoid exchanges of body fluids") and moralisms ("When it comes to preventing AIDS, don't medicine and morality teach the same lessons?" asked Reagan of the American College of Physicians).

In the media and in political debate, the epidemiological category of *risk group* has been used to stereotype and stigmatize people already seen as outside the moral and economic parameters of "the general population." Jesse Helms's success in October 1987 in getting the Senate to prevent federal dollars from being spent on safe sex information for gay men — the hardest hit "risk group" in the US, and the only group in which reported transmission of the virus has

8.   National Association of People with AIDS, "Statement of Purpose," September 1986.

declined (to less than two percent new infections in San Francisco in 1987) due to safe sex education by gay men themselves—makes clear the social and political, as opposed to epidemiological, functions of the *risk group* concept: to isolate and condemn people rather than to contact and protect them.

risk practice This concept, which has replaced *risk group* for all but surveillance purposes in the thinking of the National Academy of Sciences, moves the emphasis away from characterizing and stigmatizing people as members of groups. The aging of the epidemic has made clear the indifference of HIV to categories such as *junkie* and *faggot*. It doesn't care whether it enters the body of a nurse or a prostitute, a Senator Paul Gann or a "Patient Zero." As heterosexual transmission increases, the only meaningful risk behaviors become intravenous injection and penetrative sex,[9] both of which are purposive activities engaged in by people of every sexual persuasion and economic class.

The continued emphasis on *risk groups* rather than *risk practices* in press and political discussions of AIDS masks the evidently unspeakable fact that functionally there *are* no differences in sexual practices engaged in by gay men and by heterosexual men and women—only in the values ascribed to them.[10]

spread The terms *carrier* and *spread* are central to popular descriptions of HIV transmission. AIDS is popularly seen as a disease that was initially *contained*, confined to identifiable "risk groups" that were not part of "the general population." *Spread* (or *leakage*, as it is sometimes called) suggests the insidious movement of the disease or infection outside its "natural" limits. *Spread* and *leakage* share common sexual and polluting connotations, which are carried over into media descriptions of gay male sexual practices and social haunts. The anus (for popular purposes regarded as an exclusively gay male orifice) becomes a cesspool, an unnatural breeding ground for the "AIDS virus." Luridly described bathhouses and bars such as the Mine Shaft become the sewers, or loci of *leakage* and *spread*.

victim Within the many self-support groups founded by people with life-threatening diseases, the term *victim* is emphatically rejected. Although it would seem argument enough for dropping the term *victim* that the people called "AIDS victims" have declared repeatedly that they prefer the designation "people with

9.   That is, voluntary as opposed to accidental behaviors such as transfusions or health workers' needle-stick injuries. Nursing an infant is another proven mode of transmission, but since it is not hedged round with the fretwork of hysteria characterizing the concept of *risk groups* (*mothers?*), I only note it here.
10.   I say *functionally* because of course there is a technical difference in anal penetrative sex when a man is the receptor. Structurally, however, this is a minor difference, a variation. Symbolically, though, this hotly contested (male) hole remains, for the heterosexual man, a site of extreme privilege, his pink badge of *virtù*, so to speak.

AIDS," so far their stated wishes have been disregarded. The term persists in the media, among health care workers, and among politicians battling for "victims' rights."

Webster's Third tells us that "*victim* applies to anyone who suffers as a result of ruthless design or incidentally or accidentally." According to this definition, it would appear that *victim* is a neutral, descriptive term for a person on whom an undeserved ill-fate is visited. Hence the cliché: we are all potential victims. A victim is someone like us, someone for whom we have empathy. What, then, is wrong with *victim*?

1) *the fatalism.* Fear and pity are the emotions raised by the victim, and, as we know, these emotions are less than useless for dealing actively with serious issues. Fear and pity are aroused in order ultimately to be cathartically disposed of, to enable the passive spectator of the AIDS "spectacle" to remain passive, and eventually to distance him- or herself from the scapegoated object of fear and pity.

Fatalism implies that nothing, or next to nothing, can be done about the cultural, social, and medical crises presented by AIDS. It denies the very possibility of all that is *in fact* being done by people living with AIDS and those working with them. The opposite of the fatalistic term, *victim*, interestingly, would be aggressor, assaulter, a role too frequently taken by those most determined to see people with AIDS as victims.

2) *the effect of cancellation.* Fatalism leads to the virtual cancellation of the person called "victim." It reduces him or her to a foredoomed conclusion, an end point, a single final word. The phrase *people living with AIDS* reveals the life, the activity, the continued and not to be forgotten existence of those who *now* have AIDS and demand our attention.

3) *the negative psychological sense.* In a modern "psychological society" we cannot live our fatalism undiluted. Fates are often joined by unconscious wishes, and victims are often seen to be in some way complicit with, to have courted, their fate. Victims of rape, for example, must constantly battle the suspicion that they were "asking for it," and women, in general, are often equated with a kind of masochism that *allows* them to be victimized. Victims always end up revealing some tragic character flaw that has invited their tragedy.

The proof that *victim* is not simply a term applied to the unlucky, to those undeserving and noncomplicit with their fate, is the frequently employed phrase, "innocent victim," which is *not* seen as redundant. "The most innocent victims" is *Newsweek*'s caption accompanying two photographs, one of two young parents with an infant, the other of a woman with a small child. The caption suggests, of course, that other people with AIDS are less innocent. The *Village Voice*'s Nat Hentoff, who has shown considerably more compassion for unborn fetuses than for people living with AIDS, has found the linguistic device that neatly captures the distinction between guilty and innocent victims, replacing the telling redundancy *innocent victims* with a less telling one: the innocent are now "victims of AIDS victims."

A patronage that simultaneously grants "victims" powerlessness and then assigns them blame for that powerlessness is nothing new. It is therefore important to make connections between the construction of AIDS victimhood and similar constructions of the poor, who also suffer the triple curse of objectification, institutionalized powerlessness, and blame for their condition.

Indeed, we must make connections, wherever and whenever possible, between the keywords of AIDS and the more general vocabulary of power struggles with which these words are inevitably linked.

AIDS, Homophobia, and Biomedical Discourse: An Epidemic of Signification*

PAULA A. TREICHLER

An Epidemic of Signification

In multiple, fragmentary, and often contradictory ways we struggle to achieve some sort of understanding of AIDS, a reality that is frightening, widely publicized, and yet finally neither directly nor fully knowable. AIDS is no different in this respect from other linguistic constructions, which, in the common-sense view of language, are thought to transmit preexisting ideas and represent real-world entities and yet, in fact, do neither. For the nature of the relationship between language and reality is highly problematic; and *AIDS* is not merely an invented label, provided to us by science and scientific naming practices, for a clear-cut disease entity caused by a virus. Rather, the very nature of AIDS is constructed through language and in particular through the discourses of medicine and science; this construction is "true" or "real" only in certain specific ways — for example, insofar as it successfully guides research or facilitates clinical control over the illness.[1] The name *AIDS* in part *constructs* the disease and helps make it intelligible. We cannot therefore look "through" language to determine what AIDS "really" is. Rather we must explore the site where such determinations *really* occur and intervene at the point where meaning is created: in language.

* Reprinted from *Cultural Studies*, vol. 1, no. 3 (October 1987), pp. 263–305; minor changes and corrections have been made for the present publication; information and references have not been updated. Research for this essay was funded in part by grants from the National Council of Teachers of English and the University of Illinois Graduate College Research Board. My thanks to Teresa Mangum, research assistant on this project; to Stephen J. Kaufman, M. Kerry O'Banion, Eve Kosofsky Sedgwick, and Michael Witkovsky for guidance and insight; and to those who have kept me in touch with AIDS developments in diverse fields. An earlier version of this essay was presented at the annual meeting of the Modern Language Association, New York, December 1986.

1.   Discussing the validity of their interpretation of everyday life in a science laboratory, Bruno Latour and Steve Woolgar claim, similarly, that the "value and status of any text (construction, fact, claim, story, this account) depend on more than its supposedly 'inherent' qualities. . . . The degree of accuracy (or fiction) of an account depends on what is subsequently made of the story, not on the story itself" (*Laboratory Life: The Construction of Scientific Facts*, Cambridge, England, Cambridge University Press, 1985, p. 284).

Of course, AIDS is a real disease syndrome, damaging and killing real human beings. Because of this, it is tempting—perhaps in some instances imperative—to view science and medicine as providing a discourse about AIDS closer to its "reality" than what we can provide ourselves. Yet the AIDS epidemic—with its genuine potential for global devastation—is simultaneously an epidemic of a transmissible lethal disease and an epidemic of meanings or signification.[2] Both epidemics are equally crucial for us to understand, for, try as we may to treat AIDS as "an infectious disease" and nothing more, meanings continue to multiply wildly and at an extraordinary rate.[3] This epidemic of meanings is readily apparent in the chaotic assemblage of understandings of AIDS that by now exists. The mere enumeration of some of the ways AIDS has been characterized suggests its enormous power to generate meanings:

1. An irreversible, untreatable, and invariably fatal infectious disease that threatens to wipe out the whole world.

2. A creation of the media, which has sensationalized a minor health problem for its own profit and pleasure.

3. A creation of the state to legitimize widespread invasion of people's lives and sexual practices.

4. A creation of biomedical scientists and the Centers for Disease Control to generate funding for their activities.

5. A gay plague, probably emanating from San Francisco.

6. The crucible in which the field of immunology will be tested.

7. The most extraordinary medical chronicle of our times.

8. A condemnation to celibacy or death.

9. An Andromeda strain with the transmission efficiency of the common cold.

10. An imperialist plot to destroy the Third World.

11. A fascist plot to destroy homosexuals.

---

2.   I use the term *epidemic* to refer to the exponential compounding of meanings as opposed to the simpler spread of a term through a population.

3.   The term *signification,* derived from the linguistic work of Ferdinand de Saussure, calls attention to the way in which language (or any other "signifying system") organizes rather than labels experience (or the world). Linking signifiers (phonetic segments or, more loosely, words) and signifieds (concepts, meanings) in ways that come to seem "natural" to us, language creates the illusion of "transparency," as though we could look through it to "facts" and "realities" that are unproblematic. Many scientists and physicians, even those sensitive to the complexities of AIDS, believe that "the facts" (or "science" or "reason") will resolve contradiction and supplant speculation; they express impatience with social interpretations, which they perceive as superfluous or incorrect. (See, for example, Richard Restak, "AIDS Virus Has No Civil Rights," *Chicago Sun-Times,* September 15, 1985, pp. 1, 57–58.) Even Jacques Leibowitch writes that, with the discovery of the virus, AIDS loses its "metaphysical resonances" and becomes "now no more than one infectious disease among many" (*A Strange Virus of Unknown Origin,* trans. Richard Howard, intro. by Robert C. Gallo, New York, Ballantine, 1985, p. xiv). The position of this essay is that signification processes are not the handmaidens of "the facts"; rather, "the facts" themselves arise out of the signifying practices of biomedical discourse.

12. A CIA plot to destroy subversives.

13. A capitalist plot to create new markets for pharmaceutical products.

14. A Soviet plot to destroy capitalists.

15. The result of experiments on the immunological system of men not likely to reproduce.

16. The result of genetic mutations caused by "mixed marriages."

17. The result of moral decay and a major force destroying the Boy Scouts.

18. A plague stored in King Tut's tomb and unleashed when the Tut exhibit toured the US in 1976.

19. The perfect emblem of twentieth-century decadence, of fin-de-siècle decadence, of postmodern decadence.

20. A disease that turns fruits into vegetables.

21. A disease introduced by aliens to weaken us before the takeover.

22. Nature's way of cleaning house.

23. America's *Ideal Death Sentence.*

24. An infectious agent that has suppressed our immunity from guilt.

25. A spiritual force that is creatively disrupting civilization.

26. A sign that the end of the world is at hand.

27. God's punishment of our weaknesses.

28. God's test of our strengths.

29. The price paid for the sixties.

30. The price paid for anal intercourse.

31. The price paid for genetic inferiority and male aggression.

32. An absolutely unique disease for which there is no precedent.

33. Just another venereal disease.

34. The most urgent and complex public health problem facing the world today.

35. A golden opportunity for science and medicine.

36. Science fiction.

37. Stranger than science fiction.

38. A terrible and expensive way to die.[4]

---

4.   These conceptualizations of AIDS come chiefly from printed sources (journals, news stories, letters to the editor, tracts) published since 1981. Many are common and discussed in the course of this essay; the more idiosyncratic readings of AIDS (e.g., as a force destroying the Boy Scouts) are cited to suggest the dramatic symbol-inducing power of this illness as well as our continuing lack of social consensus about its meaning. Sources for the more idiosyncratic views are as follows: (2) Senator Jesse Helms; (6) Gallo's introduction to Leibowitch, *A Strange Virus,* pp. xvi–xvii; (8) gay rights activist on Channel 5 television broadcast, Cincinnati, October 18, 1985 (compare the French joke that the acronym for AIDS, SIDA in French, stands for Syndrome Imaginaire pour Décourager les Amoureux [*Newsweek,* November 24, 1986, p. 47]); (9) one science writer's characterization of the popular view (John Langone, "AIDS: The Latest Scientific Facts," *Discover,* December 1985, pp. 27–52); (10) GRIA (Haitian Revolutionary Internationalist Group), "AIDS: Syndrome of an Imperialist Era," undated flyer distributed in New York City, Fall 1982 (and see Marcia Pally, "AIDS and the Politics of Despair: Lighting Our Own Funeral Pyre," *The Advocate,* no. 436, December 24,

Such diverse conceptualizations of AIDS are coupled with fragmentary interpretations of its specific elements. Confusion about transmission now causes approximately half the US population to refuse to *give* blood. Many believe you can "catch" AIDS through casual contact, such as sitting beside an infected person on a bus. Many believe that lesbians—a population relatively free of sexually transmitted diseases in general—are as likely to be infected as gay men. Other stereotypes about homosexuals generate startling deductions about the illness: "I thought AIDS was a gay disease," said a man interviewed by *USA Today* in October 1985, "but if Rock Hudson's dead it can kill anyone."

We cannot effectively analyze AIDS or develop intelligent social policy if we dismiss such conceptions as irrational myths and homophobic fantasies that deliberately ignore the "real scientific facts." Rather they are part of the necessary work people do in attempting to understand—however imperfectly—the complex, puzzling, and quite terrifying phenomenon of AIDS. No matter how much we may desire, with Susan Sontag, to resist treating illness as metaphor, illness *is* metaphor, and this semantic work—this effort to "make sense of" AIDS—has to be done. Further, this work is as necessary and often as difficult and imperfect for physicians and scientists as it is for "the rest of us."[5]

1985, p. 8); (12) Gary Lee, "AIDS in Moscow: It Comes from the CIA, or Maybe Africa," *Washington Post National Weekly Edition*, December 30, 1985, p. 16; (13) Langone, in *Discover*, citing a story in a Kenyan newspaper; (14) *National Inquirer* story cited in Brian Becher, "AIDS and the Media: A Case Study of How the Press Influences Public Opinion," unpublished research paper, College of Medicine, University of Illinois at Urbana-Champaign, 1983; (15) John Rechy, "An Exchange on AIDS," Letter to the Editor, with reply by Jonathan Lieberson, *New York Review of Books*, October 13, 1983, pp. 43–45; (16) Soviet view cited in Jonathan Lieberson, "The Reality of AIDS," *New York Review of Books*, January 16, 1986, p. 45; (17) Jonathan Gathorne-Hardy, Letter to the Editor, *New York Times Book Review*, June 29, 1986, p. 35; (18) cited in William Check, "Public Education on AIDS: Not Only the Media's Responsibility," *Hastings Center Report*, Special Supplement, vol. 15, no. 4 (August 1985), p. 28; (19) Toby Johnson, "AIDS and Moral Issues," *The Advocate*, no. 379, October 27, 1983, pp. 24–26: "Perhaps AIDS is just the first of a whole new class of diseases resulting from the tremendous changes human technology has wrought in the earth's ecology"; (20) example of AIDS "humor" cited in David Black, *The Plague Years: A Chronicle of AIDS, The Epidemic of Our Times*, New York, Simon & Schuster, 1986; (23) acronym cited in Lindsy Van Gelder and Pam Brandt, "AIDS on Campus," *Rolling Stone*, no. 483, 1986, p. 89; (24) Richard Goldstein, "Heartsick: Fear and Loving in the Gay Community," *Village Voice*, June 28, 1983; (25) Black, *The Plague Years*, citing one view of plagues; (31) cited in Pally, "AIDS and the Politics of Despair"; (37) Robert C. Gallo, "The AIDS Virus," *Scientific American*, January 1987, pp. 47–56.

5.   Sontag, in *Illness as Metaphor*, New York, Farrar, Strauss & Giroux, 1978, argues that the confusion of illness with metaphor damages people who are ill, and certainly with AIDS there is ample evidence for this argument. Laurence R. Tancredi and Nora D. Volkow, for example, in "AIDS: Its Symbolism and Ethical Implications," *Medical Heritage*, vol. 2, no. 1 (January–February 1986), pp. 12–18, arguing that "the metaphor essentially creates the framework for the individual's experience of the disease," cite studies indicating that many people with AIDS experience a variety of psychological difficulties as a result of its symbolic (as opposed to its prognostic) message. But metaphor cannot simply be mandated away. Goldstein, in "Heartsick," writes: "Since we are so vulnerable to the erotic potential of metaphor, how can we hope to be less susceptible when illness intersects with sex and death?" Sontag argues that once the cause and cure of a disease are known it

I am arguing, then, not that we must take both the social and the biological dimensions of AIDS into account, but rather that the social dimension is far more pervasive and central than we are accustomed to believing. Science is not the true material base generating our merely symbolic superstructure. Our social constructions of AIDS (in terms of global devastation, threat to civil rights, emblem of sex and death, the "gay plague," the postmodern condition, whatever) are based not upon objective, scientifically determined "reality" but upon what we are told about this reality: that is, upon *prior* social constructions routinely produced within the discourses of biomedical science.[6] (AIDS as infectious disease is one such construction.) There is a continuum, then, not a dichotomy, between popular and biomedical discourses (and, as Latour and Woolgar put it, "a continuum between controversies in daily life and those occurring in the laboratory"),[7] and these play out in language. Consider, for example, the ambiguities embedded within this statement by an AIDS "expert" (an immunologist) on a television documentary in October 1985 designed to *dispel* misconceptions about AIDS:

> The biggest misconception that we have encountered and that most cities throughout the United States have seen is that many people feel that casual contact — being in the same room with an AIDS victim — will transmit the virus and may infect them. This has not been substantiated by any evidence whatsoever. . . . [This misconception lingers because] this is an extremely emotional issue. I think that when there are such strong emotions associated with a medical problem such as this it's very difficult for facts to sink in. I think also there's the problem that we cannot give any 100 percent assurances one way or the other about these factors. There may always be some exception to

ceases to be the kind of mystery that generates metaphors. Her view that biomedical discourse has a special claim on the representation of "reality" implies as well that the entities it identifies and describes are themselves free from social construction (metaphor). But as Stephen Durham and Susan Williams insist, in "AIDS Hysteria: A Marxist Analysis," presented at the Pacific Northwest Marxist Scholars Conference, University of Washington, Seattle, April 11–13, 1986 (Freedom Socialist Publications, 5018 Rainier Ave. South, Seattle, WA 98118), despite the origins of the AIDS crisis in the domain of microbiology, the "greatest obstacles to establishing a cure for AIDS and a rational, humane approach to its ravages do not flow from the organic qualities of the [virus]."

6.   Allan M. Brandt, in *No Magic Bullet: A Social History of Venereal Disease in the United States since 1880,* New York, Oxford University Press, 1987 (expanded version of 1985 edition), p. 199, summarizes the ways in which AIDS thus far recapitulates the social history of other sexually transmitted diseases: the pervasive fear of contagion, concerns about casual transmission, stigmatization of victims, conflict between the protection of public health and the protection of civil liberties, increasing public control over definition and management, and the search for a "magic bullet." Despite the supposed sexual revolution, Brandt writes, we continue through these social constructions "to define the sexually transmitted diseases as uniquely sinful." This definition is inaccurate but pervasive, and as long as disease is equated with sin "there can be no magic bullet" (p. 202).

7.   Latour and Woolgar, *Laboratory Life,* p. 281.

the rule. Anything we may say, someone could come up with an exception. But as far as most of the medical–scientific community is concerned, this is a virus that is actually very *difficult* to transmit and therefore the general public should really not worry about casual contact — not even using the same silverware and dishes would probably be a problem.[8]

Would you buy a scientific fact from this man? Can we expect to understand AIDS transmission when this is part of what we have to work with? The point is not merely that this particular scientist has not yet learned to "talk to the media," but that ambiguity and uncertainty are features of scientific inquiry that must be socially and linguistically managed.[9] What is at issue here is a fatal infectious disease that is simply not fully understood; questions remain about the nature of the disease, its etiology, its transmission, and what individuals can do about it. It does not seem unreasonable that in the face of these uncertainties people give birth to many different conceptions; to label them "*mis*conceptions" implies what? Wrongful birth? That only "facts" can give birth to proper conceptions and only science can give birth to facts? In that case, we may wish to avert our eyes from some of the "scientific" conceptions that have been born in the course of the AIDS crisis:

> AIDS could be *anything*, considering what homosexual men do to each other in gay baths.

> Heroin addicts won't use clean needles because they would rather get AIDS than give up the ritual of sharing them.

> Prostitutes do not routinely keep themselves clean and are therefore "reservoirs" of disease.

8.   Allan Sollinger, PhD, Department of Immunology, University of Cincinnati Medical Center, speaking as an expert guest on a television documentary, Cincinnati, October 1985. By this time a number of leading authorities on AIDS had come to believe that scientists had to begin communicating to the public with greater clarity and certainty. The Centers for Disease Control issued a "definitive statement" in October 1985 that AIDS *cannot* be spread by casual contact. Mathilde Krim, PhD, director of the American Foundation for AIDS Research, discussed transmission with emphatic clarity on the *MacNeil-Lehrer Newshour*, September 4, 1985: "AIDS is contagious strictly through the transmission of a virus which passes from one person to another during sexual intercourse or with contaminated blood. It is not contagious *at all* through casual interaction with people, in normal social conditions such as living in a household with a patient or meeting patients on the bus or in the working place or in school." Interestingly, as Deborah Jones Merritt's comprehensive review makes clear, constitutional precedents for addressing public health problems give broad latitude to the state; strong scientific "evidence" is essentially not required as a basis for interventions ("Communicable Disease and Constitutional Law: Controlling AIDS," *New York University Law Review*, no. 61 [November 1986], pp. 739–799).
9.   Nathan Fain and Check discuss turning points in AIDS-related communications as scientists gained skill in reducing ambiguity. See Nathan Fain, "AIDS: An Antidote to Fear," *Village Voice*, October 1, 1985, p. 35, and Check, "Public Education on AIDS."

AIDS is homosexual; it can only be transmitted by males to males.

AIDS in Africa is heterosexual but uni-directional; it can only be transmitted from males to females.

AIDS in Africa is heterosexual because anal intercourse is a common form of birth control.[10]

The point here is that no clear line can be drawn between the facticity of scientific and nonscientific (mis)conceptions. Ambiguity, homophobia, stereotyping, confusion, doublethink, them-versus-us, blame-the-victim, wishful thinking: none of these popular forms of semantic legerdemain about AIDS is absent from biomedical communication. But scientific and medical discourses have traditions through which the semantic epidemic as well as the biological one is controlled, and these may disguise contradiction and irrationality. In writing about AIDS, these traditions typically include characterizing ambiguity and contradiction as "nonscientific" (a no-nonsense, lets-get-the-facts-on-the-table-and-clear-up-this-muddle approach), invoking faith in scientific inquiry, taking for granted the reality of quantitative and/or biomedical data, deducing social and behavioral reality from quantitative and/or biomedical data, setting forth fantasies and speculations as though they were logical deductions, using technical euphemisms for sensitive sexual or political realities, and revising both past and future to conform to present thinking.

Many of these traditions are illustrated in an article by John Langone in the December 1985 general science journal *Discover*.[11] In this lengthy review of research to date, entitled "AIDS: The Latest Scientific Facts," Langone suggests that the virus enters the bloodstream by way of the "vulnerable anus" and the "fragile urethra"; in contrast, the "rugged vagina" (built to be abused by such blunt instruments as penises and small babies) provides too tough a barrier for the AIDS virus to penetrate.[12] "Contrary to what you've heard," Langone concludes—and his conclusion echoes a fair amount of medical and scientific writing at the time—"AIDS isn't a threat to the vast majority of heterosexuals. . . . It is now—and is likely to remain—largely the fatal price one can pay for anal intercourse."[13] (This excerpt from the article also ran as the cover

10.   These conceptions and others are widespread. For specific citations and discussion, see, for example, Leibowitch, *A Strange Virus;* Langone, "AIDS: The Latest Scientific Facts"; Wayne Barrett, "Straight Shooters: AIDS Targets Another Lifestyle," *Village Voice,* October 26, 1985, pp. 14–18; Lawrence K. Altman, "Linking AIDS to Africa Provokes Bitter Debate," *New York Times,* November 21, 1985, pp. 1, 8.
11.   Langone, "AIDS: The Latest Scientific Facts."
12.   *Ibid.,* pp. 40–41.
13.   *Ibid.,* p. 52.

WHY AIDS IS LIKELY TO REMAIN LARGELY A GAY DISEASE

THE VULNERABLE RECTUM

The rectum, the lower portion *(left)* of the large intestine that ends in the anus, is lined *(below)* with fragile, easily invaded columnar cells. Moreover, the closer to the anus, the more blood vessels there are. Anal intercourse, second only to oral sex in frequency among homosexuals, can tear the lining, allowing AIDS virus–infected semen ready entry to the blood stream. This sexual practice is the commonest cause of AIDS.

THE FRAGILE URETHRA

The urethra, the thin tube *(left)* leading from the bladder through the penis, is also mostly lined with columnar cells, with numerous underlying blood vessels *(below)*.

During anal intercourse with an AIDS-infected partner, the virus can pass from the rectum into the urethra, where it is able to penetrate the delicate walls.

THE RUGGED VAGINA

Unlike the rectum, the vagina *(left)* is designed to withstand the trauma of intercourse as well as childbirth. Its lining *(below)* is composed of layers of plate-like squamous cells that resist rupture and infectious agents, presumably including the AIDS virus. Its tissue has fewer blood vessels and is usually naturally lubricated during intercourse.

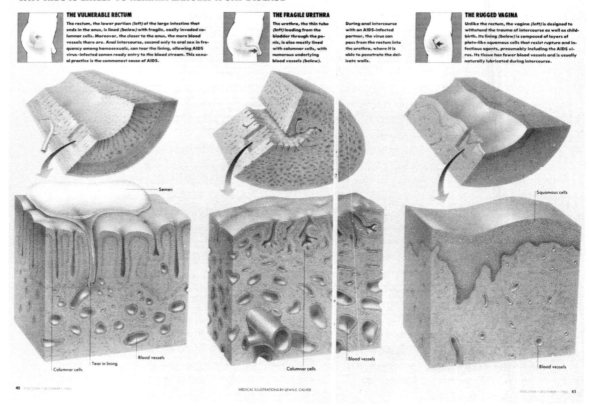

MEDICAL ILLUSTRATIONS BY LEWIS E. CALVER

Vulnerable Rectum / Fragile Urethra / Rugged Vagina.
Medical illustrations by Lewis E. Calver for Discover,
December 1985.

blurb.) It sounded plausible; and detailed illustrations demonstrated the article's conclusion.[14]

But by December 1986 the big news — what the major US news magazines were running cover stories on — was the grave danger of AIDS to heterosexuals.[15] No dramatic discoveries during the intervening year had changed the fundamental scientific conception of AIDS.[16] What had changed was not "the facts" but the way in which they were now used to construct the AIDS text and the meanings we were now allowed — indeed, at last encouraged — to read from that text.[17] The AIDS story, in other words, is not merely the familiar story of

14. Visual representations of AIDS are not the subject of this essay, yet it is worth noting that they have been a source of continuing controversy. In Watney and Gupta's textual and visual "dossier" on the rhetoric of AIDS, one writer calls the magnified electron micrograph of the HTLV-III virus "the spectre of the decade" (Simon Watney and Sunil Gupta, "The Rhetoric of AIDS: A Dossier Compiled by Simon Watney, with Photographs by Sunil Gupta," *Screen*, vol. 27, no. 1 [January–February 1986], pp. 72–85). The cover of *Time*, August 12, 1985, also treats a photograph of the virus as proof of its reality; "magnified 135,000 times," the virus is pictured "destroying T-cell"—cf. Roberta McGrath's analysis of the cultural and political role of photography in naturalizing the biomedical model ("Medical Police," *Ten*, no. 8 [1984], p. 14). Some members of the San Francisco gay community complained early that public health warnings used euphemistic language ("avoid exchange of bodily fluids") and through innocuous pictures subverted the message that AIDS was a deadly and physically ravaging disease (Frances FitzGerald, *Cities on a Hill*, New York, Simon & Schuster/Touchstone, 1987, p. 93. First published as "A Reporter at Large: The Castro-II," *The New Yorker*, July 28, 1986). On other aspects of media coverage of AIDS, see Becher, "AIDS and the Media"; Black, *The Plaque Years*; Check, "Public Education on AIDS"; Barbara O'Dair, "Anatomy of a Media Epidemic," *Alternative Media*, vol. 14, no. 3 (Fall 1983), pp. 10–13; Harry Schwartz, "AIDS in the Media," in *Science in the Streets: A Report to the Twentieth Century Task Force on the Communication of Scientific Risk*, New York, Priority Press, 1984. Controversies over graphics were not limited to popular journals: a photo published in *Science* purporting to be an isolated strain of Gallo's "AIDS virus" figured in the international dispute over its discovery (Robert C. Gallo, *et al.*, "HTLV-III Legend Correction," Letter to the Editor, *Science*, no. 232 [April 18, 1986], p. 307; Colin Norman, "A New Twist in AIDS Patent Fight," News and Comment, *Science*, no. 232 [April 18, 1986], pp. 308–309).

15. See, for example, *Newsweek*, November 3, 1986, pp. 66–67, and November 24, 1986, pp. 30–47; Erik Eckholm, "Broad Alert on AIDS: Social Battle Is Shifting," *New York Times*, June 17, 1986, pp. 19–20; Kathleen McAuliffe, *et al.* "AIDS: At the Dawn of Fear," *US News and World Report*, January 12, 1987, pp. 60–69; Mortimer B. Zuckerman, "AIDS: A Crisis Ignored," Editorial, *US News and World Report*, January 12, 1987, p. 76; Katie Leishman, "Heterosexuals and AIDS: The Second Stage of the Epidemic," *The Atlantic*, February 1987, pp. 39–58; "Science and the Citizen," *Scientific American*, January 1987, pp. 58–59.

16. The 2nd International Conference on AIDS, held in Paris in June 1986, revealed no major scientific breakthroughs (Deborah M. Barnes, "AIDS Research in New Phase," *Science*, no. 233 [July 18, 1986], p. 282); rather, answers to several crucial questions were clarified or strengthened. Check notes that, as health and science reporting on AIDS has evolved, "articles about the spread of AIDS to the so-called general public do not have to be pegged to any specific new data" ("Public Education on AIDS," p. 31).

17. The Paris conference was one of several fact-pooling and consensus-building events in 1986 that influenced new readings of existing evidence. Also influential were the *US Surgeon General's Report on Acquired Immune Deficiency Syndrome*, Washington, D.C., Public Health Service, 1986, which advocated intensified sex education in the schools; an investigation by the National Institute of Medicine and the National Academy of Sciences (David Baltimore and Sheldon M. Wolff, *Confronting AIDS: Directions for Public Health, Health Care, and Research*, Washington, D.C., National Academy Press, 1986), which emphasized the dangers of heterosexual transmission; and a World Health

heroic scientific discovery. And until we understand AIDS as both a material and a linguistic reality — a duality inherent in all linguistic entities but extraordinarily exaggerated and potentially deadly in the case of AIDS — we cannot begin to read the story of this illness accurately or formulate intelligent interventions.

Intelligent interventions from outside biomedical science have helped shape the discourse on AIDS. Almost from the beginning, members of the gay community, through intense interest and informed political activism, have repeatedly contested the terminology, meanings, and interpretations produced by scientific inquiry. Such contestations had occurred a decade earlier in the struggle over whether homosexuality was to be officially classified as an illness by the American Psychiatric Association.[18] Gay men and lesbians in the succeeding period had achieved considerable success in political organizing. AIDS, then, first struck members of a relatively seasoned and politically sophisticated community. The importance of not relinquishing authority to medicine was articulated early in the AIDS crisis by Michael Lynch:

> Another crisis exists with the medical one. It has gone largely unexamined, even by the gay press. Like helpless mice we have peremptorily, almost inexplicably, relinquished the one power we so long fought for in constructing our modern gay community: the power to determine our own identity. And to whom have we relinquished it? The very authority we wrested it from in a struggle that occupied us for more than a hundred years: the medical profession.[19]

To challenge biomedical authority — whose meanings are part of powerful and deeply entrenched social and historical codes — has required considerable tenacity and courage from people dependent in the AIDS crisis upon science and medicine for protection, care, and the possibility of cure. These contestations provide the model for a broader social analysis, which moves away from AIDS as a "life-style" issue and examines its significance for this country, at this time, with the cultural and material resources available to us. This, in turn, requires us to acknowledge and examine the multiple ways in which our social constructions guide our visions of material reality.

Organization conference that concluded that AIDS must now be considered a pandemic of catastrophic proportions. (An epidemic disease is prevalent within a specific community, geographical area, or population at a particular time, usually originating elsewhere; a pandemic disease is present over the whole of a country, a continent, or the world.) See also "AIDS: Public Health and Civil Liberties," *Hastings Center Report*, Special Supplement, vol. 16, no. 6 (December 1986); "AIDS: Science, Ethics, Policy," Forum, *Issues in Science and Technology*, vol. 2, no. 2 (Winter 1986), pp. 39–73.

18.   See Ronald Bayer, *Homosexuality and American Psychiatry: The Politics of Diagnosis*, New York, Basic Books, 1981.

19.   Michael Lynch, "Living with Kaposi's," *Body Politic*, no. 88 (November 1982).

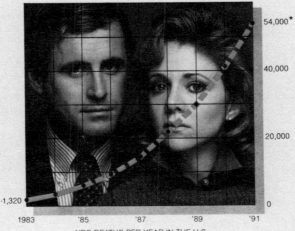

REAGAN: POLITICAL TROUBLES AHEAD

U.S.News & WORLD REPORT

JANUARY 12, 1987 $1.95

AIDS

What You Need to Know
What You Should Do

54,000*

40,000

20,000

-1,320

0

1983   '85   '87   '89   '91

AIDS DEATHS PER YEAR IN THE U.S.

*Americans killed in Vietnam: 58,135

AIDS and Homophobia:
Constructing the Text of the Gay Male Body

Whatever else it may be, AIDS is a story, or multiple stories, read to a surprising extent from a text that does not exist: the body of the male homosexual. It is a text people so want—need—to read that they have gone so far as to write it themselves. AIDS is a nexus where multiple meanings, stories, and discourses intersect and overlap, reinforce, and subvert one another. Yet clearly this mysterious male homosexual text has figured centrally in generating what I call here an epidemic of signification. Of course "the virus," with mysteries of its own, has been a crucial influence. But we may recall Camus's novel: "The word 'plague' . . . conjured up in the doctor's mind not only what science chose to put into it, but a whole series of fantastic possibilities utterly out of keeping" with the bourgeois town of Oran, where the plague struck.[20] How could a disease so extraordinary as *plague* happen in a place so ordinary and dull? AIDS, initially striking people perceived as alien and exotic by scientists, physicians, journalists, and much of the US population, did not pose such a paradox. The "promiscuous" gay male body—early reports noted that AIDS "victims" reported having had as many as 1,000 sexual partners—made clear that even if AIDS turned out to be a sexually transmitted disease it would not be a commonplace one. The connections between sex, death, and homosexuality made the AIDS story inevitably, as David Black notes, able to be read as "the story of a metaphor."[21]

20.   Albert Camus, *The Plague*, trans. Stuart Gilbert, New York, Modern Library, 1948 (first published Paris, Gallimard, 1947).
21.   "I realized . . . that any account of AIDS was not just a medical story and not just a story about the gay community, but also a story about the straight community's reaction to the disease. More than that: it's a story about how the straight community has used and is using AIDS as a mask for its feelings about gayness. It is a story about the ramifications of a metaphor" (Black, *The Plague Years*, p. 30). AIDS is typically characterized as a "story," but whose? For AIDS as a story of scientific progress, see Gallo, "The AIDS Virus"; Arnold Relman, "Introduction," *Hastings Center Report*, Special Supplement, vol. 15, no. 4 (August 1985), p. 1; Eve K. Nichols, *Mobilizing Against AIDS: The Unfinished Story of a Virus* (Conference of the Institute of Medicine/National Academy of Sciences), Cambridge, Massachusetts, Harvard University Press, 1986; Jonathan Lieberson, "Anatomy of an Epidemic," *New York Review of Books*, August 18, 1983, pp. 17–22. But for Lynch ("Living with Kaposi's"), Goldstein ("Heartsick"), FitzGerald (*Cities on a Hill*), Larry Kramer ("1,112 and Counting," *New York Native*, March 1983, pp. 14–27), D. W. McLeod and Alan V. Miller ("Medical, Social, and Political Aspects of the AIDS Case: A Bibliography," *Canadian Gay Archives*, no. 10), Thom Gunn (*Lament*, Champaign, Illinois, Doe Press, 1985), Steve Ault ("AIDS: The Facts of Life," *Guardian*, March 26, 1986, pp. 1, 8), Dennis Altman (*AIDS in the Mind of America*, New York, Doubleday, 1986), the San Francisco *A.I.D.S. Show—Artists Involved with Death and Survival* (documentary video produced by Peter Adair and Rob Epstein, directed by Leland Moss; based on theater production at Theatre Rhinoceros, San Francisco; aired on PBS, November 1986), and others, AIDS is the story of crisis and heroism in the gay community. In the tabloids, AIDS has become the story of Rock Hudson (ROCK IS DEAD, ran the headlines in the [London] *Sun* on October 3, 1985, THE HUNK WHO LIVED A LIE), Liberace, and other individuals. A documentary film about the Fabian Bridges case, a young man with AIDS in Houston, is called *Fabian's Story* (see J. Ostrow, "AIDS Documentary Addresses Agonizing Issues," *Denver Post*, March 24, 1986). For Geoff Mains (*Urban Aboriginals: A Celebration of Leathersexuality*, San Francisco, Gay Sunshine Press, 1985), AIDS inter-

Ironically, a major turning point in US consciousness came when Rock Hudson acknowledged that he was being treated for AIDS. Through an extraordinary conflation of texts, the Rock Hudson case dramatized the possibility that the disease could spread to the "general population."[22] In fact this possibility had

---

rupts the adventure story of leather sex, a "unique and valuable cultural excursion" (p. 178). And in Thom Gunn's poem, *Lament*, AIDS is a story of change and the death of friends. The stories we tell help us determine what our own place in the story is to be. FitzGerald writes that the "new mythology" about AIDS in the San Francisco gay community—that many gay men are changing their lives for the better—was "an antidote to the notion that AIDS was a punishment—a notion that . . . lay so deep as to be unavailable to reason. And it helped people act against the threat of AIDS" (*Cities on a Hill*, p. 116). But for Richard Mohr ("Of Deathbeds and Quarantines: AIDS Funding, Gay Life and State Coercion," *Raritan*, vol. 6, no. 1 [Summer 1986], pp. 38–62), this new mythology—in which the loving relationship replaces anonymous sex—is a dangerous one: "The relation typically is asked to bear more than is reasonable. The burden on the simple dyad is further weighed down by the myth, both romantic and religious, that one finds one's completion in a single other. White knights and messiahs never come in clusters" (p. 56). For discussion of AIDS as a public drama, see "AIDS: Public Health and Civil Liberties"; Ronald Bayer, "AIDS: The Public Context of an Epidemic," *Millbank Quarterly*, no. 64, Supplement 1, pp. 168–182; and McLeod and Miller, "Medical, Social, and Political Aspects."

22. Articulate voices had taken issue with the CDC position from the beginning, warning against the public health consequences of treating AIDS as a "gay disease" and separating "those at risk" from the so-called "general population." See, for example, comments by Gary MacDonald, executive director of an AIDS action organization in Washington: "I think the moment may have arrived to desexualize the disease. AIDS is *not* a 'gay disease,' despite its epidemiology. . . . AIDS is not transmitted because of who you *are*, but because of what you *do*. . . . By concentrating on gay and bisexual men, people are able to ignore the fact that this disease has been present in what has charmingly come to be called 'the general population' *from the beginning*. It was not spread from one of the other groups. It was *there* ("AIDS: What Is to Be Done?" Forum, *Harper's Magazine*, October 1985, p. 43).

One can extrapolate from Ruth Bleier's observation that questions shape answers (*Science and Gender*, London, Pergamon, 1986, p. 4), and suggest that the question "Why are all people with AIDS sexually active homosexual males?" might more appropriately have been "*Are* all people with AIDS sexually active homosexual males?" It is widely believed (not without evidence) that federal funding for AIDS research was long in coming because its chief victims were gay or otherwise socially undesirable. Black describes a researcher who made jokes about *fagocytes* (phagocytes), cells designed "to kill off fags" (*The Plague Years*, pp. 81–82). Secretary of Health and Human Services Margaret Heckler was only one of many officials who expressed concern not about existing people with AIDS but about the potential spread of AIDS to "the community at large" (with the result that Heckler was called "the Secretary of Health and Heterosexual Services" by some gay activists; see "AIDS: What Is to Be Done?" p. 51).

There is evidence that the "gay disease" myth interferes with diagnosis and treatment. Many believe that AIDS may be underdetected and underreported in part because people outside the "classic" high-risk groups are often not asked the right questions (physicians typically take longer to diagnose AIDS in women, for example). Health professionals and AIDS counselors sometimes avoid the word *gay* because for many people this implies an identity or life-style; even *bisexual* may mean a life-style. Although "homosexually active" is officially defined as including even a single same-sex sexual contact over the past five years, many who have had such contact do not identify themselves as "homosexual" and therefore as being at risk for AIDS. Nancy Shaw ("California Models for Women's AIDS Education and Services," report, San Francisco AIDS Foundation [333 Valencia St., 4th Floor, San Francisco, CA 94103], and "Women and AIDS: Theory and Politics," presented at the annual meeting of the National Women's Studies Association, University of Illinois, Urbana, June 1986) suggests that for women as well the homosexual/heterosexual dichotomy confuses diagnosis and treatment as well as the perception of risk. Pally ("AIDS and the Politics of Despair"),

been evident for some time to anyone who wished to find it: as Jean Marx summarized the evidence in *Science* in 1984, "Sexual intercourse both of the heterosexual and homosexual varieties is a major pathway of transmission."[23] But only in late 1986 (and somewhat reluctantly at that) did the Centers for Disease Control expand upon their early "4-H list" of high-risk categories: HOMOSEXUALS, HEMOPHILIACS, HEROIN ADDICTS, and HAITIANS, and the sexual partners of people within these groups.[24] The original list, developed during 1981 and 1982, has structured evidence collection in the intervening years and contributed to a view that the major risk factor in acquiring AIDS is being a particular kind of person rather than doing particular things.[25] Ann Giudici Fettner pointed out in 1985 that "the CDC admits that at least 10 percent of AIDS sufferers are gay *and* use IV drugs. Yet they are automatically counted in the homosexual and bisexual men category, regardless of what might be known —or not known—about how they became infected."[26] So the "gay" nature of AIDS was in part an artifact of the way in which data was collected and reported. Though almost from the beginning scientific papers have cited AIDS cases that appeared to fall outside the high-risk groups, it has been generally hypothesized that these cases, assigned to the categories of UNKNOWN, UNCLASSIFIED, or OTHER,

Marea Murray ("Too Little AIDS Coverage," Letter to the Editors, *Sojourner,* July 1985, p. 3), and Cindy Patton ("Feminists Have Avoided the Issue of AIDS," *Sojourner,* October 1985, pp. 19–20) all argue that AIDS is a "women's issue" and should receive more attention in feminist publications (and see COYOTE, Background Paper, 1985 COYOTE Convention Summary, May 30–June 2, 1985, San Francisco; Ellen Switzer, "AIDS: What Women Can Do," *Vogue,* January 1986, pp. 222–223, 264–265; Jane Sprague Zones, "AIDS: What Women Need to Know," *The [National Women's Health] Network News,* vol. 11, no. 6 [November–December 1986], pp. 1, 3). The persistence and consequences of the perception that AIDS is a disease of gay men and IV drug users are documented in a number of recent publications, notably Leishman, "Heterosexuals and AIDS." CDC interviews with members of two heterosexual singles clubs in Minneapolis documented that as of late 1986 this already infected population had made virtually no modifications in their sexual practices ("Positive HTLV-III/LAV Antibody Results for Sexually Active Female Members of Social/Sexual Clubs— Minnesota," *Morbidity and Mortality Weekly Report,* no. 35 [1986], pp. 697–699). Ralph J. DiClemente, Jim Zorn, and Lydia Temoshok ("Adolescents and AIDS: A Survey of Knowledge, Attitudes, and Beliefs about AIDS in San Francisco," *American Journal of Public Health,* vol. 76, no. 12 [1986], pp. 1443–1445) found that many adolescents in San Francisco, a city where public health information about AIDS has been extensive, were not well informed about the seriousness of the disease, its causes, or preventive measures.

23.   Jean L. Marx, "Strong New Candidate for AIDS Agent," Research News, *Science,* May 4, 1984, p. 147.

24.   Centers for Disease Control, "Update: Acquired Immunodeficiency Syndrome—United States," *Morbidity and Mortality Weekly Report,* no. 35 (1986), pp. 757–760, 765–766.

25.   Jeff Minson, "The Assertion of Homosexuality," *m/f,* nos. 5–6 (1981), pp. 19–39, and Jeffrey Weeks, *Sexuality and Its Discontents: Meanings, Myths, and Modern Sexualities,* London, Routledge & Kegan Paul, 1985, analyze the evolution of homosexuality as a coherent identity. Bayer, *Homosexuality and American Psychiatry,* and Ronald Bayer and Robert L. Spitzer, "Edited Correspondence on the Status of Homosexuality in DSM-III," *Journal of the History of the Behavioral Sciences,* no. 18 (1982), pp. 32–52, document the intense and acrimonious "contests for meaning" during the American Psychiatric Association's 1970s debates over the official classification of homosexuality.

26.   Fettner, in "AIDS: What Is to Be Done?" p. 43.

would ultimately turn out to be one of the four H's.[27] This commitment to categories based on stereotyped identity filters out information. Nancy Shaw argues that when women are asked in CDC protocols "Are you heterosexual?" "this loses the diversity of behaviors that may have a bearing on infection."[28] Even now, with established evidence that transmission can be heterosexual (which begins with the letter *H* after all), scientific discourse continues to construct women as "inefficient" and "incompetent" transmitters of HIV, passive receptacles without the projectile capacity of a penis or syringe — stolid, uninteresting barriers that impede the unrestrained passage of the virus from brother to brother.[29] Exceptions include prostitutes, whose discursive legacy — despite their longstanding professional knowledge and continued activism about AIDS — is to be seen as so contaminated that their bodies are virtual laboratory cultures for viral replication.[30] Other exceptions are African women, whose exotic bodies,

27.   See Nichols, *Mobilizing Against AIDS,* and Associated Press, "571 AIDS Cases Tied to Heterosexual Causes," *Champaign-Urbana News-Gazette,* December 12, 1986, p. A-7, on the reclassification in 1986 of the CDC's 571 previously "unexplained cases"; formerly classified as "none of the above" (i.e., outside the known high-risk categories), some of these cases were reclassified as heterosexually transmitted.

28.   Shaw, "Women and AIDS."

29.   Even after consensus in 1984 that AIDS was caused by a virus, there continued to be conflicting views on transmission and different explanations for the epidemiological finding that AIDS and HIV infection in the US were appearing predominantly in gay males. One view holds that this is essentially an artifact ("simple mathematics") created because the virus (for whatever reason) infected gay men first and gay men tend to have sex with each other. The second is that biomedical/physiological factors make gay men and/or the "passive receiver" more infectable. A third view is that the virus can be transmitted to anyone but that certain cofactors facilitate the development of infection and/or clinical symptoms. For more information, see Leibowitch, *A Strange Virus,* pp. 72–73, Leishman, "Heterosexuals and AIDS," and Mathilde Krim, "AIDS: The Challenge to Science and Medicine," in *AIDS: The Emerging Ethical Dilemmas: A Hastings Center Report,* Special Supplement, vol. 15, no. 4 (August 1985), p. 4. Many scientists suggest that, whatever sex the partners may be, infection, as Fain ("AIDS: An Antidote to Fear") put it, "requires a jolt injected into the bloodstream, likely several jolts over time, such as would occur with infected needles or semen. In both cases, needle and penis are the instruments of contagion." Women, having no penises, are therefore "inefficient" transmitters. For more detailed discussion, see my essay on women and AIDS, forthcoming in *AIDS: The Burdens of History,* ed. Elizabeth Fee and Daniel M. Fox, Berkeley, University of California Press.

          Evidence of heterosexual transmission was at first explained away. When R. R. Redfield, *et al.* ("Heterosexually Acquired HTLV-III/LAV Disease [AIDS-Related Complex and AIDS]: Epidemiological Evidence for Female-to-Male Transmission," *Journal of the American Medical Association,* no. 254 [1985], pp. 2094–2096; "Female-to-Male Transmission of HTLV-III," *Journal of the American Medical Association,* no. 255 [1986], pp. 1705–1706) identified infection in US servicemen who claimed sexual contact only with female prostitutes, some hypothesized "quasi-homosexual contact" or called the data into question on the grounds that servicemen would be likely to withhold information about homosexuality or drug use (some evidence for this is offered by John J. Potterat, *et al.,* "Lying to Military Physicians about Risk Factors for HIV Infections," Letter to *Journal of the American Medical Association,* vol. 257, no. 13 [April 3, 1987], p. 1727). For discussion of the relation of transmission to funding, see Barnes, "AIDS Research in New Phase," p. 283, and "AIDS Funding Boost Requested," *Daily Illini,* September 27, 1985, p. 7.

30.   Brandt, *No Magic Bullet,* and Judith Walkowitz, *Prostitution and Victorian Society: Women, Class, and the State,* New York, Cambridge University Press, 1983, review the longstanding equation of

sexual practices, or who knows what are seen to be so radically different from those of women in the US that anything can happen in them.[31] The term *exotic*, sometimes used to describe a virus that appears to have originated "elsewhere" (but "elsewhere," like "other" is not a fixed category), is an important theme running through AIDS literature.[32] The fact that one of the more extensive and visually elegant analyses of AIDS appeared recently in *National Geographic* is perhaps further evidence of its life on an idealized "exotic" terrain.[33]

The early hypotheses about AIDS, when the first cases appeared in New York, Los Angeles, and Paris, were sociological, relating it directly to the supposed "gay male life-style." In February 1982, for example, it was thought that a particular supply of amyl nitrate (poppers) might be contaminated. "The poppers fable," writes Jacques Leibowitch, becomes

> a Grimm fairy tale when the first cases of AIDS-without-poppers are discovered among homosexuals absolutely repelled by the smell of the product and among heterosexuals unfamiliar with even the words *amyl nitrate* or *poppers*. But, as will be habitual in the history of AIDS, rumors last longer than either common sense or the facts would warrant. The odor of AIDS-poppers will hover in the air a long time — long enough for dozens of mice in the Atlanta epidemiology labs to be kept in restricted cages on an obligatory sniffed diet of poppers 8 to 12 hours a day for several months, until, nauseated but still healthy, without a trace of AIDS, the wretched rodents were released — provisionally — upon the announcement of a new hypothesis: *promiscuity*.[34]

This new perspective generated numerous possibilities. One was that sperm

---

prostitutes with disease, and the conceptual separation of infected prostitutes (and other voluntarily sexually active women) from "innocent victims" (see also COYOTE, "Background Paper"; Shaw, "Women and AIDS"; Colin Douglas, *The Intern's Tale*, New York, Grove, 1975, repr. 1982; Erik Eckholm, "Prostitutes' Impact on Spread of AIDS Debated," *New York Times*, November 5, 1985, pp. 15, 18; and Nancy Shaw and Lyn Paleo, "Women and AIDS," in *What to Do about AIDS*, ed. Leon McKusick, Berkeley, University of California Press, 1986, pp. 142–154).

31.   Discussions of AIDS and heterosexual transmission in Africa include Lieberson, "The Reality of AIDS"; Treichler, forthcoming in *AIDS: The Burdens of History;* Cindy Patton, *Sex and Germs: The Politics of AIDS*, Boston, South End Press, 1985; June E. Osborn, "The AIDS Epidemic: An Overview of the Science," *Issues in Science and Technology*, vol. 2, no. 2 (Winter 1986), pp. 40–55; Jean L. Marx, "New Relatives of AIDS Virus Found," Research News, *Science*, no. 232 (April 11, 1986), p. 157; Fran P. Hosken, "Why AIDS Pattern Is Different in Africa," Letter to the *New York Times*, December 15, 1986; Douglas A. Feldman, "Role of African Mutilations in AIDS Discounted," Letter to the *New York Times*, January 7, 1987; Lawrence K. Altman, "Heterosexuals and AIDS: New Data Examined," *New York Times*, January 22, 1985, pp. 19–20; and "New Human Retroviruses: One Causes AIDS . . . and the Other Does Not," *Nature*, no. 320 (April 3, 1986), p. 385.

32.   Leibowitch, *A Strange Virus*, p. 73.

33.   Peter Jaret, "Our Immune System: The Wars Within," *National Geographic*, June 1986, pp. 702–735.

34.   Leibowitch, *A Strange Virus*, p. 5.

itself could destroy the immune system. "God's plan for man," after all, "was for Adam and Eve and not Adam and Steve."[35] Women, the "natural" receptacles for male sperm, have evolved over the millennia so that their bodies can deal with these foreign invaders; men, not thus blessed by nature, become vulnerable to the "killer sperm" of other men. AIDS in the lay press became known as the "toxic cock syndrome."[36] While scientists and physicians tended initially to define AIDS as a gay sociological problem, gay men, for other reasons, also tended to reject the possibility that AIDS was a new contagious disease. Not only could this make them sexual lepers, it didn't make sense: "How could a disease pick out just gays? That had to be medical homophobia."[37] Important to note here is a profound ambivalence about the origins of illness. Does one prefer an illness caused by who one is and therefore perhaps preventable, curable, or containable through "self-control"—or an illness caused by some external "disease" which has a respectable medical name and can be addressed strictly as a medical problem, beyond individual control? The townspeople of Oran in *The Plague* experience relief when the plague bacillus is identified: the odd happenings—the dying rats, the mysterious human illnesses—are caused by something that has originated elsewhere, something external, something "objective," something medicine can name, even if not cure. The tension between self and not-self becomes important as we try to understand the particular role of viruses and origin stories in AIDS.

But this anticipates the next chapter in the AIDS story. Another favored possibility in the early 1980s (still not universally discarded, for it is plausible so long as the cases of AIDS among monogamous homebodies are ignored) was the notion of "cofactors": no *single* infectious agent causes the disease; rather, someone who is sexually active with multiple partners is exposed to a kind of bacterial/viral tidal wave that can crush the immune system.[38] Gay men on the sexual

---

35.   Congressman William Dannemeyer, October 1985, during a debate on a homosexual rights bill (quoted in Langone, "AIDS: The Latest Scientific Facts," p. 29).

36.   Black, *The Plague Years,* p. 29.

37.   *Ibid.,* p. 40. In the gay community, the first reaction to AIDS was disbelief. FitzGerald quotes a gay physician in San Francisco: "A disease that killed only gay white men? It seemed unbelievable. I used to teach epidemiology, and I had never heard of a disease that selective. I thought, They are making this up. It can't be true. Or if there is such a disease it must be the work of some government agency—the F.B.I. or the C.I.A.—trying to kill us all" (*Cities on a Hill,* p. 98). In the San Francisco *A.I.D.S. Show,* one man is said to have learned of his diagnosis and at once wired the CIA: "I HAVE AIDS. DO YOU HAVE AN ANTIDOTE?"

38.   See Lieberson, "The Reality of AIDS," p. 43, for an example of the view that, although the virus is the "sine qua non" for AIDS, the syndrome actually develops "chiefly in those whose immune systems are already weak or defective." For broader discussion of public health issues in relation to scientific uncertainties and questions of civil liberties, see Ronald Bayer, "AIDS and the Gay Community: Between the Specter and the Promise of Medicine," *Social Research,* vol. 52, no. 3 (Autumn 1985), pp. 581–606; Mervyn F. Silverman and Deborah B. Silverman, "AIDS and the Threat to Public Health," *Hastings Center Report,* Special Supplement, vol. 15, no. 4 (August 1985), pp. 19–22; and Gene W. Matthews and Verla S. Neslund, "The Initial Impact of AIDS on Public Health Law in

"fast-track" would be particularly susceptible because of the prevalence of specific practices that would maximize exposure to pathogenic microbes. What were considered potentially relevant data came to be routinely included in scientific papers and presentations, with the result that the terminology of these reports was increasingly scrutinized by gay activists.[39] Examples from *Science* from June 1981 through December 1985 include "homosexual and bisexual men who are extremely active sexually," "admitted homosexuals," "homosexual males with multiple partners," "homosexual men with multiple partners," "highly sexually active homosexual men," and "promiscuous" versus "nonpromiscuous" homosexual males.[40] Also documented (examples are also from the *Science* collection) are exotic travels or practices: "a Caucasian who had visited Haiti," "persons born in Haiti," "a favorite vacation spot for US homosexuals," rectal insemination, "bisexual men," "increased frequency of use of nitrite inhalants," and "receptive anal intercourse."[41]

Out of this dense discursive jungle came the "fragile anus" hypothesis (tested by Richards and his colleagues, who rectally inseminated laboratory rabbits) as well as the vision of "multiple partners."[42] Even after sociological explanations for AIDS gave way to biomedical ones involving a transmissible virus, these various images of AIDS as a "gay disease" proved too alluring to abandon. It is easy to see both the scientific and the popular appeal of the "fragile anus" hypothesis: scientifically, it confines the public health dimensions of AIDS to an infected population in the millons—merely mind-boggling, that is—

the United States—1986," *Journal of the American Medical Association*, vol. 257, no. 3 (January 16, 1987), pp. 344–352.

39.   L. Altman, "Heterosexuals and AIDS," and Black, *The Plague Years*, discuss changes in specific terminology as a result of gays' objections; "sexually promiscuous" generally shifted, for example, to "sexually active" or "contact with multiple sex partners." A new classification system for AIDS and AIDS/HIV-related symptoms (adopted at the 2nd International AIDS Conference in Paris, June 1986) is based on the diverse clinical manifestations of the syndrome and its documented natural history; it avoids presumptive terminology like "pre-AIDS." J. Z. Grover's useful review of Nichols's *Mobilizing Against AIDS* ("The 'Scientific' Regime of Truth," *In These Times*, December 10–16, 1986, pp. 18–19) points out a number of problematic terms and assumptions that occur repeatedly in this book and other scientific writing on AIDS: (1) the term *AIDS victim* presupposes helplessness (the term *person with AIDS* or PWA was created to avoid this), prevention and cure are linked with a conservative agenda of "individual responsibility," sex with multiple partners and/or strangers is equated with "promiscuity," and "safe" sexual practices are conflated with the cultural practice of monogamy; (2) it differentiates "caregivers" from "victims," scientific/medical expertise from other kinds of knowledge, and "those at risk" from "the rest of us"; and (3) it notes but fails to challenge existing inequities in the health-care system. Julie Dobrow, "The Symbolism of AIDS: Perspectives on the Use of Language in the Popular Press," presented at the International Communication Association annual meeting, Chicago, May 1986, notes the dramatic and commercial appeal of common "cultural images" in popular press scenarios of AIDS.

40.   Terms are quoted from the collection *AIDS: Papers from Science 1982–1985*, ed. Ruth Kulstad, Washington, D.C., American Association for the Advancement of Science, 1986, pp. 22, 40, 49, 65, 142, and 160, respectively.

41.   *Ibid.*, pp. 47, 130, 73, 142–146, 130, 611, 611, respectively.

42.   *Ibid.*, pp. 142–146.

enabling us to stop short of the impossible, the unthinkable billions that wide-spread heterosexual transmission might infect. Another appeal of thinking of AIDS as a "gay disease" is that it protects not only the sexual practices of heterosexuality but also its ideological superiority. In the service of this hypothesis, both homophobia and sexism are folded imperturbably into the language of the scientific text. Women, as I noted above, are characterized in the scholarly literature as "inefficient" transmitters of AIDS; Leibowitch refers to the "refractory impermeability of the vaginal mucous membrane."[43] A study of German prostitutes that appeared to demonstrate female-to-male transmission of AIDS, reported in the *Journal of the American Medical Association,* was interpreted by one reader as actually representing "quasi-homosexual" transmission: Man A, infected with HIV, has vaginal intercourse with Prostitute; she, "[performing] no more than perfunctory external cleansing between customers," then has intercourse with Man B; Man B is infected with the virus via the semen of Man A.[44] The prostitute's vagina thus functions merely as a reservoir, a passive holding tank for semen that becomes infectious only when another penis is dipped into it — like a swamp where mosquitoes come to breed.

But the conception and the conclusion are inaccurate. It is not monogamy or abstention per se that protects one from AIDS infection but practices and protections that prevent the virus from entering one's bloodstream. Evidence suggests that prostitutes are at greater risk not because they have multiple sex partners, but because some of them use intravenous drugs; at this point "they may be better protected than the typical woman who is just going to a bar or a woman who thinks of herself as not sexually active but who 'just happens to have this relationship.' They may be more aware than women who are involved in serial monogamy or those whose self-image is 'I'm not at risk so I'm not going to learn more about it.'"[45] Indeed, COYOTE and other organizations of prostitutes have addressed the issue of AIDS rather aggressively for several years.[46]

43.   Leibowitch, *A Strange Virus,* p. 36.
44.   Data on female-to-male transmission presented at the 1985 International Conference on AIDS in Atlanta are summarized by Marsha F. Goldsmith, "More Heterosexual Spread of HTLV-III Virus Seen," *Journal of the American Medical Association,* no. 253 (1985), pp. 3377–3379. The hypothesis that such data reflect "quasi-homosexual contact" is suggested by Harold Sanford Kant, "The Transmission of HTLV-III," Letter to the Editor, *Journal of the American Medical Association,* no. 254 (1985), p. 1901.
45.   Shaw and Paleo, "Women and AIDS," p. 144.
46.   Kant's hypothesis in *JAMA* is quoted by Langone, "AIDS: The Latest Scientific Facts," p. 49, to support his own "vulnerable anus" hypothesis: "It is not unlikely that these prostitutes had multiple partners during a very short time, and performed no more than perfunctory external cleansing between customers." Langone does not note that the source is a Letter to the Editor. Meanwhile, reports from prostitutes in many countries, summarized in the June 1986 *World Wide Whores' News* (published by the International Committee for Prostitutes' Rights), indicate familiarity with AIDS as well as concern with obtaining better protection from infection and better health care. See also COYOTE, "Background Paper."

Donald Mager discusses the proliferation among heterosexuals of visions about homosexuality and their status as fantasy:

> Institutions of privilege and power disenfranchise lesbians and gay men because of stereotypic negative categorizations of them — stereotypes which engage a societal fantasy of the illicit, the subversive, and the taboo, particularly due to assumptions of radical sex role parodies and inversions. This fantasy in turn becomes both the object of fear and of obsessed fascination, while its status as fantasy is never acknowledged; instead, the reality it pretends to signify becomes the justification of suppression both of the fantasy itself and of those actual persons who would seem to embody it. Homophobia as a critique of societal sexual fantasy, in turn, enforces its primary location as a gay discourse, separate and outside the site of the fantasy which is normative male heterosexuality.[47]

Leibowitch comments as follows on AIDS, fantasy, and "the reality it pretends to signify":

> When they come to write the history of AIDS, socio-ethnologists will have to decide whether the "practitioners" of homosexuality or its heterosexual "onlookers" have been the more spectacular in their extravagance. The homosexual "life style" is so blatantly on display to the general public, so closely scrutinized, that it is likely we never will have been informed with such technicophantasmal complacency as to how "other people" live their lives.[48]

It was widely believed in the gay community that the connection of AIDS to homosexuality delayed and problematized virtually every aspect of the country's response to the crisis. That the response *was* delayed and problematic is the conclusion of various investigators.[49] Attempting to assess the degree to which prejudice, fear, or ignorance of homosexuality may have affected public policy and research efforts, Panem concluded that homosexuality per se would not have deterred scientists from selecting interesting and rewarding research projects. But "the argument of ignorance appears to have more credibility."[50] She quotes

47.   Donald Mager, "The Discourse about Homophobia, Male and Female Contexts," presented at the annual meeting of the Modern Language Association, New York, December 1986.
48.   Leibowitch, *A Strange Virus*, p. 3.
49.   See, for example, Schwartz, "AIDS in the Media"; Baltimore and Wolff, *Confronting AIDS*; "AIDS Hearing," Committee on Energy and Commerce, Subcommittee on Health and the Environment, US House of Representatives, September 17, 1984 (Serial No. 98–105, Washington, D.C., US Government Printing Office); and Office of Technology Assessment, *Review of the Public Health Service's Response to AIDS: A Technical Memorandum*, OTA-TM-H-24, Congress of the US, Washington, D.C., US Government Printing Office, February 1985.
50.   Sandra Panem, "AIDS: Public Policy and Biomedical Research," *Hastings Center Report*, Special Supplement, vol. 15, no. 4 (August 1985), p. 24.

James Curran's 1984 judgment that policy, funding, and communication were all delayed because only people in New York and California had any real sense of crisis or comprehension of the gay male community. "Scientists avoid issues that relate to sex," he said, "and there is not much understanding of homosexuality." This was an understatement: according to Curran, many eminent scientists during this period rejected the possibility that AIDS was an infectious disease because they had no idea how a man could transmit an infectious agent to another man.[51] Other instances of ignorance are reported by Patton and Black.[52] Physician and scientist Joseph Sonnabend attributes this ignorance to the sequestered ivory towers that many AIDS investigators (particularly those who do straight laboratory research as opposed to clinical work) inhabit and argues instead that AIDS needs to be studied in its cultural totality. Gay male sexual practices should not be dismissed out of hand because they seem "unnatural" to the straight (in both senses) scientist: "the rectum is a sexual organ, and it deserves the respect that a penis gets and a vagina gets. Anal intercourse is a central sexual activity, and it should be supported, it should be celebrated."[53] A National Academy of Sciences panel studying the AIDS crisis in 1986 cited an urgent need for accurate and *current* information about sex and sexual practices in the US, noting that no comprehensive research had been carried out since Kinsey's studies in the 1940s; they recommended, as well, social science research on a range of social behaviors relevant to the transmission and control of AIDS.[54]

It has been argued that the perceived *gayness* of AIDS was ultimately a crucial political factor in obtaining funding. Dennis Altman observes that the principle of providing adequate funding for AIDS research was institutionalized within the federal appropriations process as a result of the 1983 Congressional hearings chaired by Representatives Henry Waxman and Theodore Weiss, members of Congress representing large and visible gay communities.

> Here one sees the effect of the mobilization and organization of gays . . . ; it is salutary to imagine the tardiness of the response had IV users and Haitians been the only victims of AIDS, had Republicans controlled the House of Representatives as well as the Senate (and hence chaired the relevant oversight and appropriations committees) or, indeed, had AIDS struck ten years earlier, before the existence of an organized gay movement, openly gay professionals who could testify before the relevant committees and openly gay congressional staff.[55]

51.   *Ibid.*
52.   Patton, *Sex and Germs;* Patton, "Feminists Have Avoided the Issue of AIDS"; Black, *The Plague Years.*
53.   Joseph Sonnabend, "Looking at AIDS in Totality: A Conversation," *New York Native,* 129 (October 7–13, 1985).
54.   Baltimore and Wolff, *Confronting AIDS.*
55.   D. Altman, *AIDS in the Mind of America,* pp. 116–117.

But these social and political issues were felt by many to be essentially irrelevant. From the beginning, the hypothesis that AIDS was caused by an infectious agent was favored within the US scientific community. The hypothesis was strengthened when the syndrome began to be identified in a diversity of populations and found to cause apparently identical damage to the underlying immune system. By May 1984 a viral etiology for AIDS had been generally accepted, and the real question became precisely what kind of viral agent this could be.

Rendezvous with 007

"Interpretations," write Bruno Latour and Steve Woolgar in *Laboratory Life,* their analysis of the construction of facts in science, "do not so much *inform* as *perform.*"[56] And nowhere do we see interpretation shaped toward performance so clearly as in the issues and controversies surrounding the identification and naming of "the AIDS virus."

As early as 1979, gay men in New York and California were coming down with and dying from illnesses unusual in young healthy people. One of the actors who helped create the San Francisco *A.I.D.S. Show* recalled that early period:

> I had a friend who died way way back in New York in 1981. He was one of the first to go. We didn't know what AIDS was, there was no name for it. We didn't know it was contagious — we had no idea it was sexually transmitted — we didn't know it was anything. We just thought that he — alone — was ill. He was 26 years old and just had one thing after another wrong with him. . . . He was still coming to work — 'cause he didn't *know* he had a terminal disease.[57]

The oddness of these nameless isolated events gave way to an even more terrifying period in which gay men on both coasts gradually began to realize that too many friends and acquaintances were dying. As the numbers mounted, the deaths became "cases" of what was informally called in New York hospitals WOGS: the Wrath of God Syndrome.[58] It all became official in 1981, when five deaths in Los Angeles from *Pneumocystis* pneumonia were described in the June 5 issue of the CDC's bulletin *Morbidity and Mortality Weekly Report* with an editorial note explaining that

> the occurrence of pneumocystosis in these 5 previously healthy individuals without a clinically apparent underlying immunodeficiency is unusual. The fact that these patients were all homosexuals suggests an association between some aspect of a homosexual lifestyle or disease

56.   Latour and Woolgar, *Laboratory Life.*
57.   From *The A.I.D.S. Show.*
58.   See Sontag, *Illness as Metaphor.*

acquired through sexual contact and *Pneumocystis* pneumonia in this population.[59]

Gottlieb's 1981 paper in the *New England Journal of Medicine* described the deaths of young, previously healthy gay men from another rare but rarely fatal disease.[60] The deaths were attributed to a breakdown of the immune system that left the body utterly unable to defend itself against infections not normally fatal. The syndrome was provisionally called GRID: gay-related immunodeficiency. These published reports drew similar information from physicians in other cities, and before too long these rare diseases had been diagnosed in nongay people (for example, hemophiliacs and people who had recently had blood transfusions).[61] Epidemiological follow-up interviews over the next several months confirmed that the problem — whatever it was — was growing at epidemic rates, and a CDC task force was accordingly established to coordinate data collection, communication, and research. The name *AIDS* was selected at a 1982 conference in Washington (*GRID* was no longer applicable now that nongays were also getting sick): acquired immune deficiency syndrome ("reasonably descriptive," said Curran, "without being pejorative").[62]

Over the next two years, epidemiological and clinical evidence increasingly pointed toward the role of some infectious agent in AIDS. Researchers divided over this, with some searching for a single agent, others positing a "multifactorial cause." Most scientists affiliated with federal scientific agencies (primarily the National Institutes of Health and Centers for Disease Control) have tended toward the single-agent theory (as though "cofactors" were a kind of deuces-wild element that vulgarized serious investigation), and this view has tended to dominate scientific reporting. Although some independent researchers, clinicians, and non-US scientists protested the increasingly rigid party line of what has been called "the AIDS Mafia," multifactorial and environmental theories were subordinated to the quest for the single agent.[63] The National Cancer Institute (NCI),

59.   Centers for Disease Control, *"Pneumocystis* Pneumonia — Los Angeles," *Morbidity and Mortality Weekly Report,* vol. 30, no. 21 (June 5, 1981), pp. 250–252.
60.   M. S. Gottlieb, R. Schroff, H. M. Schanker, *et al., "Pneumocystis Carinii* Pneumonia and Mucosal Candidiasis in Previously Healthy Homosexual Men," *New England Journal of Medicine,* 305 (1981), pp. 1425–1431.
61.   See Centers for Disease Control, "Kaposi's Sarcoma and *Pneumocystis* Pneumonia among Homosexual Men — New York City and California," *Morbidity and Mortality Weekly Report,* vol. 30, no. 25 (July 3, 1981), pp. 305–308, and Keewhan Choi, "Assembling the AIDS Puzzle: Epidemiology," in *AIDS: Facts and Issues,* ed. Victor Gong and Norman Rudnick, New Brunswick, New Jersey, Rutgers University Press, 1986.
62.   Quoted in Black, *The Plague Years.*
63.   Some scientists outside the federal health care network charge that the US government — "the AIDS Mafia" — dictates a party line on AIDS. Joseph Sonnabend, MD, former scientific director of the AIDS Medical Foundation, began the *Journal of AIDS Research* to print scientific articles he believed were being suppressed because they argued for a multifactorial cause rather than a single virus. See Black, *The Plague Years,* pp. 112–118, for discussion.

for example, developed a research strategy that focused on retroviruses, essentially to the exclusion of other lines of research, while other US virology and immunology laboratories put forward their own favored possibilities.[64] By 1983 the "leading candidate" for the AIDS virus seemed to be a member of the human T-cell leukemia family of viruses (HTLV), so called because they typically infect a particular kind of cell, the T-helper cells. But these were *retroviruses,* and there was doubt that a retrovirus could cause immunosuppression in humans.[65] Yet by this time it was widely agreed that AIDS was, indeed, a "new" disease — neither a statistical fluke nor a feature of the gay life-style. This generated excitement in the medical and scientific community not only because truly new diseases are rare, but also because its *cause* might be new as well. In 1983 Luc Montagnier at the Pasteur Institute in Paris identified what he called LAV, lymphadenopathy-associated virus.[66] In 1984 Robert Gallo, at NCI, identified what *he* called HTLV-III, human T-cell lymphotropic virus type III (the third type identified by his laboratory).[67] In accordance with Koch's postulates, both

---

64.   Panem, "AIDS: Public Policy and Biomedical Research," p. 25.
65.   The scientific account of retroviruses goes something like this: A virus (from Latin *virus,* "poison") cannot reproduce outside living cells: it enters into another organism's "host" cell and uses that cell's biochemical machinery to replicate itself. These replicant virus particles then infect other cells; this process is repeated until the infection is either brought under control by the host's immune system or the infection overwhelms and kills or debilitates the host, making it susceptible to other infections (as HIV does). Alternatively, virus and host may reach a state of equilibrium in which both coexist for years. The virus's initial entry into the host cell may cause symptoms of viral infections. Certain viruses can remain inactive, or latent, inside the host cell for long periods without causing problems; they can remain integrated with the cell's DNA (genetic material) until triggered to replicate (typically when the organism is compromised by old age, immunosuppressive drug therapy, or infection by another virus or bacteria); at this point the DNA is transcribed to RNA, which in turn becomes protein.
       A retrovirus replicates "backward," transferring genetic information from viral RNA into DNA, the opposite of previously known viral actions. The retrovirus carries RNA (instead of DNA) as its genetic material along with a unique enzyme, reverse transcriptase (from which the name *retro* comes); this uses the RNA as a template to generate (transcribe) a DNA copy. This viral DNA inserts itself among the cell's own chromosomes; thus positioned to function as a "new gene" for the infected host, it can immediately start producing viral RNAs (new viruses) or remain latent until activated. In the case of HIV the latency period can be as long as fourteen years (as of this writing) followed by a very sudden explosion of replication activity that may directly kill the host's cell — chiefly the T4-lymphocyte, a white blood cell that regulates the body's immune response. The rapid depletion of T4-cells, characteristic of AIDS, leaves the human host vulnerable to many infections that a normal immune system would repel. The HTLV isolated by Gallo in 1980 was the first identified retrovirus associated with human disease (see Osborn, "The AIDS Epidemic," p. 47).
66.   F. Barre-Sinoussi, J. C. Chernann, F. Rey, *et al.,* "Isolation of a T-Lymphotropic Retrovirus from a Patient at Risk for Acquired Immune Deficiency Syndrome," *Science,* no. 220 (1983), pp. 868–871; L. Montagnier, J. C. Chernann, F. Barre-Sinoussi, *et al.,* "A New Human T-Lymphotropic Retrovirus: Characterization and Possible Role in Lymphadenopathy and Acquired Immune Deficiency Syndromes," in *Human T-Cell Leukemia/Lymphoma Virus,* ed. R. C. Gallo, M.E. Essex, and L. Gross, Cold Spring Harbor, New York, Cold Spring Harbor Laboratory, 1984, pp. 363–379.
67.   Gallo and his colleagues published four papers on the isolation of HTLV-III in *Science,* no. 224 (1984), pp. 497–508.

viruses were isolated in the blood and semen of AIDS patients; no trace was found in the healthy control population.[68]

These powerful findings — disputed and contentious though they were to be — narrowed almost at once the basic biomedical science agenda with regard to AIDS. In the construction of scientific facts, the existence of a name plays a crucial role in providing a coherent and unified signifier — a shorthand way of signifying what may be a complex, inchoate, or little-understood concept. Latour and Woolgar divide the research they studied into the long and uncertain phase that led up to the identification, synthesis, and naming of TRF (H) (the thyrotropin-releasing factor [hormone], a substance involved in neuroendocrine hormone regulation) and the subsequent narrower and more routine phase in which the concept's status as "a fact" was taken for granted (the dispute over naming is relevant to the tussle over the names LAV and HTLV).[69] So too with AIDS: before the isolation of the virus, there were considerably more universes of inquiry and open-ended speculations. Evidence for a virus as agent intensified scientific control over signification and enabled scientists to rule out less relevant hypotheses and lines of research. Of course, the existence of *two* names — LAV and HTLV-III — complicated the signification process: did two signifiers entail two distinct signifieds? Despite the wrangling over this point between the involved parties, a clearer consensus nevertheless emerged that basic research should now relate directly to the hypothesis that a single virus was "the culprit" responsible for AIDS. Important issues included (1) etiology, (2) the identification of the virus's genetic structure and precise shape, (3) clinical and other information about transmission, (4) information about the clinical expression of the disease (discovery that the virus infected brain cells encouraged its renaming, since the names LAV and HTLV both presupposed an attack on lymph cells), (5) the scope and natural history of the disease, (6) differences among "risk groups," and (7) epidemiological information including the long-term picture (circumstantial evidence but important nevertheless).

To most scientists this process of narrowing inquiry and relinquishing peripheral lines of thought is simply the way science is done, the procedural sine qua non for establishing anything that can be called a "fact." But "a statement

---

68. Koch's postulates, developed by bacteriologist Robert Koch, would require that, in order to establish a specific virus as the "cause" of the AIDS syndrome, the virus would have to be present in all cases of the disease; antibody to the virus must be shown to develop in constant temporal relation to the development of AIDS; and transmission of the same virus to a previously uninfected animal or human must be demonstrated with subsequent development of the disease and reisolation of the infective agent. With AIDS, a lethal disease, this last requirement cannot be tested on humans, but a demonstration that the virus could be used to produce an effective vaccine would more or less fulfill this requirement. See Marx, "Strong New Candidate for AIDS Agent," p. 151, and P. M. Feorino, *et al.*, "Lymphadenopathy Associated Virus Infection of a Blood Donor-Recipient Pair with Acquired Immunodeficiency Syndrome," in Kulstad, ed., *AIDS: Papers from Science*, p. 216.

69. Latour and Woolgar, *Laboratory Life*, pp. 105–150, esp. pp. 108–112.

always has borders peopled by other statements,"[70] and it is important for us to keep in mind the provisional and consensual nature of this US AIDS research agenda, each area of which exists within a heavily populated social, cultural, and ideological territory. Consider the hypothesis that AIDS originated in Africa, for example (a view supported by the research of Gallo's colleague Myron Essex, whose African viruses are genetically similar to the virus Gallo's lab identified). Not surprisingly, some "geographic buck-passing" took place among the African countries themselves (Rwanda and Zambia say AIDS originated in Zaire, Uganda says it came from Tanzania, and so on). Beneath such public maneuvering, however, many Africans privately believe AIDS may have originated somewhere else. And, despite Gallo's assertion that he cannot "conceive of AIDS coming from elsewhere into Africa," the view is by no means universal, especially among non-US researchers.[71] Further, Americans refuse to acknowledge the possibility that exports of American blood products may have spread the disease to people elsewhere. In the Soviet Union, AIDS is considered a "foreign problem," attributable to the CIA or to tribes in Central Africa.[72] In the Caribbean, and even within the US, AIDS is widely believed to come from US biological testing.[73] The French first believed AIDS was introduced by way of an "American pollutant," probably contaminated amyl nitrate (they also believed AIDS came from Morocco).[74] The Soviet Union, Israel, Africa, Haiti, and the US Armed Forces deny the existence of indigenous homosexuality and thus claim that AIDS must always have originated "elsewhere."[75]

By 1986, five years after the initial article in the *Morbidity and Mortality Weekly Report*, a Human Retrovirus Subcommittee empowered by the International Committee on the Taxonomy of Viruses was at work "to propose an appropriate name for the retrovirus isolates recently implicated as the causative agents of the acquired immune deficiency syndrome (AIDS)" — to consider, that is, what "the AIDS virus" should officially be named. After more than a year of deliberation, the nomenclature subcommittee published its recommendations in the form of a letter to scientific journals.[76] Their task has been made crucial, they note, by the widespread interest in AIDS and the multiplicity of names now in use:

70.   Michel Foucault, *The Archaeology of Knowledge,* trans. A. M. Sheridan Smith, New York, Pantheon, 1972, p. 97.
71.   African data are reviewed in L. Altman, "Linking AIDS to Africa," p. 8.
72.   Lee, "AIDS in Moscow."
73.   See Rechy, "An Exchange on AIDS."
74.   Leibowitch documents French views in *A Strange Virus.*
75.   For a fuller analysis of the theory and politics of these origin and alibi stories, see Patton, *Sex and Germs;* Weeks, *Sexuality and Its Discontents;* D. Altman, *AIDS in the Mind of America;* Ann Guidici Fettner and William Check, *The Truth About AIDS: Evolution of an Epidemic,* New York, Holt, Rinehart & Winston, 1985; and Leibowitch, *A Strange Virus.*
76.   The letter appeared in *Science,* no. 232, (May 9, 1986), p. 697.

LAV:	lymphadenopathy-associated virus (1983 — Montagnier, Pasteur)
HTLV-III:	human T-cell lymphotropic virus type III (1984 — Gallo, NCI)
IDAV:	immunodeficiency-associated virus
ARV:	AIDS-associated retrovirus (1984 — Levy, UCSF)
HTLV-III/LAV and LAV/HTLV-III:	compound names used to keep peace (the CDC's use was perhaps a reprimand to the NCI for its perceived uncooperativeness in sharing data)
AIDS virus:	popular press

The subcommittee proposes HIV, "human immunodeficiency viruses." They reason that this conforms to the nomenclature of other viruses in which the first slot signals the host species (human), the second slot the major pathogenic property (immunodeficiency), and the last slot *V* for virus. (For some viruses, though not HIV, individual strains are distinguished by the initials of the thus "immortalized" patient from whom they originally came and in whose "daughter cells" they are perpetuated.) The multiple names of "the AIDS virus" point toward a succession of identities and offer a fragmented sense indeed of what this virus, or family of viruses, "really" is. The new name, in contrast, promises to unify the political fragmentations of the scientific establishment and to certify the health of the single-virus hypothesis. The subcommittee argues in favor of its proposed name that it does not incorporate the term AIDS, on the advice of many clinicians; it is distinct from all existing names and "has been chosen without regard to priority of discovery" (not insignificantly, Montagnier and Levy signed 'the subcommittee letter but Gallo and Essex did not); and it distinguishes the HI viruses from those with distinctly different biological properties, for example, the HTLV line (HTLV-I and HTLV-II), which this subcommittee calls "human t-cell leukemia viruses," perhaps to chastise Gallo for changing the *L* in the nomenclature of the HTLVs from *leukemia* to *lymphotropic* so that HTLV-III (the AIDS virus) would appear to fit generically into the same series (and bear the stamp of his lab). In the same issue of *Science,* the editors chose to discuss this letter in their "News and Comment" column: "Disputes over viral nomenclature do not ordinarily command much attention beyond the individuals immediately involved in the fray"; but the current dissension, part of the continuing controversy over who should get credit for discovering the virus, "could provide 6 months of scripts for the television series 'Dallas.'"[77]

Why such struggles over naming and interpretation? Because, as the *Science*

---

77.   Jean L. Marx, "AIDS Virus Has New Name — Perhaps," News and Comment, *Science,* no. 232 (May 9, 1986), pp. 699–700.

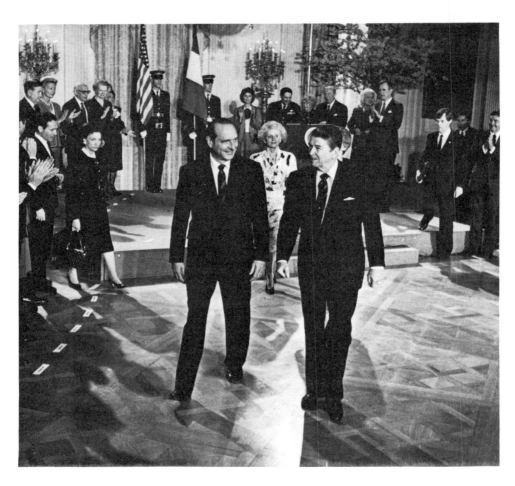

*The dispute over nomenclature of "the AIDS virus,"
called LAV by Luc Montagnier and HTLV-III by Robert
Gallo, led to the international adoption in May 1986 of
a new name—HIV; in April 1987, Prime Minister
Chirac and President Reagan met to announce an
agreement for shared paternity of the virus. (Photo: José
R. Lopez.)*

editors point out, there are high stakes where this performance is concerned—
not only patent rights to the lucrative test kits for the "AIDS virus" (Gallo fears
that loss of the HTLV-III designation will weaken his claims) but the future and
honor of immunology. Modern immunology, as Donna Haraway observes,
moved into the realm of high science when it reworked the military combat
metaphors of World War II (battles, struggle, territory, enemy, truces) into the
language of postmodern warfare: communication command control—coding,
transmission, messages—interceptions, spies, lies.[78] Scientific descriptions for
general readers, like this one from the *National Geographic* article on the immune
system, accentuate this shift from combat to code:

> Many of these enemies [of the body, or self] have evolved devious
> methods to escape detection. The viruses that cause influenza and the
> common cold, for example, constantly mutate, changing their finger-
> prints. The AIDS virus, most insidious of all, employs a range of
> strategies, including hiding out in healthy cells. What makes it fatal is
> its ability to invade and kill helper T cells, thereby short-circuiting the
> entire immune response.[79]

No ground troops here, no combat, not even generals: we see here the evolution
of a conception of the "AIDS virus" as a top-flight secret agent—a James Bond
of secret agents, armed with "a range of strategies" and licensed to kill. "Like
Greeks hidden inside the Trojan horse," 007 enters the body concealed inside a
helper T-cell from an infected host;[80] but "the virus is not an innocent passenger
in the body of its victims":[81]

> In the invaded victim, helper T's immediately detect the foreign T
> cell. But as the two T's meet, the virus slips through the cell mem-
> brane into the defending cell. Before the defending T cell can mobi-
> lize the troops, the virus disables it. . . . Once inside an inactive T
> cell, the virus may lie dormant for months, even years. Then, perhaps
> when another, unrelated infection triggers the invaded T cells to
> divide, the AIDS virus also begins to multiply. One by one, its clones
> emerge to infect nearby T cells. Slowly but inexorably the body loses
> the very sentinels that should be alerting the rest of the immune

78.   Donna J. Haraway, "The Biological Enterprise: Sex, Mind, and Profit from Human Engineer-
ing to Sociobiology," *Radical History Review*, no. 20 (Spring–Summer 1979), pp. 206–237, and "A
Manifesto for Cyborgs: Science, Technology, and Socialist Feminism in the 1980s," *Socialist Review*,
no. 80 (March–April 1985), pp. 65–108.
79.   Jaret, "Our Immune System," p. 709.
80.   *Ibid.*, p. 723; and see D. J. Anderson and E. J. Yunis, "'Trojan Horse' Leukocytes in AIDS,"
New England Journal of Medicine, no. 309 (1983), pp. 984–985.
81.   Krim, "AIDS: The Challenge to Science and Medicine."

system. Phagocytes and killer cells receive no call to arms. B cells are not alerted to produce antibodies. The enemy can run free.[82]

But on no mundane battlefield. The January 1987 *Scientific American* column "Science and the Citizen" warns of the mutability—the "protean nature of the AIDS virus"—that will make very difficult the development of a vaccine, as well as the perfect screening of blood. "It is also possible," the column concludes, "that a more virulent strain could emerge"; even now "the envelope of the virus seems to be changing."[83] Clearly, 007 is a spy's spy, capable of any deception: evading the "fluid patrol officers" is child's play. Indeed, it is so shifting and uncertain we might even acknowledge our own historical moment more specifically by giving the AIDS virus a postmodern identity: a terrorist's terrorist, an Abu Nidal of viruses.[84]

So long as AIDS was seen as a battle for the body of the gay male—a battle linked to "sociological" factors at that—the biomedical establishment was not tremendously interested in it. The first professionals involved tended to be clinicians in the large urban hospitals where men with AIDS first turned up, epidemiologists (AIDS, writes Black, is an "epidemiologist's dream"; a mystery disease that is fatal),[85] and scientists and clinicians who were gay themselves. Although from the beginning some saw the theoretical implications of AIDS, the possibility that AIDS was "merely" some unanticipated side-effect of gay male sexual practices (about which, as I've noted above, there was considerable ignorance) limited its appeal for basic scientists. But with the discovery that the agent associated with AIDS appeared to be a virus—indeed, a *novel retrovirus*—what

82.   Jaret, "Our Immune System," pp. 723–724.
83.   "Science and the Citizen," pp. 58–59.
84.   Leibowitch, in *A Strange Virus*, describes the scientific effort to identify the AIDS virus as a "medico-biological Interpol" on the trail of an international "criminal" charged with "breaking and entering" (pp. 41–42), and asks "Who is HTLV?" (p. 48). Mervyn B. Silverman, describing the mechanism of AIDS transmission at the Congressional AIDS hearing in 1983, testified in comparable language that "many believe that the virus does not act alone" ("AIDS Hearing," p. 125). In an article on a related finding in immunological research, Jos Van ("Cell Researchers Aim to Flush Out Body's Terrorists," *Chicago Tribune*, October 5, 1986) refers to cells called "free radicals," which serve as the body's "terrorists." A *Consumer Reports* article entitled "AIDS: Deadly but Hard to Catch" inadvertently invokes the structural ambiguity of "catching" the virus (who is the catcher, who is the catchee?). The policing metaphor (and the connection between *policy* and *police* has not gone unnoticed) carries over to efforts to control the spread of the virus. Lieberson ("The Reality of AIDS," p. 47) reports that some gay clubs have created "fluid patrol officers" who try to ensure that no "unsafe sex" takes place. Mohr argues that such attempts to promote "safe" sexual behavior, like recommendations for celibacy, seem "remote from reality and quite oblivious to the cussedness of sex and culture." Further, Mohr argues, "though in midcrisis it is politically injudicious to say so, safe-sex is poor sex" ("Of Deathbeds and Quarantines," p. 52); as an epigram for his essay he quotes a former gay "reprobate," now reformed: "Who wants to suck a dick with a rubber on it?" (See also Richard Goldstein, "The New Sobriety," *Village Voice*, December 30, 1986, pp. 23–28.)
85.   Black, *The Plague Years*.

SCIENTIFIC AMERICAN

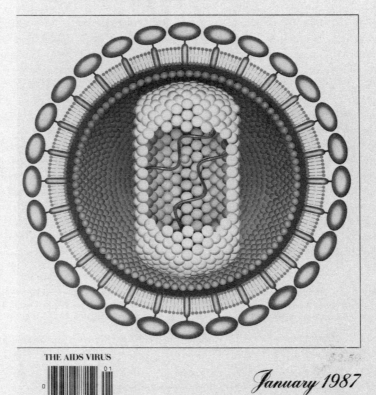

THE AIDS VIRUS

January 1987

Virus as grenade. In the cover article for Scientific American *by Robert Gallo, AIDS is inevitably a story of his own "discovery" of what he called "the HTLV-III virus." The stylized graphic encourages us to see the virus as a perfect inorganic military mechanism, primed for detonation.*

had seemed predominantly a public health phenomenon (clinical and service-oriented) suddenly could be rewritten in terms of high theory and high science. The performance moved from off-off Broadway to the heart of the theater district and the price of the tickets went way up. Among other things, identifying the viral agent made possible the development of a "definitive test" for its presence; not only did this open new scientific avenues (for example, in enabling researchers to map precise relationships among diverse AIDS and AIDS-like clinical manifestations), it also created opportunities for monetary rewards (for example, in revenue from patents on the testing kits). For these reasons, AIDS research became a highly competitive professional field.[86] Less-established assistant professors who had been working on the AIDS problem out of commitment suddenly found senior scientists peering at their data, while in the public arena the triumphs of pure basic science research were proclaimed. "Biomedical science is going brilliantly well," was how Dr. June Osborn summarized AIDS progress in mid-1986.[87] "Indeed," writes one science reporter, "had AIDS struck 20 years ago, we would have been utterly baffled by it."[88] Ten years ago we had not even confirmed the *existence* of human retroviruses, notes *Scientific American*. Asked whether NCI's strategy of focusing exclusively on retrovirus research was appropriate (considering that it might not have paid off), an official said this wouldn't have mattered: basic retroviral research was NCI's priority in any case.[89] Because it *did* pay off, it can now be said (as it could not have been said before 1984) that "AIDS may be a disease that has arrived at the right time."[90] In the words of one biomedical scientist, we face "an impending Armageddon of AIDS, and the salvation of the world through molecular genetics."[91]

86.   For discussion and analysis of the growing competition in AIDS research as the funding increased, see D. Altman, *AIDS in the Mind of America;* Black, *The Plague Years;* Patton, *Sex and Germs;* Panem, "AIDS: Public Policy and Biomedical Research"; Schwartz, "AIDS in the Media"; Office of Technology Assessment, *Review; Hastings Center Report,* Special Supplements. For an account of the case of French physician Willy Rozenbaum, see Paul Raeburn, "Doctor Faces Politics of AIDS Research," *Champaign-Urbana News-Gazette,* January 25, 1986, p. A-8.
87.   Cited in Eckholm, "Broad Alert on AIDS," p. 19.
88.   Jaret, "Our Immune System," p. 23.
89.   Panem, "AIDS: Public Policy and Biomedical Research," p. 25.
90.   "Science and the Citizen," p. 59.
91.   Quoted in Morton Hunt, "Teaming Up against AIDS," *New York Times Magazine,* March 2, 1986, p. 78. Despite whatever criticisms biomedical scientists may have had about AIDS research, an ideology of heroism, progress, and faith in ultimate scientific conquest pervades discussions. Examples include Choi, "Assembling the AIDS Puzzle"; Relman, "Introduction"; Gallo, "The AIDS Virus"; Donald S. Frederickson, "Where Do We Go from Here?" in *The AIDS Epidemic,* ed. Kevin M. Cahill, New York, St. Martin's Press, 1983, pp. 151–161; Donald P. Francis, "The Search for the Cause," in *The AIDS Epidemic;* American Medical Association Council on Scientific Affairs, "The Acquired Immunodeficiency Syndrome: Commentary," *Journal of the American Medical Association,* vol. 252, no. 15 (October 19, 1984), pp. 2037–2043; Sheldon H. Landesman, Harold M. Ginzburg, and Stanley H. Weiss, "The AIDS Epidemic," *New England Journal of Medicine,* vol. 312, no. 8 (February 21, 1985), pp. 521–525; and Merle A. Sande, "Transmission of AIDS: The Case against Casual Contagion," *New England Journal of Medicine,* vol. 314, no. 6 (February 6, 1986), pp. 380–382. Sonnabend ("Looking at AIDS in Totality") criticizes the assumptions of heroic science,

Reconstructing the AIDS Text: Rewriting the Body

There is now broad consensus that AIDS—"plague of the millennium," "health disaster of pandemic proportions"—is the greatest public health problem of our era.[92] The epidemic of signification that surrounds AIDS is neither simple nor under control. AIDS exists at a point where many entrenched narratives intersect, each with its own problematic and context in which AIDS acquires meaning. It is extremely difficult to resist the lure, familiarity, and ubiquitousness of these discourses. The AIDS virus enters the cell and integrates with its genetic code, establishing a disinformation campaign at the highest level and ensuring that replication and dissemination will be systemic. We inherit a series of discursive dichotomies; the discourse of AIDS attaches itself to these other systems of difference and plays itself out there:

self and not-self

the one and the other

homosexual and heterosexual

---

while Leibowitch (*A Strange Virus*) is distinctive in his irony and political self-consciousness about the nature of the scientific enterprise.

92. As of December 1986, ten million people were estimated to carry the virus worldwide; at least a quarter of these people are expected to develop AIDS within the next five years and many more to develop illnesses ranging from mildly disabling to lethal. By the end of 1986, almost 30,000 people in the US had been diagnosed with AIDS, and half of them had already died. The number of diagnosed cases is expected to reach 270,000 by the end of 1991, with a cumulative death toll of 179,000. There will be a heavy financial toll. With repeated hospitalizations, a person with AIDS may have medical costs of up to $500,000. The cases of AIDS diagnosed in 1986 alone will eventually cost the nation $2.25 billion in health care costs and $7 billion in lost lifetime earnings. Its expenses are seventy-five times what we are currently spending on it. (Costs vary greatly from city to city: the CDC estimated in 1986 that each case would average $147,000; the US Army estimated that a case could cost as much as $500,000 to treat; but in San Francisco, use of nonphysician caretakers, home care, and nursing home services can bring the cost of a comparable case down to $42,000. See "AIDS Hearing"; Patton, *Sex and Germs;* D. Altman, *AIDS in the Mind of America;* David L. Wheeler, "More Research Is Urged in Fight against AIDS," *Chronicle of Higher Education,* November 5, 1986, pp. 7, 10; and David Tuller, "Trying to Avoid an Insurance Debacle," *New York Times,* February 22, 1987, sec. 3, pp. 1, 8, for discussion of the politics of AIDS funding. The National Academy of Sciences Report [Baltimore and Wolff, *Confronting AIDS*] judges recent federal allocations to be "greatly improved" but still "woefully inadequate" and calls for spending $2 billion per year by 1990 for education and the development of drugs and vaccines.) See American Medical Association Council on Scientific Affairs, "Commentary," Centers for Disease Control, "Update"; Edward S. Johnson and Jeffrey Vieira, "Cause of AIDS: Etiology," in *AIDS: Facts and Issues,* ed. Victor Gong and Norman Rudnick, New Brunswick, New Jersey, Rutgers University Press, 1986, pp. 25–33; Redfield *et al.,* "Heterosexually Acquired HTLV-III/LAV," and "Female-to-Male Transmission"; Katie Leishman, "Two Million Americans and Still Counting," review of Black, *The Plague Years,* and Nichols, *Mobilizing Against AIDS, New York Times Book Review,* July 27, 1986, p. 12; Gong and Rudnick, eds., *AIDS: Facts and Issues;* and Warren Winkelstein, Jr., *et al.,* "Sexual Practices and Risk of Infection by the Human Immunodeficiency Virus: The San Francisco Men's Health Study," *Journal of the American Medical Association,* vol. 257, no. 3 (January 16, 1987), pp. 321–325, for predictions based on current distribution of HIV antibodies.

homosexual and "the general population"

active and passive, guilty and innocent, perpetrator and victim

vice and virtue, us and them, anus and vagina

sins of the parent and innocence of the child

love and death, sex and death, sex and money, death and money

science and not-science, knowledge and ignorance

doctor and patient, expert and patient, doctor and expert

addiction and abstention, contamination and cleanliness

contagion and containment, life and death

injection and reception, instrument and receptacle

normal and abnormal, natural and alien

prostitute and paragon, whore and wife

safe sex and bad sex, safe sex and good sex

First World and Third World, free world and iron curtain

capitalists and communists

certainty and uncertainty

virus and victim, guest and host

As Christine Brooke-Rose demonstrates, one must pay close attention to the way in which these apparently fundamental and natural semantic oppositions are put to work.[93] What is self and what is not-self? Who wears the white and who the black hat? (Or, in her discussion, perhaps, who wears the pants and who the skirt?) As Bryan Turner observes with regard to sexually transmitted diseases in general, the diseased are seen not as "victims" but as "agents" of biological disaster. If Koch's postulates must be fulfilled to identify a given microbe with a given disease, perhaps it would be helpful, in rewriting the AIDS text, to take "Turner's postulates" into account: (1) disease is a language; (2) the body is a representation; and (3) medicine is a political practice.[94]

93.   Christine Brooke-Rose, "Woman as a Semiotic Object," in *The Female Body in Western Culture: Contemporary Perspectives*, ed. Susan Rubin Suleiman, Cambridge, Massachusetts, Harvard University Press, 1986, pp. 305–316. See also Teresa de Lauretis, *Alice Doesn't: Feminism, Semiotics, Cinema*, Bloomington, Indiana University Press, 1984.
94.   Bryan A. Turner, *The Body and Society*, New York, Basil Blackwell, 1984, pp. 221, 209.

There is little doubt that for some people the AIDS crisis lends force to their fear and hatred of gays; AIDS appears, for example, to be a significant factor in the increasing violence against them, and other homophobic acts in the US.[95] But to talk of "homophobia" as though it were a simple and rather easily recognized phenomenon is impossible. When we review the various conceptions of the gay male body produced within scientific research by the signifier *AIDS*, we find a discourse rich in signification as to what AIDS "means." At first, some scientists doubted that AIDS could be an infectious disease because they could not imagine what gay men could do to each other to transmit infection. But intimate knowledge generated quite different conceptions:

AIDS is caused by multiple and violent gay sexual encounters: exposure to countless infections and pathogenic agents overwhelms the immune system.

AIDS is caused by killer sperm, shooting from one man's penis to the anus of another.

Gay men are as sexually driven as alcoholics or drug addicts.

AIDS cannot infect females because the virus can't penetrate the tough mucous membranes of the vagina.

Women cannot transmit AIDS because their bodies do not have the strong projectile capacity of a penis or syringe.

Prostitutes can transmit the virus because their contaminated bodies harbor massive quantities of killer microbes.

Repeated hints that the male body is sexually potent and adventurous suggest that homophobia in biomedical discourse might play out as a literal "fear of the same." The text constructed around the gay male body—the epidemic of signification so evident in the conceptions cited above and elsewhere in this essay—is driven in part by the need for constant flight from sites of potential identity and thus the successive construction of new oppositions that will barricade self from not-self. The homophobic meanings associated with AIDS continue to be layered into existing discourse: analysis demonstrates ways in which the AIDS virus is linguistically identified with those it strikes: the penis is "fragile," the urethra is "fragile," the virus is "fragile"; the African woman's body is "exotic," the virus is "exotic." The virus "penetrates" its victims; a carrier of

95.   William R. Greer, "Violence against Homosexuals Rising, Groups Say in Seeking Protections," *New York Times*, November 23, 1986, p. 15.

death, it wears an "innocent" disguise. AIDS is "caused" by homosexuals; AIDS is "caused" by a virus. Homosexuality exists on a border between male and female, the virus between life and nonlife. This cross-cannibalization of language is unsurprising. What greater relief than to find a final refuge from the specter of gay sexuality where the language that has obsessively accumulated around the body can attach to its substitute: the virus. This is a signifier that can be embraced forever.

The question is how to disrupt and renegotiate the powerful cultural narratives surrounding AIDS. Homophobia is inscribed within other discourses at a high level, and it is at a high level that they must be interrupted and challenged. Why? The following scenario for Armageddon (believed by some, desired by many) makes clear why: AIDS will remain confined to the original high-risk groups (primarily gay males and IV drug users) because of their specific practices (like anal intercourse and sharing needles). At the Paris International AIDS Conference in June 1986, the ultimate spread of the disease was posed in terms of "containment" and "saturation." "Only" gay males and drug addicts will get infected—the virus will use them up and then have nowhere to go—the "general population" (who are also in epidemiological parlance a "virgin" population) will remain untouched. Even if this view is correct (which seems doubtful, given growing evidence of transmission through plain old everyday heterosexual intercourse), and the virus stops spreading once it has "saturated" the high-risk population, we would still be talking about a significant number of US citizens: 2.5 million gay men, 7 million additional men who have at some time in the last ten years engaged in homosexual activity, 750,000 habitual IV drug users, 750,000 occasional drug users, 10,000 hemophiliacs already infected, the sex partners of these people and the children of infected women—in other words, a total of more than 10 million people (the figures are from the June 1986 Paris conference). And "saturation" is currently considered a *best*-case scenario by the public health authorities.

The fact is that any separation of not-self ("AIDS victims") from self (the "general population") is no longer possible. The US Surgeon General and National Academy reports make clear that "that security blanket has now been stripped away."[96] Yet the familiar signifying practices that exercise control over meaning continue. The *Scientific American* column goes on to note fears that the one-to-one African ratio of females with AIDS to males may foreshadow US statistics: "Experts point out, however, that such factors as the prevalence of other venereal diseases that cause genital sores, the use of unsterilized needles in clinics, and the lack of blood-screening tests may explain the different epidemiology of AIDS in Africa."[97] Thus the African data are reinterpreted to reinstate

96.   "Science and the Citizen," p. 58.
97.   *Ibid.*, p. 59.

the "us"/"them" dichotomy and project a rosier scenario for "us" (well, maybe it improves on comic Richard Belzer's narrative: "A monkey bites some guy on the ass in Africa and *he* balls some guy in Haiti and now we're all gonna fuckin' die. THANKS A LOT!").[98]

Meanwhile on the home front monogamy is coming back into its own, along with abstention, the safest sex of all. The virus in itself—by whatever name— has come to represent the moment of truth for the sexual revolution: as though God has once again sent his only beloved son to save us from our high-risk behavior. Who would have thought He would take the form of a virus: a viral Terminator ready to die for our sins.[99]

The contestations pioneered by the gay community over the past decade offer models for resistance. As old-fashioned morality increasingly infects the twentieth-century scenario, whether masquerading as "preventive health" or spiritual transformation, a new sampler can be stitched to hang on the bedroom wall: BETTER WED THAN DEAD. "It's just like the fifties," complains a gay man in San Francisco. "People are getting married again for all the wrong reasons."[100] One disruption of this narrative occurs in the San Francisco *A.I.D.S. Show*: "I *like* sex; I like to get drunk and smoke grass and use poppers and sleep with strangers:

98.   Though Lieberson insists that a "heterosexual pandemic [comparable to Africa's] has not occurred in the United States" and criticizes those who suggest it is going to ("The Reality of AIDS," p. 44), current data based on tests for antibodies to HIV among 1986 army recruits (nongay, non-drug-using, so far as researchers could determine) argue for increasing heterosexual transmission (Redfield, *et al.,* "Female to Male Transmission"). For discussion and analysis, see L. Altman, "Heterosexuals and AIDS"; D. Altman, *AIDS in the Mind of America;* Marx, "New Relatives of AIDS Virus Found"; Osborn, "The AIDS Epidemic"; Patton, *Sex and Germs;* Hosken, "Why AIDS Pattern Is Different in Africa"; Feldman, "Role of African Mutilations in AIDS Discounted"; and Robert Pear, "Ten-Fold Increase in AIDS Death Toll Is Expected by '91," *New York Times,* June 13, 1986, pp. A-1, A-17. See also Potterat, *et al.,* "Lying to Military Physicians." It has been suggested that malnutrition plays an important role in the rapid spread of AIDS in Africa (worldwide, malnutrition is the most common cause of acquired immune deficiency).

99.   We must even, perhaps, identify with the virus, an extraordinarily successful structure that has been comfortably making the acquaintance of living organisms for many more millions of years than we have. A virus that enters the human bloodstream and circulates through the body may ultimately negotiate with the host some mutually livable equilibrium. The relationship may be a close one: it is difficult to separate the effects of the virus from those of the body's defenses; and any poison intended for the guest may kill the host as well. Any given species, including human beings, may sometimes prove to be an inhospitable, even unnatural host. To speak teleologically for a moment, it is obvious that to kill the host is not in the microorganism's best interests; this sometimes happens, however, when a virus adapted to a nonhuman host shifts, through some untoward turn of events, to the human body. For the human immunodeficiency virus, believed to be a relative newcomer on earth (the presence of antibodies in stored blood now goes back to 1959 samples collected in Africa, to 1973 in US blood) and to have first inhabited African monkeys, we might have turned out to be inhospitable. But though from our perspective the virus is indeed virulent, killing quickly, in fact the long latency between infection and the appearance of clinical damage provides plenty of time—often years—for the virus to replicate and infect a new host. For the time being we are sufficiently hospitable for this virus to live off us relatively "successfully"; if mutation occurs, our relationship to the AIDS virus could evolve into something relatively benign or mutually disastrous.

100.   FitzGerald, *Cities on a Hill,* p. 115.

Call me old-fashioned, but that's what I like!" A gay pastor in San Francisco tells Frances FitzGerald that the moral transformation being forced upon the gay community reminds him of the days before Stonewall: "If I had to go back to living in the closet, I'd have to think very clearly about whether or not I'd rather be dead."[101] For Michel Foucault, the "tragedy" of AIDS was not intrinsically its lethal character, but rather that a group that has risked so much—gays—are looking to standard authorities—doctors, the church—for guidance in a time of crisis. "How can I be scared of AIDS when I could die in a car?" Foucault asked a year or so before he died. "If sex with a boy gives me pleasure. . . . " And he added: "Don't cry for me if I die."[102]

For AIDS, where meanings are overwhelming in their sheer volume and often explicitly linked to extreme political agendas, we do not know whose meanings will become "the official story." We need an epidemiology of signification—a comprehensive mapping and analysis of these multiple meanings—to form the basis for an official definition that will in turn constitute the policies, regulations, rules, and practices that will govern our behavior for some time to come. As we have seen, these may rest upon "facts," which in turn may rest upon the deeply entrenched cultural narratives I have been describing. For this reason, what AIDS signifies must be democratically determined: we cannot afford to let scientists or any other group of "experts" dismiss our meanings as "misconceptions" and our alternative views as noise that interferes with the pure processes of scientific inquiry. Rather, we need to insist that many voices contribute to the construction of official definitions—and specifically certain voices that need urgently to be heard. Although the signification process for AIDS is by now very broad—just about everyone, seemingly, has offered "readings" of what AIDS means—one excluded group continues to be users of illegal intravenous drugs. Caught between the "first wave" (gay men) and the "second wave" (heterosexuals), drug users at high risk for AIDS remain silent and invisible. One public health official recently challenged the rush to educate heterosexuals about their risk when what is needed (and has been from the beginning) is "a massive effort directed at intravenous-drug abusers and their sex partners. This means treatment for a disease—chemical dependence on drugs. We have to prevent and treat one disease, drug addiction, to prevent another, AIDS."[103]

101. *Ibid.,* p. 104.
102. Philip Horvitz, "Don't Cry for Me, Academia," Interview with Michel Foucault, *Jimmy and Lucy's House of K* (Berkeley), no. 2 (August 1985), pp. 78–80. This interview, conducted in Berkeley (and scrutinized, it's said, like the Watergate transcripts, to find out what did he know and when did he know it), concludes as Foucault enters the BART station: "Good luck," he tells Horvitz. "And don't be scared!"
103. See also Barrett, "Straight Shooters"; Stephen C. Joseph, "Intravenous-Drug Abuse Is the Front Line in the War on AIDS," Letter to the Editor, *New York Times,* December 22, 1986, p. 18. Though Check writes that "it sometimes appears that the only risk group that hasn't raised a ruckus

If AIDS's dual life as both a material and linguistic entity is important, the emphasis on *dual* is critical. Symbolic and social reconceptualizations of AIDS are necessary but not sufficient to address the massive social questions AIDS raises. The recognition that AIDS is heterosexually as well as homosexually transmitted certainly represents progress, but it does not interrupt fantasy. It is fantasy, for example, to believe that "safer sex" will protect us from AIDS; it may save us from becoming infected with the virus — New York City has instituted Singles Night at the Blood Bank, where people can meet and share their seropositivity status before they even exchange names.[104] But AIDS is to be a fundamental force of twentieth-century life, and no barrier in the world can make us "safe" from its complex material realities. Malnutrition, poverty, and hunger are unacceptable, in our own country and in the rest of the world; the need for universal health care is urgent. Ultimately, we cannot distinguish self from not-self: for "plague is life," and each of us has the plague within us; "no one, no one on earth is free from it."[105]

The discursive structures I have discussed in this essay are familiar to those of us in "the human sciences." We have learned that there is a disjunction between historical subjects and constructed scientific objects. There is still debate about whether, or to what extent, scientific discourse can be privileged — and relied upon to transcend contradiction. My own view is unequivocal: it cannot be privileged in this way. Of course, where AIDS is concerned, science can usefully perform its interpretive part: we can learn to live — indeed, *must* learn to live — as though there are such things as viruses. The virus — a constructed scientific object — is also a historical subject, a "human immunodeficiency virus," a real source of illness and death that can be passed from one person to another under certain conditions that we can apparently — individually and collectively — influence. The trick is to learn to live with this disjunction, but the lesson is imperative. Dr. Rieux, the physician-narrator of Camus's novel, acknowledges that by dealing medically with the plague he is allowing himself the luxury of "living in a world of abstractions." But not indefinitely; for "when abstraction sets to killing you, you've got to get busy with it."

But getting busy with it may require us to relinquish some luxuries of our own: the luxury of accepting without reflection the "findings" science seems

---

is the IV drug users, who are not organized" ("Public Education on AIDS," p. 28), a few commentators are beginning to draw attention to this critical problem: Barrett, "Straight Shooters"; Joseph, "Intravenous Drug Abuse"; Shaw and Paleo, "Women and AIDS"; Peg Byron, "Women with AIDS: Untold Stories," *Village Voice*, September 24, 1985, pp. 16–19; and Francis X. Clines, "Via Addicts' Needles, AIDS Spreads in Edinburgh," *New York Times*, January 4, 1987, p. 8. In the last year, the Gay Men's Health Crisis in New York, aware that many drug users may avoid information centers as well as medical authorities, has taken responsibility for going to "shooting galleries," clinics, and drug treatment centers to provide AIDS education and training to these people so that they can in turn work with other drug users.

104. "A 'Social Card' to Reassure Sex Partners," *San Francisco Chronicle*, October 17, 1985, p. 30.
105. Camus, *The Plague*, p. 229.

effortlessly able to provide us, the luxury of avoiding vigilance, the luxury of hoping it will all go away. Rather, we need to use what science gives us in ways that are selective, self-conscious, and pragmatic ("as though" they were true). We need to understand that AIDS is and will remain a provisional and deeply problematic signifier. Above all, we need to resist, at all costs, the luxury of listening to the thousands of language tapes playing in our heads, laden with prior discourse, that tell us with compelling certainty and dizzying contradiction what AIDS "really" means.

The Spectacle of AIDS

SIMON WATNEY

> And now what shall become of us without
> any barbarians? Those people were a kind
> of solution.
>
> —C. P. Cavafy,
> *Expecting the Barbarians*

> The question of identity—how it is consti-
> tuted and maintained—is therefore the
> central issue through which psychoanalysis
> enters the political field.
>
> —Jaqueline Rose, "Feminism and the
> Psychic"

The "Truth" of AIDS

As I write, there have been "about" a thousand cases of AIDS in the United Kingdom. Writing on the subject of statistics, the great Polish poet Zbignev Herbert describes the fundamentally shameful nature of the word *about* when used in circumstances of disaster. For, in such matters,

> accuracy is essential
> we must not be wrong
> even by a single one
>
> we are despite everything
> the guardians of our brothers
>
> ignorance about those who have disappeared
> undermines the reality of the world.[1]

---

1.   Zbignev Herbert, "Mr. Cogito on the Need for Precision," in *Report from the Besieged City*, New York and Oxford, Oxford University Press, 1987, p. 67.

Five years have passed since the isolation of the HIV retrovirus responsible for AIDS. Millions of pounds have been spent by the British government on public information campaigns. AIDS education workers have been appointed by local authorities throughout Britain. Tens if not hundreds of thousands of lives have been directly affected by the consequences of HIV. Yet even the most fundamental medical facts concerning HIV and AIDS remain all but universally misunderstood. The entire subject continues to be framed by a cultural agenda that is as medically misinformed as it is socially misleading and politically motivated.[2] For those of us living and working in the various constituencies most devastated by HIV, it seems, as Richard Goldstein has pointed out, as if the rest of the population were tourists, casually wandering through the very height of a blitz of which they are totally unaware. This is hardly surprising at a time when the only sources of AIDS information are themselves so profoundly polluted and unreliable. Thus in England recently *The Guardian* noted that "by the end of August 1,013 cases had been reported, of whom 572 had died," while on the same day *The Star* informed *its* readers that "AIDS has now killed more than 1,000 people in Britain."[3]

Misreporting on such a scale has been regular and systematic since the earliest days of the epidemic, and is indicative of the values and priorities of an international information industry that continues to oscillate daily between meretricious gloating over the fate of those deemed responsible for their own misfortune, and the supposed "threat" of a "real" epidemic. Currently in the United States, someone dies of AIDS every half hour. An estimated six percent of all Africans have been infected by HIV, including nearly a quarter of the entire populations of Malawi and Uganda.[4] If statistics teach us anything, it is the sheer scale and efficiency of the cultural censorship within and between different countries and continents, which guarantees that the actual situation of the vast majority of people with HIV and/or AIDS is rarely if ever discussed. Moreover, this disappearance is strategic, and faithfully duplicates the positions the social groups most vulnerable to HIV found themselves in even before the epidemic began. Thus the Latino population of the two continents of America, IV drug users, workers in the sex industry, black Africans, and gay men are carefully confined in the penal category of the "high-risk group," from which position their experience and achievements may be safely ignored. In this manner a terrible ongoing human catastrophe has been ruthlessly denied the status of tragedy, or even natural disaster.

The British government's AIDS information campaign, which has been widely admired overseas, dutifully exhorted the "general public" not to die of

2.   See Simon Watney, "The Subject of AIDS," *Copyright*, vol. 1, no. 1 (Fall 1987).
3.   Andrew Veitch, "AIDS Cases Exceed 1,000," *The Guardian*, September 8, 1987; Anthony Smith, "AIDS Death Toll Hits 1,000," *The Star*, September 8, 1987.
4.   Andrew Veitch, "'Up to 10 Million' Have AIDS Virus," *The Guardian*, June 24, 1986.

ignorance.[5] Yet this campaign has still found itself unable to address one single word to British gay men, who constitute almost ninety percent of people with AIDS in Britain. At every level of "public" address and readership, ignorance is sustained on a massively institutionalized scale by British and American media commentary. The modes of address of such commentary reveal much about the ways in which the state and the media industry "think" the question of population. Indeed, the relentless monotony and sadism of AIDS commentary in the West only serve to manifest a sense of profound cultural uneasiness concerning the fragility of the nationalistic fantasy of an undifferentiated "general public," supposedly united above all divisions of class, region, and gender, yet totally excluding everyone who stands outside the institution of marriage. Popular perceptions of all aspects of AIDS thus remain all but exclusively informed by a cultural agenda that seriously and culpably impedes any attempt to understand the complex history of the epidemic, or to plan effectively against its future. In this context it is impossible to separate individual perceptions of risk, and endlessly amplified fears concerning the "threat" of "spread," from the drastically miniaturized "truth" of AIDS, which has remained impervious to challenge or correction since the syndrome was first identified in the ideologically constitutive and immensely significant name GRID (gay-related immunodeficiency) in 1981.[6]

In this manner a "knowledge" of AIDS has been uniformly constituted across the boundaries of formal and informal information, accurately duplicating the contours of other, previous "knowledges" that speak confidently on behalf of the "general public," viewed as a homogenous entity organized into discrete family units over and above all the fissures and conflicts of both the social and the psychic. This "truth" of AIDS also resolutely insists that the point of emergence of the virus should be identified as its *cause*. Epidemiology is thus replaced by a moral etiology of disease that can only conceive homosexual desire within a medicalized metaphor of contagion. Reading AIDS as the outward and visible sign of an imagined depravity of will, AIDS commentary deftly returns us to a premodern vision of the body, according to which heresy and sin are held to be scored in the features of their voluntary subjects by punitive and admonitory manifestations of disease. Moreover, this rhetoric of AIDS incites a violent siege mentality in the "morally well," a mentality that locks only too easily into other rhetorics of preemptive "defense."[7] Thus an essentially modern universalizing discourse of "family values," "standards of decency," and so on, recruits subjects to an ever more disciplinary "knowledge" of themselves and "their" world. This "knowledge" is effortlessly stitched in the likeness of an always-already-familiar *broderie Anglais* picture of seemingly timeless "national values"

5.   See Simon Watney, "AIDS: How Big Did It Have to Get?" *New Socialist*, March 1987.
6.   See Dennis Altman, *AIDS in the Mind of America*, New York, Doubleday, 1986, p. 33.
7.   See Simon Watney, "AIDS USA," *Square Peg*, no. 17 (Autumn 1987).

and the "national past."[8] At the same time, secular institutions appropriate and refashion an equally sober discourse of "promiscuity," which drifts out across the Mediterranean to incorporate the entire African subcontinent and beyond, recharging "the Orient" with a deadly cargo of exoticism that reminds "us" that negritude has always been, for whites, a sign of sexual excess and death.

The Government of the Home

All discussion of AIDS should proceed from the known facts concerning the modes of transmission of HIV in relation to lay perceptions of health and disease that mediate and "handle" this information. That this is far from the case in contemporary AIDS commentary remains in urgent need of explanation. To begin with, an overly rational model of health education continues to ignore all questions of cultural and psychic *resistance*. Similarly, the study of risk perception lacks a theory of the subject, even in its explicitly antieconomistic "culturalist" modes.[9] Both disciplines recognize that the localization of HIV infection in particular communities is no more intrinsically remarkable than the localization of any other infectious agent in any other specific constituencies. Yet the heavily concentrated and disseminated image of AIDS as a species of "gay plague" cannot be adequately explained by available sociological theories of scapegoating, boundary protection, or "moral panics." What is at stake here is the capacity of particular ideological configurations to activate deep psychic anxieties that run far beneath the tangible divisions of the social formation. In particular, we should consider the active legacy of eugenic theory, which is as much at work within the sociobiological dogmatics of contemporary familialism as it was in the biomedical politics of National Socialism. This is not to posit a crude parallel of objectives or identities between Thatcherite Britain and Nazi Germany, but merely to observe that whenever history is biologized with recourse to the authority of seemingly unquestionable and innate laws, "the perception of a natural order of social structure and stratification" is always "thought to be readily available in the evidence of the human body."[10] It is the sense of a *totalized* threat to a biologized identification of self with nation that characterizes both Nazi medical politics and modern familialism. Thus Jews, antifascists, gypsies, and "degenerates" (including, of course, large numbers of lesbians and gay men) were postulated as intrinsic and self-evident threats to the perceived unity and the very existence of the German *Volk*, and the policy of killing them all "as a therapeutic imperative" only emerged in relation to the deeply felt danger of

8.   See Patrick Wright, *On Living in an Old County*, London, Verso, 1985.
9.   See, for example, Mary Douglas, *Risk Acceptability According to the Social Sciences*, London, Routledge & Kegan Paul, 1986.
10.   David Green, "Veins of Resemblance: Photography and Eugenics," in Holland, Spence, and Watney, eds., *Photography/Politics: Two*, London, Commedia, 1987, p. 13.

Volkstod, or "death of the people" (or "nation," or "race").[11] It is in precisely this sense that people with HIV infection, usually misdescribed as "AIDS carriers," are widely understood to threaten the equally spurious unity of "the family," "the nation," and even "the species."[12] Hence the overriding need to return to the pressing question of the contemporary government of the home, especially in the light of Foucault's argument that in the modern period

> the family becomes an instrument rather than a model: the privileged instrument for the government of the population and not the chimerical model for good government: this shift from the level of the model to that of the instrument is, I believe, absolutely fundamental, and it is from the middle of the 18th century that the family appears in this dimension of instrumentality with respect to the population: hence the campaigns on morality, marriage, vaccinations, etc.[13]

This is why it is so important to avoid any temptation to think of the ongoing AIDS crisis as a form of "moral panic," which carries the implication that it is an entirely discrete phenomenon, distinct from other elements and dramas in the perpetual moral management of the home. On the contrary, homosexuality, understood by AIDS commentary as the "cause" of AIDS, is always available as a coercive and menacing category to entrench the institutions of family life and to prop up the profoundly unstable identities those institutions generate. The felt "problem" of sexual diversity is not established and imposed externally by the state, but rather internally, by the categorical imperatives of the modern organization of sexuality. The state, of course, responds to this situation, but it is not its originator. This, after all, is what sexuality *means.* Thus, consent to social policy is grafted from desire itself, as political prescriptions are understood to "protect" heterosexual identities, which are stabilized by an ever proliferating sense of permanent personal threat, with corresponding emotional responses ranging from "outrage" to actual violence against imaginary adversaries. Hence, as I have written elsewhere,

> We can begin to understand the seeming obsession with homosexuality in contemporary Britain, whether it is presented as a threat *within* the home, in the form of deviant members of the family who must be expelled, or as deviant images invading the "innocent" space of domesticity via TV or video; or as a supposedly *external* threat in the

11.   See Robert Jay Lifton, *The Nazi Doctors: Medical Killing and the Psychology of Genocide,* New York, Basic Books, 1986, p. 25. This book should be read by anyone interested in the archeology of AIDS commentary.
12.   For an example, see William E. Dannemeyer, "AIDS Infection Must Be Reportable," *Los Angeles Times,* June 12, 1987.
13.   Michel Foucault, "On Governmentality," *Ideology & Consciousness,* no. 6 (Autumn 1979), p. 17.

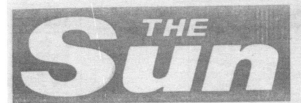

URI GELLER aims to beam in to your mind at 3pm

Thursday, August 27, 1987   20p   TODAY'S TV IS ON PAGE 14

TRINGO BINGO Page 18

TODAY!

What to do and when—see Centre Pages

EXCLUSIVE: Ryan's kinky secret revealed

MANIAC RAMBO WAS MY GAY LOVER

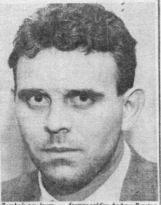

Rambo's gay lover . . . former soldier Andrew Preston

By VICTOR CHAPPLE

A HANDSOME ex-soldier last night revealed to The Sun that he was the gay lover of Rambo killer Michael Ryan.

Bi-sexual Andrew Preston, 26, gave the world a first glimpse inside the mind of the Hungerford madman who shot 16 dead in one afternoon.

The rugged ex-squaddie said: "It was clear I wasn't the first man he had slept with."

He claimed Ryan, 27, **DID** fancy women—but was simply terrified of chatting them up.

And Ryan's dilemma was made even worse by his doting mother Dorothy—who became one of his victims. Preston says she pestered her son to find a girl and get married.

And while Preston and Ryan carried on their sordid affair, Mrs Ryan believed her son was out chasing the girls.

HUMAN

Preston—who has a year-old daughter by a girlfriend—decided he must tell all after "a week of agonising"

He said: "People must know that there was another, human side, to him.

"I knew him as a gentle man who wouldn't hurt a fly."

I KISSED AND CUDDLED A KILLER - SEE PAGES 4 and 5

form of explicit sex education in schools, the (homo)sexuality of public figures, and above all, now, in the guise of AIDS.[14]

Homosexuality has lately come to occupy a most peculiar and centrally privileged position in the government of the home—homosexuality ideologically constructed as a regulative admonitory sign throughout the field of "popular" culture in the likeness of the ruthless pervert, justifying any amount of state intervention in the cause of "family values" and so on. Yet at the same time, the male homosexual becomes an impossible object, a monster that can only be engendered by a process of corruption through seduction, which is itself inexplicable, since familialism lacks any theory of desire beyond the supposed "needs" of reproduction. It is this rigorously anti-Freudian scenario that actively encourages the forward slippage from corruption theories of homosexuality to contagion theories of AIDS. In this manner the axiomatic identification of AIDS as a sign and symptom of homosexual behavior reconfirms the passionately held view of "the family" as a uniquely vulnerable institution. It also sanctions the strongest calls for "protectionist" measures, of an ever intensified censorship that will obliterate the evidently unbearable cultural evidence of that sexual diversity which stalks the terra incognita beyond the home.

Hence the incomparably strange reincarnation of the cultural figure of the male homosexual as a predatory, determined invert, wrapped in a Grand Guignol cloak of degeneracy theory, and casting his lascivious eyes—and hands—out from the pages of Victorian sexology manuals and onto "our" children, and above all onto "our" sons. Undoubtedly there is a real threat in the above scenario, which only serves to reveal the full extent to which the home is always a site of intense sexual fantasy. But the unspeakable that lurks in the very bosom of "the family" is not so much the real danger of child-molestation from *outside*, but the more radical possibility of acknowledging that the child's body is invariably an object of *parental* desire, and further, that the child itself is not only *desirable* but *desiring*. Calls for the quarantining of people infected with HIV, or the compulsory HIV testing of all gay men, immigrants, and other extra-familial categories, clearly derive from this prior, unconscious compulsion to censor and expel the signs of sexual diversity from the domestic field of vision, which is always equated with the child's point of view. Identifying with the child, the "good" parent is thus protected from troubling disturbances of adult identities, taking refuge in a projective fantasy of childhood "innocence" that significantly de-sexualizes all the actors involved. The utter violence of AIDS commentary suggests much about the force with which these repressed sexual materials return, and the forms of hysteria and hysterical identification that are responsi-

---

14.   Simon Watney, "AIDS: The Cultural Agenda," paper presented at the conference Homosexuality, Which Homosexuality? at the Free University, Amsterdam, December 1987; conference papers forthcoming.

ble for successfully paralyzing the family ensemble into the rigidly stereotyped routines of "respectable" domesticity.

It is from this perspective that we may glimpse something of the political unconscious of the visual register of AIDS commentary, which assumes the form of a diptych. On one panel we are shown the HIV retrovirus (repeatedly misdescribed as the "AIDS virus") made to appear, by means of electron microscopy or reconstructive computer graphics, like a huge technicolor asteroid. On the other panel we witness the "AIDS victim," usually hospitalized and physically debilitated, "withered, wrinkled, and loathsome of visage" — the authentic cadaver of Dorian Gray.[15] This is the *spectacle of AIDS*, constituted in a regime of massively overdetermined images, which are sensitive only to the values of the dominant familial "truth" of AIDS and the projective "knowledge" of its ideally interpellated spectator, who already "knows all he needs to know" about homosexuality *and* AIDS. It is the principal and serious business of this spectacle to ensure that the subject of AIDS is "correctly" identified and that any possibility of positive sympathetic identification *with* actual people with AIDS is entirely expunged from the field of vision. AIDS is thus embodied as an exemplary and admonitory drama, relayed between the image of the miraculous authority of clinical medicine and the faces and bodies of individuals who clearly disclose the stigmata of their guilt. The principal target of this sadistically punitive gaze is the body of "the homosexual."

The Homosexual Body

Psychoanalysis understands identification as a psychological process whereby the subject "assimilates an aspect, property, or attribute of the other and is transformed, wholly or partially, after the model the other provides." Further, "it is by means of a series of identifications that the personality is constituted and specified."[16] But the substantive process of identifying operates in two modes: the transitive one of identifying the self in relation to the *difference* of the other, and the reflexive one of identifying the self in a relation of *resemblance* to the other. The homosexual body is an object that can only enter "public" visibility in the transitive mode, upon the strictly enforced condition that any possibility of identification *with* it is scrupulously refused. In the register of object-choice, the homosexual body inescapably evidences a sexual diversity that it is its ideological "function" to restrict. In the register of gender, it exposes the impossibility of the entire enterprise. Feminized in contempt, the homosexual body speaks too much of male "heterosexual" misogyny. Masculinized, it

15.   Oscar Wilde, *The Picture of Dorian Gray* (1891), New York and Oxford, Oxford University Press, 1974, p. 224.
16.   J. Laplanche and J.-B. Pontalis, *The Language of Psycho-Analysis*, London, The Hogarth Press, 1983, p. 205.

simply disappears. It is thus constituted as a *contradictio in objecto*, an objective contradiction. Psychoanalysis will pose this "problem" in a very different way, since the body with which it deals is "not some external realm but something that is internal to the psyche. . . . For psychoanalysis does not conceive of perceptions as unmediated registrations of the reality of a pregiven body. Rather, it has a libidinal theory of perception."[17]

The "problem," then, is the body itself, radically mute, yet rendered garrulous by projective, desiring fantasies all around it, which, as Leo Bersani reminds us, are "a frantic defence against the return of dangerous images and sensations to the surface of consciousness."[18] More precisely, these "desiring fantasies are by no means turned only towards the past; they are projective reminiscences."[19] Indeed, the very notion of a "homosexual body" only exposes the more or less desperate ambition to confine mobile desire in the semblance of a stable object, calibrated by its sexual aim, regarded as a "wrong choice." The "homosexual body" would thus evidence a fictive collectivity of perverse sexual performances, denied any psychic reality and pushed out beyond the furthest margins of the social. This, after all, is what the category of "the homosexual" (which we *cannot* continue to employ) was invented to do in the first place. The social sight lines of sexuality are thus permanently tensed against "mistakes" that might threaten to undermine the fragile stability of the heterosexual subject of vision. Hence the inestimable convenience of AIDS, reduced to a typology of signs that promises to identify the dreaded object of desire in the final moments of its own apparent self-destruction. AIDS is thus made to rationalize the impossibility of the "homosexual body," and reminds us only of the dire consequences of a failure to "forget". . . . Hence the social *necessity* of the "homosexual body," disclosed in the composite photography of nineteenth-century penal anthropology and sexology, and contemporary journalism. Hence also the voice of a contemporary English ex-police pathologist in a London teaching hospital, inviting his students, in the familiar pedagogic manner, to identify the physical symptoms of homosexuality, especially the "typical keratinized funnel-shaped rectum of the habitual homosexual."[20] Other constitutional symptoms of the "habitual homosexual" include softening of the brain. It is this order of "knowledge" of the "homosexual body" that precedes most clinical AIDS commentary and seeps out into the domestic register through the mediating services of medical correspondents, who report back from the clinical front lines on "our" behalf and ceaselessly refer us to the diagnostic AIDS diptych. In these densely coded *tableaux mourants* the body is subjected to extremes of casual cruelty and

17.   Parveen Adams, "Versions of the Body," *m/f*, nos. 11–12 (1986), p. 29.
18.   Leo Bersani, *Baudelaire and Freud*, Berkeley, University of California Press, 1977, p. 129.
19.   *Ibid.*, pp. 41–42.
20.   Meyrick Horton, "General Practices," paper presented at the second annual Social Meanings of AIDS conference, South Bank Polytechnic, London, November 1987.

violent indifference, like the bodies of aliens, sliced open to the frightened yet fascinated gaze of uncomprehending social pathologists. Here, where the signs of homosexual "acts" have been entirely collapsed into the signs of death-as-the-deserts-of-depravity, there is still some chance that reflexive identification *with* the merely human fact of death might interrupt the last rites of psychic censorship, with the human body in extremis.

Thus, even and especially in the *clair-obscur* of death itself, the "homosexual body," which is also that of the "AIDS victim," must be publicly seen to be humiliated, thrown around in zip-up plastic bags, fumigated, denied burial, lest there be any acknowledgment of the slightest sense of *loss*. Thus the "homosexual body" continues to speak after death, not as a memento mori, but as its exact reverse, for a life that must at all costs be seen to have been devoid of value, unregretted, unlamented, and—final indignity—effaced into a mere anonymous statistic. The "homosexual body" is "disposed of," like so much rubbish, like the trash it was in life. Yet, as always, it is the very *excess* of the psychic operations informing this terminal "truth" of AIDS that signifies far beyond its own intentions. And, in these circumstances, ironically, the psychic consequences of the savage social organization of "sexuality" in the modern world can only serve ultimately to make instruments to plague us all. For it is precisely the displacement of epidemiology by a moralized etiology of disease, which regards AIDS as an intrinsic property of the fantasized "homosexual body," that is likely actively to encourage the real spread of HIV by distracting attention away from the well-proven means of blocking its transmission. Such attention would require listening to the voices of the "guilty" ones, would run the grave risk of acknowledging that HIV is no respector of persons or even bodies. But the spectacle of AIDS continues to protect us against any such ghastly eventuality, as we settle down before our TV screens to watch and to celebrate the long-prophesied and marvelous sight of the degenerates finally burning themselves out, comfortable and secure in our *gesundes Volksempfinden*—our healthy folk feelings.

The Spectacle of AIDS

In all its variant forms the spectacle of AIDS is carefully and elaborately stage-managed as a sensational didactic pageant, furnishing "us," the "general public," with further dramatic evidence of what "we" already "know" concerning the enormity of the dangers that surround us on all sides and at all times. It provides a purgative ritual in which we see the evildoers punished, while the national family unit—understood as the locus of "the social"—is cleansed and restored. Yet, as Jacques Donzelot has argued, "In showing the emergence of 'the social' as the concrete space of intelligibility of the family, it is the social that suddenly looms as a strange abstraction."[21]

21.   Jacques Donzelot, *The Policing of Families: Welfare Versus the State*, London, Hutchinson & Co., 1979, p. xxvi.

EXCLUSIVE! LIBERACE AND PAL WHO DIED OF AIDS

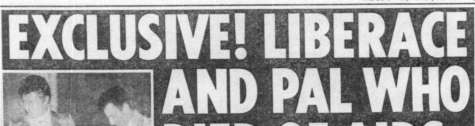

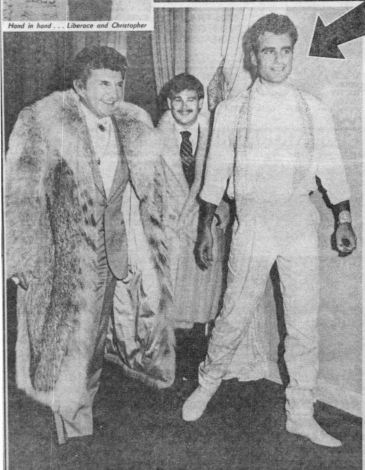

Hand in hand . . . Liberace and Christopher

Pals at a party. . fur-coated Liberace with lover Wyman and flamboyant Christopher, soon to die

Gay night out before tragedy

From **WENDY LEIGH** in **NEW YORK**

● THIS was Liberace's gay life before it turned sour—enjoying himself at a swell party with two homosexual pals. But now one of them, songwriter Christopher Adler, is dead from AIDS and Liberace himself is dying of the disease.

● There were no such worries when Liberace and his lover Carey James Wyman joined Adler at the Limelight Club in New York to mark actress Shirley MacLaine's fiftieth birthday. But just months after these exclusive pictures were taken, Christopher was complaining to Shirley: "I am having ghastly pains."

● Christopher, 30, told her: "I have a high fever and no energy at all." Friends revealed afterwards that he had died from a lymph disease brought on by AIDS. Now, two years later, Liberace is close to death at his millionaire mansion in Palm Springs, California.

● The 67-year-old master showman is being treated round the clock by a team of doctors. Close friends visit him every day and hundreds of get-well messages have been sent by fans. Last night a friend said: "There is no change in Liberace's gravely-ill condition despite the vigorous efforts of his doctors."

● In his 30-year career as one of the most successful personalities in showbiz, Liberace is reported to have averaged earnings of more than £3 million a year and has built up a fortune in jewellery, paintings, a string of lavishly decorated homes, a museum, 20 cars and 18 pianos.

Venerealizing AIDS, the spectacle reduces "the social" to the scale of "the family," from which miniaturized and impoverished perspective all aspects of consensual sexual diversity are systematically disavowed. We are thus returned to the question of "sexuality" in the modern world, but with a wholly different point of view from that which sustained earlier twentieth-century campaigns—conceived in terms of a right to privacy—on behalf of "sexual minorities." For it is precisely the concept of privacy that is the central term of familialism, now used to challenge the authority of the traditional liberal distinction between "public" and "private," which has defined the consensus view of how the space of "the social" has been thought for well over a century. That consensus is now up for grabs.[22]

The category of "homosexuality" has always in any case constituted a serious "problem" in relation to laws and social policies drawn up in the terms of a supposedly physical public/private distinction. Legitimated, to some extent, in the technical sphere of the private, it has been all the more problematized in the public domain. AIDS commentary demonstrates this very clearly, insofar as it is invariably addressed to a "family" that is also "the nation." Hence the extraordinary fact that even after 1,000 cases of AIDS, the British government has yet to direct a single item of information, advice, or support to the constituency most directly affected by the consequences of HIV since the early 1980s—gay men. This is evidently because we are not recognized as a part of "the social," from which we are paradoxically excluded by virtue of our partially legalized "private" status. And let us not forget that we are talking here about *at least* ten percent of the overall population of the United Kingdom. The spectacle of AIDS is thus always modified by the fear of being too "shocking" for its domestic audience, while at the same time it amplifies and magnifies the collective "wisdom" of familialism. AIDS commentary thus provides a unique perspective on the contemporary government of the home, which is experienced from within as a refuge of "privacy," and in the defense of which its members agree that it can hardly be sufficiently regulated. In this manner all aspects of "public" life are gradually annexed and subsumed by the precepts and "etiquette" of privacy at the very moment that its most eloquent advocates are drawing their curtains against what they perceive as a hostile and dangerous outside world.

Yet, as we have seen, the home itself is also recognized as a site of potential *inner* corruption, and the prosecution of the "public" by the "private" is ideally personified in the fantasy of the "homosexual body," whose sexual object-choice is displaced into the calibrated signs of AIDS. This body is as repulsive as the task of policing recalcitrant desire requires it to be. The spectacle of AIDS is thus placed in the service of the strongly felt need for constant domestic surveillance and the strict regulation of identity through the intimate mechanisms of sexual

22.   See Simon Watney, *Policing Desire: Pornography, AIDS, and the Media*, Minneapolis, University of Minnesota Press, 1987, chapter 4.

guilt, sibling rivalries, parental favoritism, embarrassment, hysterical modesty, house-pride, "keeping-up-with-the-Joneses," hobbies, diet, clothes, personal hygiene, and the general husbandry of the home. These are the concrete practices that authorize consent to "political" authority, and it is in relation to them that the entire spectacle of AIDS is unconsciously choreographed, with its studied emphasis on "dirt," "depravity," "license," and above all "promiscuity." Yet the proliferating agencies and voices that offer their "expertise" on behalf of "the family" are inevitably as uneven and inept as is the actual maintenance of power in the home itself. "The family" is thus frequently provided with mutually conflicting and contradictory messages from the very experts to which it has granted authority. Hence, for example, the glaring contemporary British conflict between popular consent for sex education in schools and an imperative against any form of education that is held to "advocate" homosexuality. "Public" sex education thus comes to duplicate the "knowledge" of "the family," which is duly inscribed in the national curriculum with the full force of law. In a very similar way, the strong lobby in favor of "AIDS education" in schools, and far beyond, is equally compelled to ignore the actual experience of most people with AIDS, or the communities most vulnerable to HIV infection, lest they also be accused of "advocating" homosexuality. Here, as in all similar instances, the concept of "advocacy" speaks from a discourse of sexual "acts" by which the "innocent" might become "corrupted" and turned into "habitual homosexuals." Such a concept functions within the powerful anti-Freudian project that aspires to erase all notions of desire from the epistemological field of "family," that is, "public," life.

In these circumstances, the spectacle of AIDS operates as a public masque in which we witness the corporal punishment of the "homosexual body," identified as the enigmatic and indecent source of an incomprehensible, voluntary resistance to the unquestionable governance of marriage, parenthood, and property. It is at precisely this point that opposition to the familial sovereignty of AIDS commentary can be posed most effectively. For, as I have argued, the overall spectacle of AIDS places its own audience at direct risk of HIV infection by distracting attention away from the demonstrably effective means of preventing its transmission. At the same time, the tremendous discursive responsibility that is placed upon the notion of "promiscuity" throughout AIDS commentary renders it especially vulnerable to challenge when it is isolated from the propping imagery of venerealized death. It can easily be demonstrated, for example, that HIV is not a venereal condition, since it is not necessarily or exclusively sexually transmitted. It is not difficult to grasp the fact that if every disease that can or may be sexually transmitted were classified as venereal, the list would include all the most common known medical ailments, as Kaye Wellings has pointed out in relation to the earlier venerealizing of herpes in the 1970s.[23] It must also be

23. Kaye Wellings, "Sickness and Sin: The Case of Genital Herpes," paper presented to the

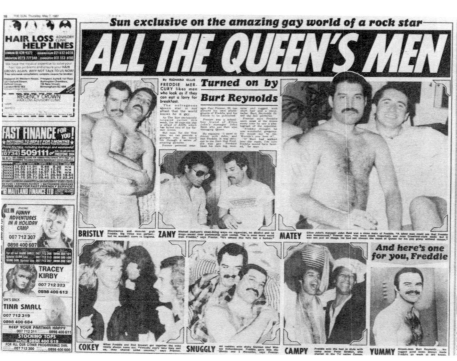

Sun exclusive on the amazing gay world of a rock star

ALL THE QUEEN'S MEN

By RICHARD ELLIS

Turned on by Burt Reynolds

BRISTLY

ZANY

MATEY

And here's one for you, Freddie

COKEY

SNUGGLY

CAMPY

YUMMY

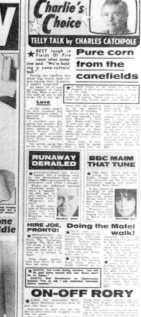

A People investigation on the eve of the church's great debate

SECRETS OF THE GAY VICARS

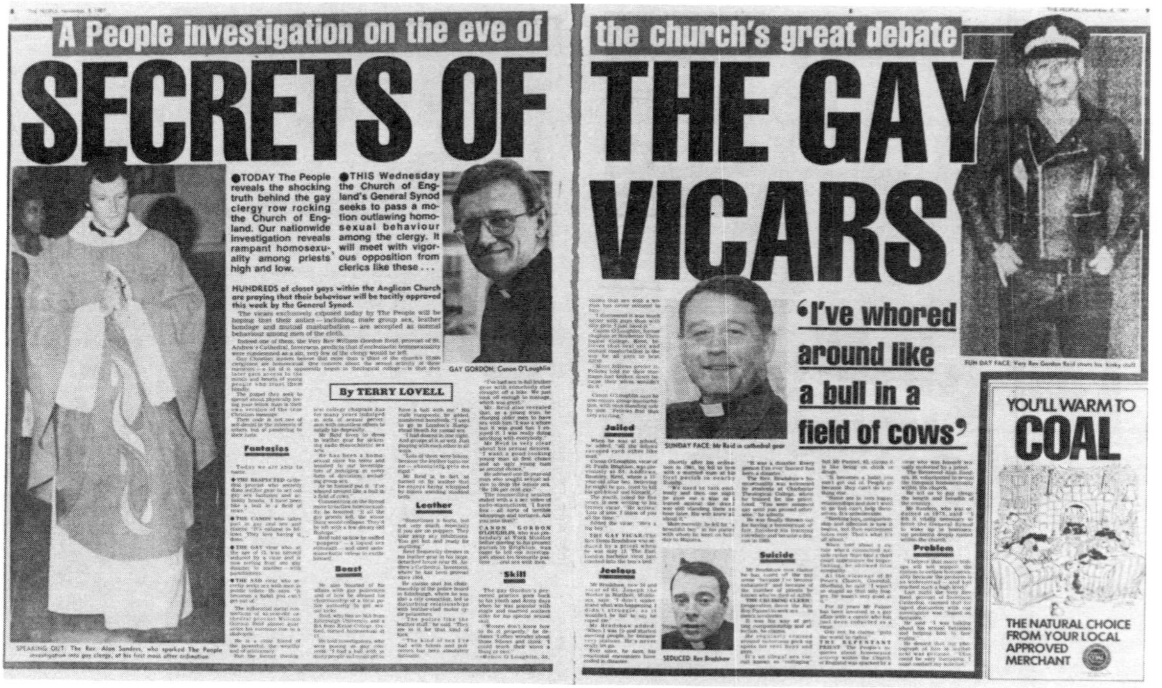

By TERRY LOVELL

'I've whored around like a bull in a field of cows'

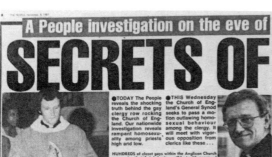

SPEAKING OUT: The Rev. Alan Sanders, who sparked The People investigation into gay clergy, at his first mass after ordination

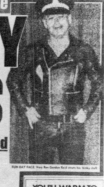

GAY GORDON: Canon O'Loughlin

SUNDAY FACE: Mr Reid in cathedral gear

Fantasies

Leather

Beast

Skill

Jailed

Suicide

Jealous

SEDUCED: Rev Bradshaw

FUN DAY FACE: Very Rev Gordon Reid sports his kinky stuff

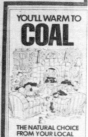

forcefully pointed out on every available occasion that those posing "monogamy" as a preferable alternative to prophylactic information are in turn responsible for increasing the spread of HIV by mischievously suggesting that monogamy affords some kind of intrinsic "moral" defense against a retrovirus. In such ways the entire authority of the spectacle of AIDS could be undermined by the protectionist rhetoric of the spectacle itself. This also permits the wider affirmation of sexual desire and diversity in the presentation of safer sex as an emancipatory and life-saving protectorate for the nation, posed in actively democratic terms that enlarge conceptions of the self beyond the narrowing confines of "citizenship." In these respects the challenge of AIDS reeducation exemplifies the insight of Ernesto Laclau and Chantal Mouffe that what is being exploded in the postmodern period

> is the idea and the reality itself of a unique space of constitution of the political. What we are witnessing is a politicisation far more radical than any we have known in the past, because it tends to dissolve the distinction between the public and the private, not in terms of the encroachment on the private by a unified public space, but in terms of a proliferation of radically new and different political spaces. We are confronted with the emergence of a *plurality of subjects* whose forms of constitution and diversity it is only possible to think if we relinquish the category of "subject" as a unified and unifying essence.[24]

By insisting on the psychoanalytic perception of the *psychic reality* of desire, we may avoid the shortcomings of a sexual politics that continues to see "gay oppression" as a unitary and distinct phenomenon that might easily be rectified and remedied through direct political and legislative interventions, however intrinsically expedient these may be in relation to the only too concrete institutions that currently secure the meaning and practice of "justice." The spectacle of AIDS teaches us, however, that it is the structure, epistemology, and "decorum" of "sexuality" itself that have inexorably led us to the tragic impasse in which we find ourselves, where seemingly unified "sexual minorities" are widely and routinely regarded, in their entirety, as disposable constituencies. This point cannot be sufficiently emphasized. For let there be no mistake: the spectacle of AIDS calmly and constantly entertains the possible prospect of the death of all western European and American gay men from AIDS—a total, let us say, of some twenty million lives—without the slightest flicker of concern, regret, or grief. Psychoanalysis may alert us to the psychological processes that can be activated in particular, complex historical circumstances in order to endorse an

British Sociological Association, Medical Sociology Group, 1983, p. 10.
24.   Ernesto Laclau and Chantal Mouffe, *Hegemony and Socialist Strategy: Towards a Radical Democratic Politics*, London, Verso, 1985, p. 181.

indifference that casually dehumanizes whole categories of persons. To turn back now to the prospect of a politics rooted in the subjectivity of public/private space can only serve to strengthen the powerful emergent forms of a secularized fundamentalism that will not cease to prosecute its own "projective reminiscences," picked out in the spotlights of its own displaced desires. In the meantime, all those who threaten to expose the brutal, hypocritical, and degrading implications of contemporary "family values" and "standards of decency" will undoubtedly continue to be stridently denounced — quite accurately — as "enemies of the family."

AIDS is increasingly being used to underwrite a widespread ambition to erase the distinction between "the public" and "the private," and to establish in their place a monolithic and legally binding category — "the family" — understood as the central term through which the world and the self are henceforth to be rendered intelligible. Consent to this strategy is sought by tapping into lay perceptions of health, sickness, and disease, unevenly accreted down the centuries, and sharing only the common human fear and disavowal of death. Health education thus emerges as the central site of hegemonic struggle in the coming decades — a struggle that refuses and eludes all known lines of previous party-political allegiance and observance. A new and essentially talismanic model of power is emerging, offering to protect subjectivities carefully nurtured in folklore and superstition, now rearticulated in a discourse of ostensibly medical authority. We are witnessing the precipitation of a moralized bio-politics of potentially awesome power — a cunning combination of leechcraft and radiotherapy, eugenics and a master narrative of "family health" — with social policies that aspire with sober fanaticism to the creation of a modernity in which *we* will no longer exist. The spectacle of AIDS thus promises a stainless world in which *we* will only be recalled, in textbooks and carefully edited documentary "evidence," as signs of plagues and contagions averted — intolerable interruptions of the familial, subjects "cured" and disinfected of desire, and "therapeutically" denied the right to life itself.

AIDS and Syphilis:
The Iconography of Disease

SANDER L. GILMAN

Images without End

In the summer of 1986, *Newsweek* published a cover story on Gerald Friedland of Montefiore Medical Center. Written in the informal and personal style of the "new journalism," "The AIDS Doctor" is an example of the attempt by the mainstream media to alter the dominant image of the "AIDS patient."[1] The opening sentence of the essay sets not only its tone but its agenda: "One day in April 1985, Dr. Gerald H. Friedland found himself at the bedside of a young woman named Maria, letting her know as gently as he could that she was going to die." Disregarding the self-conscious echo of the opening of Dante's *Inferno*, we can read in this sentence a clear desire to shift the image of the person with AIDS from that of the gay man to that of the heterosexual woman. The authors introduce us to an "exemplary" person with AIDS (PWA) who is nevertheless both a woman and a medical anomaly: "Nothing in her medical history marked her as a candidate for AIDS, not at first glance." She should have been a noncombatant in the "AIDS invasion" of North America, since she was not one of the "4-H's" — homosexuals, heroin addicts, hemophiliacs, and Haitians — the four groups labeled as being "at risk" through the early '80s.[2] Maria was an "incidental victim," infected by her former husband, an IV drug user, who had subsequently died of AIDS.

The *Newsweek* cover story both reflects and works to shape the public image of the person with AIDS, an image that has been constructed by the media over the past several years in ways that are contradictory and confusing.[3] It is vital that

1.   Peter Goldmand and Lucille Beachy, "The AIDS Doctor," *Newsweek*, July 21, 1986.
2.   See Michael S. Gottlieb and Jerome E. Groopman, eds., *Acquired Immune Deficiency Syndrome: Proceedings of a Shering Corporation-UCLA Symposium* (held in Park City, Utah, February 5–10, 1984), New York, Liss, 1984.
3.   See H. Schwartz, "AIDS in the Media," in *Science in the Streets*, New York, Priority Press, 1984, pp. 30ff.; and Andrea J. Baker, "The Portrait of AIDS in the Media: An Analysis of the *New York Times*," in Douglas A. Feldman and Thomas M. Johnson, eds., *The Social Dimension of AIDS: Method and Theory*, New York, Prager, 1986, pp. 179–197. For general background on the image of PWAs, see Caspar G. Schmidt, "The Group-Fantasy Origins of AIDS," *Journal of Psychohistory*, no.

we understand this social construction of AIDS, because it has directly affected the lives of so many. People have been stigmatized (and destroyed) as much by the "idea" of AIDS as by its reality. Since each of us has the potential of stigmatizing and being stigmatized, since the construction of images of disease is a dynamic process to which the sufferers, real and imagined, consistently respond, it is in our best interest to recognize the process. Not that we can expect to eliminate it, but we can at least become aware of the regularity with which it recurs historically.

Icons of disease appear to have an existence independent of the reality of any given disease. This "free-floating" iconography of disease attaches itself to various illnesses (real or imagined) in different societies and at different moments in history. Disease is thus restricted to a specific set of images, thereby forming a visual boundary, a limit to the idea (or fear) of disease. The creation of the image of AIDS must be understood as part of this ongoing attempt to isolate and control disease.

My approach to the image of PWAs is rooted in an attempt to plumb the meaning of specific representations of disease. These icons of disease overtly link the visual representation of the sufferer with the "ground" or context in which such images function.[4] My interest is in understanding the iconographic references of such images, and through these references, the extraordinary power the images have to reflect (and shape) society's response to individuals suffering with disease.

---

12 (1984), pp. 37–78; Dennis Altman, *AIDS in the Mind of America: The Social, Political, and Psychological Impact of a New Epidemic*, New York, Doubleday, 1986; David Black, *The Plague Years: A Chronicle of Aids, the Epidemic of Our Times*, New York, Simon & Schuster/London, Picador, 1986; Graham Hancock and Enver Carim, *AIDS: The Deadly Epidemic*, London, Gollanz, 1986; Richard Liebmann-Smith, *The Question of AIDS*, New York, New York Academy of Sciences, 1985; Eve K. Nicols, *Mobilizing against AIDS: The Unfinished Story of a Virus*, Cambridge, Massachusetts, Harvard University Press, 1986; Lon G. Nungasser, *Epidemic of Courage: Facing AIDS in America*, New York, St. Martin's, 1986; Earl E. Shelp, Ronald H. Sunderland, and Peter W. H. Mansell, *AIDS: Personal Stories in Pastoral Perspective*, New York, Pilgrim Press, 1986; Barbara Peabody, *The Screaming Room: A Mother's Journal of Her Son's Struggle with AIDS: A True Story of Love, Dedication and Courage*, San Diego, Oak Tree, 1986. For a sense of the cultural context of much of this literature, see George L. Mosse's brilliant study *Nationalism and Sexuality: Respectability and Abnormal Sexuality in Modern Europe*, New York, Howard Fertig, 1985.

4.   An icon is a sign that represents objects through a relationship of similarity, by exemplifying some property associated with the object. I use the term in the sense suggested by C. S. Peirce; see Charles Hartshorne, Paul Weiss, and Arthur W. Burks, eds., *Collected Papers of C. S. Peirce*, Cambridge, Massachusetts, Harvard University Press, 1931–58, vol. 2, p. 282. Peirce argues that the properties of the sign that underlie its iconic nature are intrinsic, i.e., independent of the actual existence of the object (vol. 4, p. 447). He also argues, and I follow him in this, that icons therefore cannot represent particular individuals, but only general classes of things (vol. 3, p. 434). Thus the representation of a patient suffering from a disease has iconic character, even if the patient and disease are "real," i.e., existing apart from the icon in time and space.

The First Image of AIDS

The construction of the image of AIDS has, by now, a seven-year history. In 1979 Alvin Friedman-Kien of New York University Medical Center identified a group of patients suffering from a rare form of cancer, Kaposi's sarcoma (KS), which presents striking symptoms, bluish or purple-brown lesions on the skin. Although the normal course of the disease is seldom fatal, these young patients were dying within eight to twenty-four months of their diagnoses. Other physicians reported similar patterns,[5] and by June 1981, twenty-six such cases were reported by the Centers for Disease Control (CDC) in their *Morbidity and Mortality Weekly Report (MMWR)*.[6] During this same period, five cases of *Pneumocystis carinii* pneumonia (PCP), an illness caused by a ubiquitous protozoan parasite that usually manifests itself only in individuals with depressed immune systems, appeared in Los Angeles. By the time of the report, two of these patients had died. Shortly thereafter, ten new cases of PCP were diagnosed, and two of these patients also had KS.[7]

The initial appearance of this pattern in the United States led investigators at the CDC to try to comprehend its nature by constructing an image of the patient.[8] The epidemiologists found a common cluster of attributes. These patients were living in large urban areas (New York, Miami, Los Angeles, and San Francisco), and they were all young men. In addition, all of them were homosexual: as early as the June 5, 1981, report in the *MMWR*, the patients' sexual orientation, and more importantly its "quality," had been noted: "Two of the five [patients] reported having frequent homosexual contacts with various partners." The centrality of sexual orientation in the early picture of AIDS can be further seen in the designation of the disease during the first quarter of 1982 as GRID (gay-related immunodeficiency). This label structured the understanding of AIDS in such a marked manner that PWAs were not only stigmatized as carriers of an infectious disease, but also placed within a very specific category. For AIDS (a term officially coined only in the fall of 1982) was understood as a specific subset of the larger category of sexually transmitted diseases (STDs), as a disease from which homosexuals suffered as a direct result of their sexual practices and related "life-style" — for example, the use of "poppers" (amyl or butyl

5.   A detailed chronology of scientific findings about AIDS from 1981 to 1985 has been worked out by Robert C. Gallo and Luc Montagnier, scientists who were both involved in many of the initial discoveries concerning the disease. It details the disease from 1981 to 1985. See *The Chronicle of Higher Education*, April 8, 1987, p. 8, for that chronology.
6.   A. Friedman-Kien, et al., "Kaposi's sarcoma and *Pneumocystis* pneumonia among homosexual men — New York City and California," *MMWR*, no. 30 (1981), p. 305–308.
7.   M. S. Gottlieb, et al., "*Pneumocystis* pneumonia — Los Angeles," *MMWR*, no. 30 (1981), pp. 250–252; and S. M. Friedman, et al., "Follow-up on Kaposi's sarcoma and *Pneumocystis* pneumonia," *MMWR*, no. 30 (1981), pp. 409–410.
8.   See the initial editorial by J. A. Sonnabend, "The Etiology of AIDS," in *AIDS Research*, 1 (1984–85), pp. 1–12.

nitrate).[9] The idea of the person afflicted with an STD, one of the most potent in the repertory of images of the stigmatized patient, became the paradigm through which people with AIDS were understood and categorized. Even though the *MMWR* began, in late 1982, to record the appearance of the syndrome among such groups as hemophiliacs and IV drug users, sexual orientation persisted as the defining characteristic of the person with AIDS.[10]

The fact that AIDS appeared in the late 1970s served to link the disease to two unrelated social concerns: first, the perception of an increase in STDs in the US (following a period of perceived decline), signalled in 1975 by the declaration of the National Institute for Allergy and Infectious Diseases that research into STDs was its number one priority; and second, the growth of public awareness —at least in large urban areas—of the gay liberation movement, which followed in the wake of the Stonewall riots in Greenwich Village in 1969.[11] From the beginning, the person with AIDS was seen as a male homosexual with a sexually transmitted disease and thus as different from the perceived normal spectrum of patients.

We must stress that AIDS is thought to be caused by a retrovirus, now labeled HIV, spread by direct contact with infected body fluids, including blood and semen. Sexual contact is not necessary to contract the virus.[12] But AIDS was characterized not as a viral disease, such as Hepatitis B, but as a sexually transmitted disease, such as syphilis.

The Iconography of Syphilis

The initial categorization of AIDS as an STD (albeit in a very specific— homosexual—context) strongly marked the initial picture of the disease. Let us examine a series of visual images of people with AIDS—taken from the popular press during the past few years—in relation to historical images of people suffering from syphilis. The images of PWAs are taken from a press presumed to be sympathetic to these people, not from the papers and journals of the religious

---

9.   See Liebmann-Smith, *Question of AIDS*, pp. 84–86, and M. M. Lederman," Transmission of the Acquired Immuno-Deficiency Syndrome through Heterosexual Activity," *Annals of Internal Medicine*, 104 (1986), pp. 115–117.
10.   See Jacques Leibowitch, *A Strange Virus of Unknown Origin*, trans. Richard Howard, New York, Ballantine, 1985, pp. 3–9, and J. W. Curran, W. M. Morgan, E. T. Starcher, A. M. Hardy, and H. W. Jaffe, "Epidemiological Trends of AIDS in the United States," *Cancer Research*, no. 45 (1985), pp. 4602s–4604s.
11.   June E. Osborn, "The AIDS Epidemic: An Overview of the Science," *Issues in Science and Technology*, no. 2 (1986), p. 56–65.
12.   J. Seale, "AIDS and Hepatitis B Cannot Be Venereal Diseases," *Journal of the Canadian Medical Association*, no. 130 (1984), pp. 109–110. See also L. D. Grouse's editorial, "HTLV-III Transmission," *Journal of the American Medical Association*, no. 254 (1985), pp. 2130–2131. It is not, as Helen Mathews Smith notes, that "syphilis presents a paradigm for our latest venereal epidemic," but rather that AIDS is not a sexually transmitted disease though it has been so categorized (Helen Mathews Smith, "AIDS: Lessons from History," *MD Magazine*, no. 30 [1986], pp. 43–51).

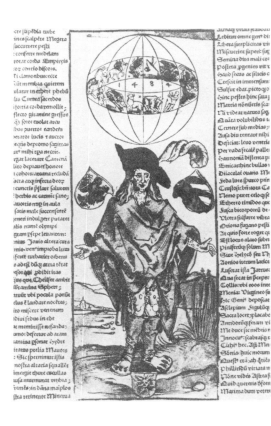

Albrecht Dürer. Syphilitic. 1496.

right, which have, since the nineteenth century, seen such people, as Allan Brandt observed, "as [suffering from] an affliction of those who willfully violated the moral code [and suffering] a punishment for sexual irresponsibility."[13] And yet the stigma of STDs persists, even in self-consciously liberal journals of public opinion.

As background to the iconographic history of these images of PWAs, however, I wish to examine a series of images taken from the nearly five-hundred-year-old iconography of syphilis in order to see how the boundaries of syphilis were constructed at its initial outbreak and during its subsequent history. The visual image of the syphilitic has its roots in the first years of the spread of an especially virulent form of syphilis, just after Charles VIII of France entered the besieged city of Naples in 1495. Carried by the retreating French armies, the *Mal de Naples, Morbus Gallicus, Malafranzcos,* or *Franzosenkrankheit* soon appeared in

13.   Allan Brandt, *No Magic Bullet: A Social History of Venereal Disease in the United States Since 1880,* New York, Oxford University Press, 1985, p. 134.

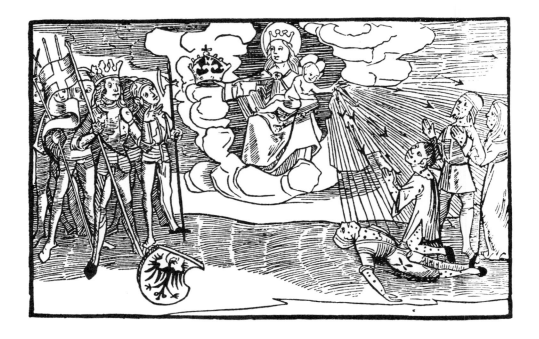

the German states.[14] On August 1, 1496, the first visual representation of the syphilitic appeared in a broadside written by Theodoricus Ulsenius and illustrated by Albrecht Dürer. The broadside locates the origin of the disease (for then, as now, there was an obsession with discovering the origin of disease rather than the means of controlling it) in the ill-fated appearance of five planets in the sign of the Scorpion (the zodiacal sign that rules the genitalia) in 1484. Dürer depicts an isolated male sufferer, who bears the signs and symptoms of syphilis like stigmata. Although echoing the position of the suffering Christ, exemplum of masculinity, the figure wears an enormous, plumed hat; an abundant cloak; broad-toed, slashed shoes; and long, flowing hair. This is thus a German carica-ture of the sufferer as fop, as outsider, as *Frenchman*, already associated in German myth with sexual excess and deviance. Nevertheless he is portrayed as a victim of the signs of the zodiac, which determine his affliction.[15] From the very

14.   On a general history of syphilis see Iwan Bloch, *Der Ursprung der Syphilis*, 2 vols., Jena, Gustav Fischer, 1901–1911. While Bloch supports the "Columbian" thesis, he does summarize the other literature as well. On the modern history of the disease see Brandt, *No Magic Bullet*, as well as H. L. Arnold, Jr., "Landmark Perspective: Penicillin and Early Syphilis," *Journal of the American Medical Association*, no. 251 (1984), pp. 2011–2012.

15.   Erwin Panofsky, "Homage to Fracastoro in a Germano-Flemish Composition of About 1590," *Nederlands Kunsthistorisch Jaarboek*, no. 12 (1961), pp. 1–33. On the iconographic significance of the scorpion as a sign of perverse sexuality, see Luigi Aurigemma, *La signe zodiacal du scorpion dans les*

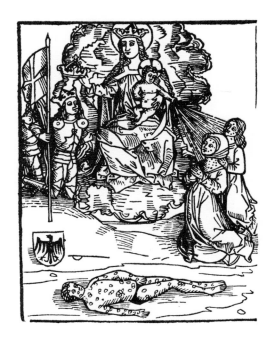

Left: Title page vignette for Sebastian Brant's pamphlet on syphilis. 1496.

Right: Vignette from Joseph Grünpeck's commentary on Brant's pamphlet. 1496.

first image, then, the syphilitic is seen as isolated, visually recognizable by his signs and symptoms, and sexually deviant.

That both men and women suffered from the new epidemic of syphilis is reflected in many early images, but a distinction is always drawn between the active and exemplary suffering of the male and the passive suffering of the female. The privileging of the male sufferer can be seen in a reworking of one of the earliest images of the syphilitic. A woodcut on the title page of a broadside on the new epidemic by the famed jurist and author of *The Ship of Fools* (1496), Sebastian Brant, shows a closed community of syphilitics, three male and one female, being punished by the *flaggellum Dei* (the whip of God) for their sexual transgressions.[16] Arrows signify the martyrdom of the victims, who suffer as a consequence of Adam and Eve's fall. The figure of the Christ child indicates, however, the potential for cure. In a reworking of this image, appearing in Joseph Grünpeck's 1496 commentary on Brant, the male sufferer is brought forward and isolated, a shift in emphasis that creates the illusion of the male as

---

traditions occidentales de l'antiquité grèco-latine à la Renaissance, Paris, Mouton 1976, p. 92. On the more general problem of disease and art in the Renaissance, see Millard Meiss, *Painting in Florence and Siena after the Black Death,* Princeton, Princeton University Press, 1951.

16.   Karl Sudhoff, *Zehn Syphilis-Drucke aus den Jahren 1495–1498,* Milan, R. Lier, 1924, p. xxii.

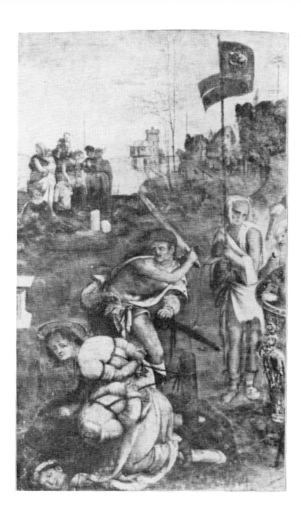

Amico Aspertini. Decapitation of St. Valerian and His Brother. *1506.*

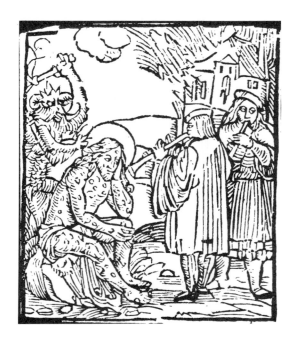

Illustration for broadside "On the Pox Called Malafrantzosa." 1500.

exemplary sufferer.[17] He is portrayed as the primary victim of the disease, not as its harbinger.

Amico Aspertini's painting, in the Oratoria of Saint Cecilia in Bologna, of the decapitation of St. Valerian and his brother (dated 1506), depicts a syphilitic in the long-established iconographic tradition of the leper, who bears the signs of his disease to the world. The change of signification to include a specific sexual reference is indicated by the emblem of the scorpion on his banner. Although, by the sixteenth century, leprosy was no longer endemic in Western Europe, its iconography remained as part of the popular storehouse of images of disease and pollution and was immediately attached to the new disease of syphilis.

But it is not merely "vacant" constructions of disease that influence the representation of the new illness. In a broadside prayer from about 1500, the image shows the syphilitic as embodied in the prefiguration of Job "smote . . . with sore boils from the sole of his foot unto his crown" (Job 2:7) by Satan.[18] But this figure is also presented in the classic pose of melancholia, elbow on knee, head on hand, a gesture of passive submission and reflection as well as despair.[19] Also central to this image, as in the earlier images found in Brant and Grünpeck, is the image of cure, but in this case a cure for melancholia. The syphilitic's friends play their instruments, attempting, as David did for Saul, to cure his melancholy madness with music.

The conflation of such images of earlier, known "diseases" — for which there was a perceived cure — with the new disease of syphilis provided a vocabulary through which to understand and, thus, to limit the disease. But the anonymous author of this broadside also suggests another contemporary understanding of the source of the disease, once again in a biblical prefiguration: he prays "that You [God] remember Abraham's prayer for Sodom and Gomorrah and save me from such a painful, horrible plague." Abraham's prayer was that, if ten righteous men be found in these sinful cities, God would spare them. Of course, they were not to be found (Genesis 18 and 19). Given the implications of the phrase "Sodom and Gomorrah" for the Renaissance, it is evident that the author is indicating the sexual source of the new pollution. But it is the male, the Job figure who represents the sufferer, and even with this notion of the sexual source of the disease, the male is understood simply as the victim.

Only during the Enlightenment does the image of the syphilitic shift from male to female, and with this shift comes another: from victim to source of infection. Already in the high Middle Ages, woman was shown as both seductive and physically corrupt — for example in the sculpture of *Madam World* from the St. Sebaldus Church in Nuremberg. Female beauty only serves as a mask for

17.   *Ibid.*, p. 71.
18.   Reproduced in the *Archiv für die Geschichte der Medizin*, no. 1 (1907), plate 8.
19.   See Moshe Barasch, *Gestures of Despair in Medieval and Early Renaissance Art*, New York, New York University Press, 1976.

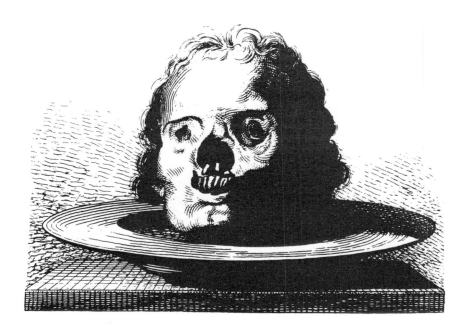

Head of a syphilitic prostitute. 18th century.

corruption and death, demonstrated by the contrast between the front and back of the sculpture. By the eighteenth century, the corrupt female is associated with the signs of a specific disease, syphilis—for example, in a late eighteenth-century popular print of the decayed head of a syphilitic prostitute. The change here is also from the innate corruption of the female to her potential for corrupting the male. The shift in the image of the syphilitic from the male "victim" of the disease to its female "source" took more than two hundred years to occur. In the baroque period, for example, the victim is still male, as is the case in Luca Giordana's *Allegory of Syphilis* (1664). But by the time of William Hogarth's *Marriage à la Mode* (1745), both the money-hungry aristocrat and the title-hungry alderman's daughter are represented as syphilitics. The popular image of the woman as exemplary syphilitic eventually permeates even medical literature in the early nineteenth century. In his great atlas of skin diseases of 1806, Jean-Louis Alibert, one of the founders of modern dermatology, represents all of his syphilitics as women.[20]

20.   Jean-Louis Alibert, *Description des maladies de la peau . . . ,* Paris, n.p., 1806–14. See the general discussion of Alibert in Susanne Dahm, *Frühe Krankenbildnisse: Alibert, Esquirol, Baumgärtner,* Cologne, Arbeiten der Forschungsstelle des Instituts für Geschichte der Medizin der Universität zu

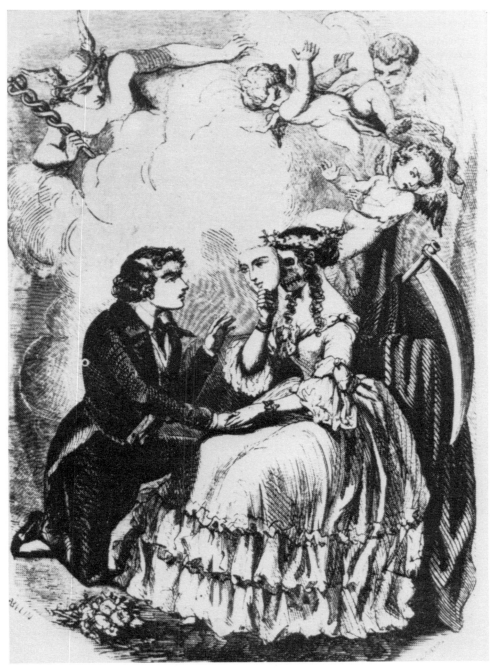

Title page vignette for 19th-century French translation of Francastoro's Syphilis.

The image of the seductress as the source of pollution can be seen even more strikingly on the title page of a mid-nineteenth-century French edition of Francastoro's "Syphilis," the poem that gave the disease its name in the sixteenth century. This image is a nineteenth-century variation of the baroque emblem representing the choice of Hercules, tempted by the vice of luxury, *Voluptas,* who hides her ugliness behind a mask. The difference here, of course, is that by the nineteenth-century "vice" has become "disease," seduction has become infection. We find, then, a continuity in the representation of the sufferer of a sexually transmitted disease as an outsider (present in the very first image by Dürer); by the Enlightenment the image of the outsider, the other, the deviant, is that of woman as source of pollution.

The Iconography of AIDS

The appropriation of the iconography of syphilis for the representation of people with AIDS is not random; it is, rather, a result of the perception that the sexual orientation of people with AIDS was determinant, and that these people suffered from a sexually transmitted disease. In addition, the "taming" of syphilis and other STDs with the introduction of antibiotics in the 1940s left our culture with a series of images of mortally infected and infecting people suffering a morally repugnant disease — without a sufficiently powerful disease to function as the referent of these images. During the 1970s there was an attempt to associate this iconography with genital herpes, but the symptomology of this viral disease was too trivial to warrant such an association over the long run. AIDS appeared then as the perfect referent, even if it was not a "typical" STD.

In a photograph that appeared in the *New York Times* on December 23, 1985, we see an image of the PWA as a patient isolated from the supposed act of healing (parallel to the images of the exemplary syphilitic in the broadsides of Brant and Grünpeck). The sense of physical distance is palpable; the observers are as far removed from the patient as they can be without being in another room. While this is a standard representation of medical treatment — like many late nineteenth- and twentieth-century photographs of physicians at work — the ground provided for the observer of this image is the tension communicated, not by the treatment of the patient, but by the implications of the disease. In 1985 (and subsequently), the *New York Times* was full of articles on the anxiety of health workers treating people with AIDS. The anxiety conveyed by the image thus corresponded, for the reader of the *Times,* to that of a "general public" worried about the transmission of AIDS. Moreover, by 1985, the significance of the

---

Köln, 1981. On the image of the prostitute as source of pollution in a nineteenth-century model of public health, see Charles Bernheimer, "Of Whores and Sewers: Parent-Duchatelet, Engineer of Abjection," *Raritan,* no. 6 (1987), pp. 72–90.

single male patient for the readers of the *New York Times* was self-evident: This is a homosexual male, both victim and cause of his own pollution. Already feminized in the traditional view of his sexuality, the gay man can now also represent the conflation of the images of the male sufferer and the female source of suffering traditionally associated with syphilis.

A group of photographs printed in the Long Island newspaper *Newsday* on August 4, 1985, represents an attempt on the part of the liberal media to soften the image of PWAs. The uppermost photograph in the group shows a hemophiliac; like the central figure in Brant's broadside, he is part of a mixed-sex group, in this case the family. The heterosexual male is seen here as both victim (of a polluted blood supply) and source of pollution (for his family). But the next three photographs return to the traditional iconography of STDs and the resultant despair of contagion and death. These are images of marginal men — marginal sexually or "racially" — presented visually as isolated, especially in the context of the first photograph of the hemophiliac with his family. In addition, these men, as in Dürer's broadside or Grünpeck's revision of the Brant image, show us their stigmata, KS lesions.

The final photograph in the series also represents the PWA as isolated, his very position once again echoing the classical iconographic position of melancholia. This association of the "AIDS victim" with the traditional iconography of melancholy is an extraordinarily powerful one; it reappeared as the first illustration for an update on AIDS in the popular scientific journal *Discover* in September 1986.[21] In an essay subtitled "Still No Reason for Hysteria," John Langone's agenda was to dispel the growing fear that AIDS was a potential danger for everyone, including heterosexuals. The iconography of depression, with its emphasis on the body, stresses the age-old association of the nature of the mind (here, homosexuality as "mental illness") with the image of the body (here, homosexuality as sexual deviance). The image of the body is made to "portray" the state of mind. The person with AIDS remains the suffering, hopeless male, shown as depressed and marginal. But there is an additional dimension to the use of the image of the melancholic in this image from *Discover*. For the purpose of the essay is to condemn — as unfounded — the media's "hysteria" about the possibility that AIDS will spread to heterosexuals. The photograph of the "AIDS victim" associates the PWA with the stigma of mental illness by means of iconographic association with the figure of the melancholic who has capitulated to despair. But the *Discover* photograph not only draws the analogy with the despair of impending death. Through a broader analogy extended to the "general population," which is seen to suffer from "unwarranted" AIDS phobia, it intends the PWA to function as a stand-in for the mental illness (read: fearful fantasy) of an entire nation. It is this broader association that works to counter

21.   John Langone, "AIDS Update: Still no Reason for Hysteria," *Discover*, no. 7 (September 1986), pp. 28–47.

the claim that AIDS is a danger to the entire community. Thus is the boundary between the "normal" and the hysterically feared "abnormal" drawn.

The Geographical Image of AIDS

The desire to locate the origin of a disease is the desire to be assured that we are not at fault, that we have been invaded from without, polluted by some external agent. In the late fifteenth century, syphilis was first understood as resulting from the malevolent influence of the zodiac. But it quickly came to be linked to another major event of the 1490s, Columbus's voyages of discovery to the Americas. Syphilis was seen as society's punishment for transgressing the God-given boundaries of human endeavor, a divine scourge that punished Europe for the collapse of the feudal system, the rise of capitalism, and the desire to find new worlds to feed this new economic system. Sebastian Brant labels it thus in *The Ship of Fools*.[22] But the geographical locus of the disease shifted with time and circumstances. In the nineteenth century, during an age of expanded colonialism and black slavery, a new argument placed the origin of syphilis in Africa, prior to the voyage of Columbus.

A similar story can be told about AIDS in the 1980s. In the United States, AIDS has been labeled an "African" or "Haitian" disease.[23] This presumed origin is, of course, very much in line with the white American notion that blacks, being inherently different, have a fundamentally different relationship to disease. For more than a century, blacks were assumed, for example, to have a much higher rate of mental illness because of their inability to cope with civilization.[24] It was also assumed that American blacks had a greater immunity to syphilis because of the "African" origin of the disease, leading to the horrors of the Tuskegee syphilis experiment, in which blacks infected with the disease were observed, without any medical intervention, until their deaths.[25]

The irony is that a polluted blood supply put American blacks—at least

22.   See Edwin H. Zeydel's translation of *The Ship of Fools*, New York, Dover, 1962, pp. 220–223. Brant's is the first German text to indicate the source of the disease in the New World. It quickly becomes a commonplace, partially because the "cure" proposed for the disease in early sixteenth-century German tracts, such as that by Ulrich von Hutten, is also seen to come from the New World. The cure, said to be found in the wood and bark of the *guaiacum* tree, becomes an important import into Germany through the efforts of the German trading family, the House of Fugger. The view is that, given the inherent balance of nature, if the disease comes from the New World, so too must its cure. This is an attempt to re-create a sense of the balance lost with the opening of the New World and the spread of syphilis. Many contemporary writers, among them Paracelsus, reject this analogy as spurious.
23.   Liebowitch, *A Strange Virus*, pp. 77–80.
24.   Sander L. Gilman, *Difference and Pathology: Stereotypes of Sexuality, Race, and Madness*, Ithaca, Cornell University Press, 1985, pp. 131–149.
25.   James H. Jones, *Bad Blood: The Tuskegee Syphilis Experiment: A Tragedy of Race and Medicine*, New York, The Free Press, 1981.

those suffering from such genetically transmitted diseases as sickle-cell anemia, which is treated with blood transfusions—at special risk for AIDS.[26] They were not, however, understood as being in a similar category with hemophiliacs. Blacks were deemed to be at risk because of their perceived sexual difference—their "hypersexuality"—as well as their "sociopathic" use of drugs. Black sexuality, associated with images of sexually transmitted disease, became a category of marginalization, as it had in the past.[27] But in the 1980s, after the intolerable state of blacks in this country was made visible by the civil rights movement in the '60s and '70s, it was no longer so easy to locate the source of disease among American blacks, as had been done in the Tuskegee experiment. Instead, the source of pollution was perceived to be foreign blacks, black Africans and Haitians, and thus American "liberal" sensibilities were assuaged even while speculations about the origin of AIDS continued to be determined by American racist ideology.

For the French, at least initially, AIDS was an American disease. With the increased adoption of American cultural models and practices by the French gay community (which even adopted the Anglicism *gai*), it was believed that the disease was the result of the excessive use of contaminated "poppers" imported from North America.[28] Even today, AIDS is popularly perceived in Europe as born, along with jeans and rock music, in the USA. In a recent title story on AIDS in the German weekly news magazine *Der Spiegel* (February 9, 1987), the central images are taken from American political cartoonists, even though the essay purports to be about AIDS in the Federal Republic.

For the Soviets the geographic origin of the disease is also the US: the HIV virus was man-made by the biological warfare specialists at Fort Detrick, Maryland, in conjunction with the scientists at the CDC. In the Soviet view, AIDS is an American biological weapon gone berserk and destroying its creator.[29] A cartoon published in *Pravda* reflects the complexity of national images of AIDS: an American general is shown paying for a test tube of AIDS virus supplied to him by a venal-looking scientist. Swimming about in the test tube, representing the power of the "AIDS virus," are tiny swastikas; the dead, casualties of AIDS, appear in the cartoon as concentration camp victims, their bare feet showing. This attempt to place the blame for AIDS on the United States worked only until the spring of 1987, when the Soviets, in the climate of *glasnost,* admitted that they, too, had indigenous cases of the disease. But during 1985 and 1986, the Soviets simply updated the old image of the US as degenerate and therefore sick. Indeed, the "orthodox" view was that homosexuality—and thus AIDS—was a

26.   S. Piomelli, "Chronic Transfusions in Patients with Sickle Cell Disease: Indications and Problems," *American Journal of Pediatric Hematology and Oncology,* no. 7 (1985), pp. 51–55.
27.   Gilman, *Difference and Pathology,* pp. 76–108.
28.   Leibowitch, *A Strange Virus,* p. 5.
29.   J. Seale, "AIDS Virus Infection: A Soviet View of Its Origin," *Journal of the Royal Society of Medicine,* no. 79 (1986), pp. 494–495.

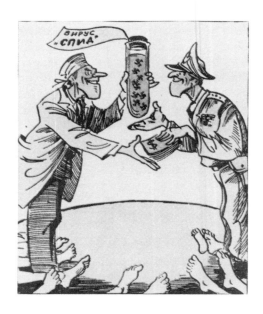

D. Ageva. AIDS as an American biological weapon.
Pravda, *November 1, 1986.*

pathological reflex of the late forms of capitalism which would (and did) vanish once the Soviet state was created.

One aspect of the construction in the United States of a geography of AIDS focused, as I have said, on its "African" or "Haitian" origins. Indeed, the withdrawal of the "risk group" label from Haitians followed a period of severe persecution, both direct and indirect, of Haitians in the US. To be Haitian and living in New York City meant that you were perceived as an AIDS "carrier." The irony is that it seems evident, given the most recent epidemiology of the disease in Haiti, that the disease, limited to the large urban areas on the island, was a result of contact between HIV seropositive North American tourists and Haitians, who passed the disease to their sexual partners and children.[30] In the US, however, the fact that AIDS was found among heterosexuals in Haiti could only be evidence that Haiti was the *source* of the disease. Heterosexual transmission was labeled by investigators a more "primitive" or "atavistic" stage of the development of AIDS. The pattern of infection in the US, where the disease existed only among marginal groups (including blacks), was understood as characterizing a later phase of the disease's history. It was only in "higher" cultures,

30.   On the Haitian question see J. W. Pape, et al., "The Acquired Immuno-Deficiency Syndrome in Haiti," *Annals of Internal medicine,* no. 103 (1985), pp. 774–778. On the "African" connection see the exchange of letters in the *British Medical Journal [Clinical Research],* no. 290 (1985), pp. 1284–1285, 932, 1006; no. 291 (1986), p. 216.

such as the United States, that the disease was limited to such specific groups as could be immediately and visually identifiable. This creation of a boundary between the infected—labeled and literally seen as different—and the healthy rested on the need to make a clear distinction between the heterosexual, non-IV drug using, white community and those at risk. Thus Anthony Pinching cogently observed in his September 1986 essay on the Western fantasy of a perverted and diseased black population as "originators" of AIDS:

> Rumours have circulated about the use of anal intercourse as a common means of birth control in Africa; this idea represents a carry-over from the initial perceptions of AIDS as something intrinsically to do with homosexual behavior. The widespread acceptance of these alternative explanations seems to indicate a remarkable ignorance about the countries in question; more disturbingly they have shown that many observers are unwilling to accept the obvious, if unpleasant, conclusion that AIDS, or rather HIV, is heterosexually transmitted.[31]

While heterosexual transmission is the primary means of the spread of the disease, another means for the transmission of HIV in black Africa has its roots in the imposition of models of Western medicine. The status of Western medicine and its association with inoculation is so high that no medical treatment, even by indigenous medical practitioners, is considered complete without an injection.[32] Due to the prohibitive cost of needles and syringes, blood is passed from patient to patient as the needle is used and reused. It is thus not the fantasized perverted nature of black sexuality that is at the core of the transmission of the disease in Africa, but the results of a wholesale exportation of Western medical practices without knowledge of or sensitivity to local conditions.

The geography of AIDS in North America, the drawing of the boundaries of risk, has had yet another dimension. AIDS is perceived as endemic to cities, which have traditionally been seen as harborers of disease and degeneracy.[33] AIDS is the plague of cities, as seen in the biblical image of Sodom and Gomorrah: righteous Abraham, who dwells in a tent, is contrasted in Genesis with the sinful dwellers in the city. Thus arises the seemingly natural association among three quite distinct groups perceived as corrupt city-dwellers: homosexuals, IV drug users, and Haitians. And purity lives, in this fantasy, where nature (and therefore goodness) dominates: on the farm and in the small town. This Rous-

31.   Anthony Pinching, "AIDS and Africa: Lessons for Us All," *Journal of the Royal Society of Medicine*, no. 79 (1986), pp. 501–503.

32.   John R. Seale and Zhores A. Medvedev, "Origin and Transmission of AIDS: Multi-Use Hypodermics and the Threat to the Soviet Union: Discussion Paper," *Journal of the Royal Society of Medicine*, no. 80 (1987), pp. 301–304.

33.   On theories of degeneration and the city see Sander L. Gilman and J. Edward Chamberlin, eds., *Degeneration: The Dark Side of Progress*, New York, Columbia University Press, 1985.

seauian view of the city inflects the image of the PWA, constructing for us an image of an urban deviant: a black IV drug user or a homosexual.

The Borders of the Image

What might have happened if AIDS had appeared in a different context? What if it had first been identified in IV drug users or hemophiliacs? Among the latter it would have been seen as an iatrogenic illness, not the fault of the patient but of the system, and the group stigma would surely have been less. Among IV drug users, AIDS would still have been stigmatized as a disease of a marginal group, but it would have been seen as a product of a sociopathic act associated with a specific class and race, and it would, therefore, be limited in its perceived locus. For in 1981 it was not the yuppies with their drug of choice, cocaine, who would have been infected, but the blacks of Harlem and the South Bronx, shooting heroin with shared needles. But these were not the groups that defined the illness.

What happened instead is that these two groups inherited the stigmatization of the sexually transmitted disease: IV drug users continued to be defined through this paradigm as dangerous sociopaths, and hemophiliacs as a marginalized, genetically disordered minority. This stigmatization became so widespread that it permeated social categories ordinarily exempt from stigma. In 1985, two community school boards in Queens sued the New York City Board of Education in order to exclude a seven-year old child, diagnosed as having AIDS, from the school system. (At the time the case was brought there were about seventy-eight children under the age of twelve in New York City who had been diagnosed with AIDS; fifty-two had already died.) The child in question had most probably contracted the disease *in utero*.

The attorney for the local school board, Robert Sullivan, observed concerning this child that "in many instances children who have AIDS are the children . . . of parents who are not as responsible as we would like them to be. . . . They may be the children of an IV drug user or a victim of sexual abuse." They are, in short, "not in the best family setting a child should be in . . . not a recommended family setting."[34] Even the dying child, the exemplary innocent within our pantheon of images of disease (think of the death of Dickens's Little Nell or Harriet Beecher Stowe's Little Eva), has become infected with the unclean image of the sexually transmitted disease. Nowhere is this often unconscious pollution of the image of the child clearer than in the caption to an Associated Press photograph of the central figure in a parallel court case, Ryan

34.   Dorothy Nelkin and Stephen Hilgartner, "Disputed Dimensions of Risk: A Public School Controversy over AIDS," *Milbank Memorial Fund Quarterly*, no. 64, Supplement 1 (1986), pp. 118–142. Compare K. M. Shannon and A. J. Amman, "Acquired Immune Deficiency Syndrome in Childhood," *Journal of Pediatrics*, no. 106 (1985), pp. 332–342.

White, whose attempts to enter the Kokomo, Indiana, school system led to a massive boycott by his schoolmates' parents, afraid of the potential for infection. In the *Ithaca Journal* of May 1, 1986, a photograph of Ryan White showed him, as the caption stated, and "his sister Andrea . . . [meeting] cast members of 'Cats' at a star-studded gala in New York Tuesday night to raise money for AIDS research. Ryan . . . is a homophiliac [*sic*] who contracted AIDS through a blood transfusion." The conflation of *hemophiliac* and *homosexual* by the caption is an extraordinarily simple one given the construction of the image of the PWA. In an attempt to work against this conflation, many images of children with AIDS show the child in the family setting, which contrasts radically with the imposed isolation of the gay man or IV drug user with AIDS. The presence of the family serves to signal the "normality" of the child and the low risk of transmission, in spite of the child's radical stigmatization. The media wishes to maintain society's image of the pure, dying child. But such an iconographic device is rarely sufficient to overcome the stigma of AIDS.

The irrational reaction to children with AIDS has had disastrous consequences for children and family alike. The hysteria crescendoed in the much publicized case of the Ray family in Arcadia, Florida. On August 24, 1987, the three hemophiliac sons, ages eight, nine, and ten—after having been barred from school the previous year when it was discovered that they had tested HIV-positive—were readmitted by court order to the local elementary school. The community quickly organized a boycott of the school, and the family's home was burned down on August 28. The irony of this event's taking place the week before the Labor Day weekend, when many Americans watch the annual telethon for "Jerry's kids," children suffering from muscular dystrophy, cannot be overstated. For the enormous power of this annual telethon depends on the appearance of the handicapped children as objects of the viewers' sympathy. One can well imagine the same individuals who burned down the Ray house sitting in their own homes a week later, watching the Jerry Lewis telethon with tears of sympathy in their eyes.

To understand the need for the continuation of this stigmatization even after it has become evident that AIDS is not solely a sexually transmitted disease, it is important to note that there is a powerful secondary effect of the stigma. It clearly defines the boundaries of pollution, limiting the risk to the homosexual (and those other groups now stigmatized), and thus confines heterosexuals' fears about their own vulnerability. The more heterosexual transmission of AIDS becomes a media "fact," the greater the need for heterosexuals to retain the image of AIDS as a disease of socially marginal groups.

There have been some attempts by the media to make the public aware of the risk to all members of society of acquiring AIDS. But the association of AIDS with homosexuality and with sexually transmitted disease has proven more powerful than anticipated. And this association is often guaranteed by the image of the person who has AIDS. Recall the *Newsweek* story published in the summer of

1986, in which the editorial intent was to change the image of the typical person with AIDS from male to female in order to stress the risk for the "general population." Accompanying this essay were three photographs of PWAs: all of them are of men, and all are shown in the traditional guise of the isolated male sufferer that dominated the early history of images of syphilis. The first image the reader sees upon opening this cover story is not only male but also black. The black gay man thus becomes the icon of the PWA even in the context of a story that explicitly stresses the potential widespread heterosexual transmission of the disease.

By the spring of 1987 the public understanding of AIDS as a disease not limited to specific marginal groups had begun to grow. The statement of Surgeon General C. Everett Koop in support of extending information about condoms, together with increased media attention to heterosexual transmission, meant that by March 1987 the majority of those tested in the public AIDS clinics in New York and San Francisco were heterosexuals. But even this awareness of the reclassification of AIDS did not mitigate the need to maintain strict boundaries. In a cartoon of mid-March 1987, J. D. Crowe of the San Diego *Tribune* depicted the source of heterosexual transmission as a group of prostitutes

J. D. Crowe. Cartoon for San Diego Tribune. *1987.*

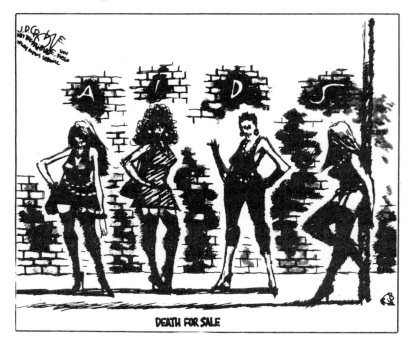

DEATH FOR SALE

proffering death. This shift—from male victim to female source of pollution—clearly repeats the history of the iconography of syphilis. A new group has now been labeled as the source of disease: women, but not all women, only those considered to be outside the limits of social respectability. Even while acknowledging heterosexual transmission, the attempt is made to maintain clear and definite boundaries so as to limit the public's anxiety about their own potential risk.

It is evident that the study of the verbal and visual images of its sufferers reveals many of the contradictions in our understanding of a disease. With society's attempt to categorize and limit AIDS still in its first decade, the construction of the image of the person with AIDS can already be seen both to parallel and to deviate from earlier models. While the powerful iconography of the sexually transmitted disease haunts our understanding of AIDS, other images, such as those of depression, have also entered into the construction of the image of the PWA, as it did in the image of the syphilitic. With the representation of AIDS, as with other diseases, it is the historically determined variations that mark the function and place of the sufferer in relationship to the society in which he or she dwells. Through their study, we can begin to understand how such models of disease evoke the most deep-seated sense of the self's fragility. The construction of various boundaries of disease, of images of the patient as the container and transmitter of the disease, depends on our sense of our own mortality and our consequent desire to distance and isolate those we designate as ill. Those suffering from the very diseases about which such fantasies are spun are themselves not immune to these representations; they respond to the isolation and stigmatization that is the social boundary of their disease, not part of the disease itself. It is in the world of representations that we manage our fear of disease, isolating it as surely as if we had placed it in quarantine. But within such isolation, these icons remain visible to all of us, proof that we are still whole, healthy, and sane; that we are not different, diseased, or mad.

Stuart Marshall. Bright Eyes, *Part I. 1984.*

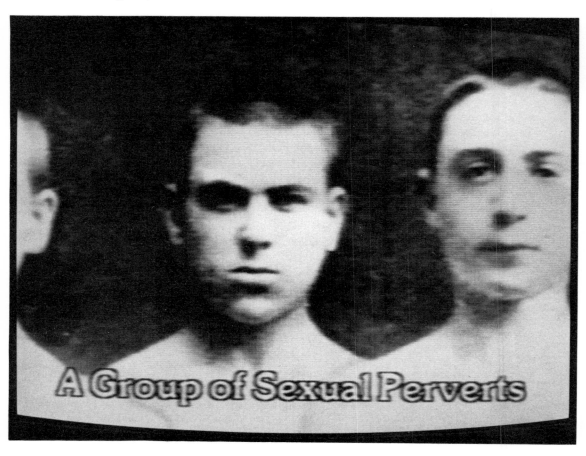

Pictures of Sickness:
Stuart Marshall's *Bright Eyes**

MARTHA GEVER

> *Female doctor: "Are some symptoms easier to see than others?"*
> *Male doctor: "Yes, I think that they are."*
> *Female doctor: "Which symptoms do you think are the most easily seen?"*
> *Male doctor: "Those that we recognize, those that are familiar to us, those that we've seen before."*
> *Female doctor: "Are they always self-evident?"*
> *Male doctor: "Sometimes a symptom is invisible, which means that it must be aggressively hunted out. Sometimes it is visible and we do not see it. . . ."*
>
> —*Bright Eyes,* Part One

It isn't necessary to read every word published or to watch television regularly to know that mass-media coverage of AIDS usually takes the form of news of "medical breakthroughs" and government pronouncements, statistics offered by "experts," or discussions of the "social impact" of the epidemic (for the latter, projections of health care costs and the economic effect on the insurance industry are common). The only notable exception is coverage of celebrities with AIDS, beginning with Rock Hudson. Aside from news reporting, television's attention to AIDS is generally limited to "social problem" programs. Whether documentary or dramatic in format, these latter are usually described

* I would like to thank the friends who discussed *Bright Eyes* with me or who generously read earlier versions of this essay, or both, and offered many provocative, useful suggestions: Terri Cafaro, Douglas Crimp, Rosalyn Deutsche, Carlos Espinosa, Tim Landers, Ernie Larsen, and Eileen O'Neill.

as sensitive, poignant, or tragic — adjectives that indicate not the seriousness of AIDS but rather the presumptions such programs carry in the first place. It is, of course, predictable that television producers and programmers would rely on conventional forms to publicize a major health crisis. The containment of knowledge about AIDS within familiar structures functions as reassurance for those worried about a "disease" that seems out of control.

Each news story, investigative report, panel discussion, talk show, or "realistic" drama about AIDS circulated by the mass media contributes to the shape of the narrative by which the epidemic is made comprehensible to "the public." And the impetus of this narrative is fear — a generalized fear that is alternately incited and allayed, again and again. (Picking up a newspaper, I read the headline, "AIDS Virus: Always Fatal?" The article proposes no answer to this question. In the meantime a TV newscaster promises, "Tonight at eleven: a new vaccine against the AIDS virus that scientists are ready to test.") Although scenarios painted with fear and propagated by the mass media are common devices used by public officials to promote support for their policies, which depend on such sentiments as a xenophobia and anticommunism, the manipulation of the fear of AIDS is of another order.[1] Unlike the typical crises proclaimed in the media — the "Middle East crisis," "the Sandinistas' threat to our national security," or, on the domestic front, the "drug crisis" — the AIDS crisis is not the invention of policymakers. Indeed, it is the *absence* of public policy concerning AIDS that has determined responses to the epidemic and has left the mass media to its own devices.[2] And what the mass media has produced reveals its complicity in constructing the very fears it presumes judiciously to mediate. From the beginning, when it was announced that AIDS was a syndrome that primarily affected gay men, the full machinery of homophobia — a particular sexual fear characterized by denial — went into action.

Almost every social crisis induced or supported by the mass media — teenage pregnancy or the disintegration of the family, for example — relies at least in part on a moral argument. But the battleground upon which the "war on AIDS"[3] is waged is morality itself. In the US, morality has become the rallying

1.   When early reports of AIDS in the US linked the syndrome with Haitian immigrants, however, the mass-media presentation of this information was redolent with the racism characteristic of our immigration policies.
2.   As has been well documented in the gay press, the mainstream press and television practically ignored AIDS for several years after the syndrome was first discovered in the US, and there is continuing censorship of news critical of the inertia of government and medical institutions — again regularly reported in the gay press.
3.   President Reagan and most of his appointed officials have repeatedly delayed and at times obstructed funding measures for research, medical care, and social services for PWAs since the epidemic began. Now, however, the Reagan Administration has adopted the rhetoric of warfare in issuing announcements about its concern for public health. In spite of this fact, continuing in the tradition of activism in the US, some AIDS activists also favor military metaphors, conflating militarism with militancy and, unfortunately, reinforcing the war-mongering mentality that pervades

cry for conservatives, who berate the media for undermining the established order of patriarchy and capitalism and accuse the public affairs departments of television stations and networks of being incorrigibly liberal and amoral.[4] But the reticence concerning sexual matters evident in reporting on AIDS confirms that in news, as in entertainment, the television industry adheres to restricted, normalizing standards of morality, even when advocating tolerance of those whose "sexual orientation" is "different." That the decision to permit advertising condoms on TV was, and still is, considered morally questionable by many industry executives, whose business nevertheless depends on sexual come-ons to sell other products, reveals both the limits and the contradictions of their liberal postures. Even the national Public Broadcasting Service (PBS), which pretends to take greater risks in programming, has taken up the topic of AIDS only gingerly.[5]

PBS first broached the subject in a 1985 broadcast of an intensely homophobic, racist, and inflammatory documentary in their *Frontline* series. Purportedly a profile of a man with AIDS, Fabian Bridges, *AIDS: A Public Inquiry* portrayed an unemployed black, gay protagonist as a dangerous criminal irresponsibly roaming the country and engaging in sex with unsuspecting victims. The *Frontline* producers tracked the man down, pretended to befriend him in order to elicit personal information, then turned him in to the health authorities after they got their footage. As one of the first prime-time productions about AIDS in the US, with the imprimatur of public television further validated by documentary veracity, the program confirmed the most irrational, rabid fears of the promiscuous homosexual threatening public health.

Subsequently, PBS aired a segment of the science series *Nova* devoted to AIDS, featuring a pantheon of scientists and computerized animations of viruses and blood cells. The discussion focused on the methods being used to develop drugs that might alleviate, if not cure AIDS, and the likelihood of a vaccine against the HIV virus. Nothing was said, however, about the US government's

---

our culture. Other AIDS activists, however, have criticized the use of military analogies. For example, Maxine Wolfe, a member of ACT UP, spoke out eloquently against the horrifying analogy in a proposed Human Rights Campaign Fund petition that would have called for a "Manhattan Project on AIDS." The petition ultimately called for an "emergency life-saving project."

4.   The most prominent to hold this position have been Presidents Nixon and Reagan and their henchmen. But its most consistent proponent is *New York Times* television critic John Corry, who has repeatedly insinuated this line into his regular reviews of political programs on network and public television. In a booklet published by the right-wing Media Institute, Corry outlines his critique of what he calls "the dominant culture," ruled by left-leaning journalists, lamenting, "The old consensus morality has disappeared. Once it was understood that the United States was generally right and its enemies generally wrong" (John Corry, *TV News and the Dominant Culture*, Washington, D.C., The Media Institute, 1986, p. 25).

5.   The public television system is composed of autonomous stations, however, and some of these—notably KQED in San Francisco and WNET and WNYC in New York City—have regularly aired, and sometimes produced, programs on AIDS.

reluctance to fund such research, to speed treatment drugs through the FDA approval process, or their insistence on the cruel use of double-blind testing procedures for people with a fatal disease. The drug featured in the program was AZT, the only drug to have achieved government approval; again *NOVA* failed to raise the relevant questions about the relationship between the FDA and Burroughs-Wellcome, AZT's manufacturer: Why was this highly toxic drug rushed through the process when no others were? Why was the company allowed to charge up to $13,000 per year for each patient? Why were ninety-eight percent of the patients in the studies conducted by the government's designated AIDS Treatment Evaluation Units being given AZT, even after this drug was available on the market?

In 1986 PBS aired *The A.I.D.S. Show*, a documentary by Peter Adair and Robert Epstein based on a gay theater review staged by San Francisco's Theatre Rhinoceros. Because the theater production and the tape feature a number of gay characters — men with AIDS, their lovers and friends — this broadcast represented a departure from the commercial networks' offerings, which only show visibly debilitated, pathetically ill gay men and other PWAs. *The A.I.D.S. Show*'s emphasis on coping with death, however, replaces homophobic responses to AIDS with exemplary tales of personal suffering and strength.

And finally, last fall, with great fanfare, and with warnings to parents that they might want to exercise "discretion," PBS broadcast a special program, entitled *AIDS: Changing the Rules,* on safe sex practices for heterosexuals. Introduced with the punning promise of "straight talk" on AIDS, the program is exactly the opposite. It begins with the assumption that gay people have already learned about safe sex (from PBS?) and repeatedly asserts that "heterosexuals haven't really been at risk until now," with no apparent awareness of the smugness and naiveté of this insupportable statement. Because the program's agenda only includes advice for those deemed respectable, responsible citizens — that is, straight adults — the fluidity of sexual desire is not even considered a possibility. Fear of sex determines even "straight talk" about it: When Rubén Blades demonstrates the proper use of a condom by putting one on a banana — "I sure wish there were an easier way of showing you this" — he explains coyly, "Leave a little slack at the end, you know, for what 'comes' [wink] later." And when Beverly Johnson speaks with obvious embarrassment about oral sex, she says, "When a man goes down on a woman, there's some danger, especially if a woman is menstruating. Unfortunately there's not much you can do to protect yourself." Is it really possible that the makers of a safe sex video are unaware of the availability of dental dams to provide just such protection?

And that, to date, is as much as PBS has been willing or has dared to show, despite the fact that AIDS has been known to be a major public health problem in the US for *over six years.*

*

> *In traveling from the known world to the unknown world, the seeker of truth will encounter many strange phenomena as yet unclassified by science, and upon his shoulders rests the responsibility of discovering order within this chaos. The light of scientific knowledge must be brought to play upon the twilight world of nature and the exotic species which inhabit its dark corners. Our guiding law must be the classification and categorization of all that is yet unknown, in order that the truth of human society be thrown sharply into relief.*
>
> —*Bright Eyes*, Part Two

Until my first viewing of Stuart Marshall's videotape *Bright Eyes*, I had intentionally avoided much of the mass-media coverage of AIDS, whether that of the lurid tabloid press or of respectable public television. Like most people, I am prone to anxiety about illness that no amount of scientific explanation can ease. And what I saw on television or read in the mass press either attempted precisely that—to pacify me with scientific data—or conveyed a picture of collective panic manifesting itself in overt, vicious homophobia, leaving me with feelings of both outrage and depression and affirming my impulse to steer clear. Nor have I revised my assessment of what the mass media will allow in its coverage of AIDS. But my willful avoidance was mitigated by Marshall's tape, not simply because it offers an intelligent political and historical analysis of the underpinnings of the current discourse on AIDS, but because the tape was conceived to contest the homophobia that has permeated the dominant media's representation of AIDS.

Bright Eyes was produced for Britain's Channel Four, a commercial broadcast channel founded in 1979 by an act of Parliament with provisions for funding and programming innovative television.[6] Marshall's video was broadcast in December 1984 in *The Eleventh Hour* series, a showcase for independent work whose title refers to its late-night time slot. Despite the fact that it received high ratings and repeated requests for a rebroadcast, Channel Four has thus far

---

6.   Though the grass on the other side of the Atlantic might seem greener, Channel Four has not always honored its obligations to gay audiences. They refused to air Caroline Sheldon's film *17 Rooms; or, What Do Lesbians Do in Bed?*, which had been slated for a 1986 gay and lesbian series. Their reluctance in this case had nothing to do with what the film shows—in fact, nothing explicitly sexual—but rather with anticipated objections to the film's title.

refused. Nevertheless, Channel Four has subsequently acquired and broadcast other work on AIDS, including the US production *Chuck Solomon: Coming of Age*, made by San Francisco filmmakers Marc Huestis and Wendy Dallas and turned down by PBS. After seeing the results of PBS's policies regarding programs on AIDS (as well as other topics deemed controversial), it seems reasonable to assume that PBS will never show *Bright Eyes*, or any other work that offers a serious critique of the association of AIDS and homosexuality. Thus far, Marshall's tape has been shown in this country only at closed-circuit screenings,[7] although the conditions of its original exhibition, as well as the source of production funds for *Bright Eyes*, place the tape within the boundaries of the mass media.

Marshall's consciousness of the terms operating in this arena becomes obvious in the first few minutes of *Bright Eyes*. The tape opens with the desultory exchange quoted here as the opening epigraph. The two doctors' conversation about diagnostic dilemmas is repeatedly interrupted by shots of an approaching ambulance — the sort of images that might appear in *St. Elsewhere* — and culminates in close-ups of an orderly wheeling a patient on a gurney through a hospital corridor and shouting, "Stand back! This man has AIDS! He's highly infectious! Stand back!" Staged with a high-pitched tension common to television drama, the lines are convincing — until the action stops abruptly and the words "Moral Panic Productions Presents" appear, followed by the program's title superimposed on a freeze-frame close-up of the faces of two anxious hospital workers wearing surgical masks. The orderly's fallacious statement is thus accentuated, and Marshall replaces the familiar but terrible specter of viral contagion with a reference to the infectious appeal of dramatic clichés.

When the action resumes, the hospital setting has disappeared, the tone of emergency evaporated. After a rapid montage of newspaper headlines composed of phrases such as "The Gay Plague," "Sex Killer Bug," and "Gay Bug," together with photos from a tabloid spread topped by a banner that reads "Pictures that Reveal the Disturbing Truth of AIDS Sickness," one of the doctors from the previous segment reappears, now dressed as a late nineteenth-century gentleman. As his speech indicates, he acts the part of another doctor, this time reading an article on the advantages of photography for medical study published in an 1893 issue of the British medical journal *The Lancet*.

In these short sequences, Marshall reveals his method. The rapid cuts from realistic melodrama to still images to the cool recitation of a historical text typifies the disjunctive technique used throughout. This functions to reframe and examine the meanings of myriad pictures signifying sickness and deviance, and, in the process, to demonstrate the historical construction of both. Three

---

7.   In 1987 *Bright Eyes* was included in exhibitions at the New Museum of Contemporary Art, the Museum of Modern Art, and the Kitchen in New York City; and in the programs of the San Francisco Lesbian and Gay Film Festival, the Los Angeles Lesbian and Gay Film and Video Festival, and the American Film Institute's National Video Festival in Los Angeles.

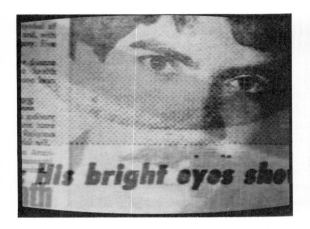
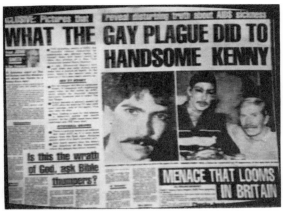

Stuart Marshall. Bright Eyes, *Part I. 1984.*

historical moments provide the basic structure of the three-part tape: the late nineteenth-century consolidation of scientific authority in rationalizing, classifying, and regulating social subjects; the Third Reich's conscription of eugenic theories to justify policies of persecution and genocide of members of undesirable social groups; and the present, in which the effects of definitions of sexual pathology are again evident in the general complacency about the cruel, dehumanizing treatment of people with AIDS. The movement of the tape, however, never follows the uninterrupted course of a simple chronological progression or logical academic argument. Rather, present and past mingle, mediated by television artifice, which is likewise the object of analysis.

The tape's title derives from one such telling instance of historical reverberation. Marshall intercuts an illustrated text from a late nineteenth-century sociological treatise with two photos of PWA Kenny Ramsaur from a spread in the British tabloid *Sunday People*. These latter are the photographs—"before and after"—said to "reveal the disturbing truth about AIDS sickness" by showing "what the gay plague did to handsome Kenny." An off-screen voice reads excerpts from Havelock Ellis's *The Criminal* detailing characteristics attributed to certain criminal types, including "sexual offenders," accompanied by caricatures and photographic studies from the same book. As Ellis is quoted saying, "In those guilty of sexual offences [Cesare] Lombroso finds the eyes nearly always bright," the image cuts to a close-up of Ramsaur's eyes in the "before AIDS" photo; the camera then pans to the caption: "Handsome Kenny: His bright eyes show no hint of the agony to come." On the sound track, Ellis's words continue: ". . . the voice either rough or cracked; the face generally delicate, except in the development of the jaws, and the eyelids and lips swollen." The photo of a healthy Ramsaur reappears and the camera pans again, stopping when the second photo of Ramsaur, his face swollen, fills the screen. Ellis again: "Occasionally they are humpbacked or otherwise deformed."

Marshall's presentation of the photos of Ramsaur in *Sunday People* demonstrates the continuation of a tradition where deviance—or nature's presumed punishment for it—is revealed as visible physical "deformity." The movement is easy, says an off-screen voice, since, "for more than a hundred years homosexuality has been described as a disease." Then, another picture from *The Criminal*, a photograph captioned "A Group of Perverts." Thus introduced, the young men posed together for this illustration become examples of the category of sexual offenders, a legal term employed by jurists and social scientists in the nineteenth century to describe, collectively, prostitutes, rapists, and homosexuals. Today, the classification *sexual offender* remains on the books, but now the three previously related types are legally separated. Prostitution remains an illegal (or state-regulated), although selectively prosecuted occupation;[8] rape is treated as a violent crime; and the offense of homosexuality is more a target for social disapprobation than grounds for imprisonment or internment in mental hospitals.[9] This latter observation may, however, soon be reversed, given currently intensified demands for mandatory HIV testing, contact tracing, and even tatooing or quarantining of HIV antibody positive individuals, many of whom are likely to be gay men. The persistence of attempts to link homosexuality and criminality are also confirmed in statements by homophobic politicians such as Jesse Helms and William Dannemeyer and pundits such as Nat Hentoff and Pete Hamill of the *Village Voice*.[10]

All such proposals and policies lean heavily on medical science, which

8.   It is no accident that, in the mass-media commentary on AIDS, the figure of the prostitute serves as the emblem of the pernicious female carrier of AIDS, the embodiment of threat to heterosexual men who are not IV drug users.
9.   The 1986 Supreme Court ruling in *Bowers v. Hardwick* upholding state laws prohibiting sodomy, however, appears to signal a reversal in the trend away from criminalizing homosexual acts that had prevailed in the late '70s and early '80s in the US.
10.   Helms's and Dannemeyer's antigay bigotry is legion, and their statements and actions concerning AIDS have surprised no one. Hentoff and Hamill, on the other hand, are established liberal columnists writing for one of the most widely read liberal publications in the country. Hamill's proposal that the law treat seropositive individuals who transmit the virus to others as murderers is only quantitatively more insidious than the positions held by Hentoff, who advocates the scientifically dubious practice of mandatory HIV testing and persistently differentiates between the "innocent" and "guilty victims" of AIDS. At the same time, Hentoff, the self-proclaimed champion of civil rights, seems utterly unconcerned with the persecution of those deemed "guilty" of AIDS, all gay men and black and Latino IV drug users. See Pete Hamill, "The Secret Sharers," *Village Voice*, June 23, 1987, p. 10; and Nat Hentoff, "AIDS: A Failure of Intelligence," *Village Voice*, June 23, 1987, p. 34; "The New Priesthood of Death," *Village Voice*, June 30, 1987, p. 35; "Playing Russian Roulette with AIDS," *Village Voice*, July 7, 1987, p. 37; and "The AIDS Debate: A Breakthrough," *Village Voice*, November 17, 1987, p. 38. Hentoff has directly aligned himself with such moral conservatives in the Reagan Administration as Secretary of Education William Bennett and Presidential Assistent Gary Bower in calling for mandatory testing.

performs an ideological function similar to that of Western legal discourse, conflating homosexuality, deviance, perversion, and sexual pathology with one another and with abnormality. Representations that claim to reproduce reality are used by doctors and lawyers alike to identify and classify physical phenomena, thus isolating the components that constitute disease — either individual or social — in the form of visible evidence. As Marshall demonstrates in the first section of *Bright Eyes*, the images of illness produced and reproduced within the larger project of empirical, instrumental science function as concrete proof. The utility of photography in this regard, precociously argued by the doctor-author of the *Lancet* text quoted at the outset of *Bright Eyes*, established the camera as an instrument of presumed objectivity.[11] Marshall tracks one of the historical ramifications of this concept in Part Two of the tape.

Again in reenactment, photographs and books fuel a bonfire in a fictionalized newsreel of the Nazis' destruction of the Institute for Sexual Science in Berlin in 1933. A woman's voice relates a first-person account of the event to the institute's founder, Magnus Hirshfeld, who is shown as the sole spectator in a theater in Paris where the pseudo-newsreel plays on the screen. At intervals, Hirshfeld narrates, with no apparent emotion, the political history of the homosexual rights movement in Germany dating back to 1897 — including his efforts to enlist support from the medical and psychological professions in affirming the legitimacy of homosexuality — and the various attacks he and his allies endured. Marshall renders the facts of Nazi brutality at a distance — in past tense — as projected images of burning photographs and books, a symbolic act of annihilation that stands for the systematic extermination of gay men during the Third Reich (lesbians were not routinely arrested for sexual crimes, since lesbianism was not acknowledged in German law).[12]

Central to this narrative is Hirshfeld's passionate faith in photographic and scientific objectivity — the institute's collection of material on anatomy and sexual theories and practices numbered some 12,000 books and 35,000 photographs — and the corresponding passion of the Nazis' manic hatred, mobilized as a eugenic purge of the German population. The scientific credo of the Enlightenment, to which Hirshfeld ardently subscribed and which he regarded as the foundation of a rational, tolerant society, was easily conscripted by Heinrich Himmler and the SS to provide them with ideological ammunition for their murderous campaign against gay men.[13]

11.   For a sustained discussion of instrumental uses of photography, see Allan Sekula, "The Body and the Archive," *October*, no. 39 (Winter 1986), pp. 3–64.
12.   For many years the history of Nazi persecutions of gay men was regularly ignored in literature about the Third Reich. One helpful corrective is Richard Plant, *The Pink Triangle: The Nazi War against Homosexuals*, New York, Henry Holt and Company, 1986. Much of the material Marshall relates in this regard is also chronicled in Plant's book.
13.   In his study of contemporary debates concerning sexuality and their precedents in the nine-

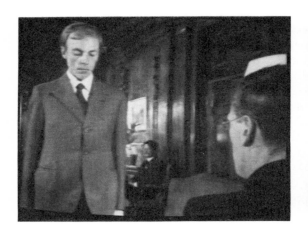 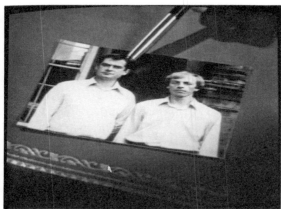

Stuart Marshall. Bright Eyes, *Part II. 1984.*

In the scene following the Hirshfeld story, a young man in Vienna is summoned to Gestapo headquarters, where he is shown a snapshot of himself and a friend, with an affectionate inscription on the back. This photograph is presented as evidence of his "unnatural" desires, sufficient proof to condemn him to a Nazi work camp. The horrifying details of gay men's experiences in these camps are reported, once again, retrospectively. The actor who played the sentenced man is now shown as a passenger in a car traveling on the autobahn in contemporary Germany. He has not aged, as the rules of historical realism would dictate, but nevertheless gives a first-person account of the conditions in the camps, where gay men were simultaneously starved and worked to death, or shot by SS guards who forced them to attempt escape. While he summarizes aspects of the little known and rarely acknowledged history of the Nazi persecutions of homosexuals, the woman driving the car periodically asks questions and interjects an equally disturbing story of two lesbians imprisoned and tortured by the SS. As an epilogue to this history lesson, Marshall contrasts shots of the overgrown, abandoned Nuremberg stadium, famous site of Nazi spectacles, with glimpses of the prosaic but well-maintained granite bridges traversing the autobahn. The male actor draws attention to what would otherwise pass unnoticed:

---

teenth century, Jeffrey Weeks quotes Hirshfeld: "I believe in Science, and I am convinced that Science, and above all the natural Sciences, must bring to mankind, not only truth, but with truth, Justice, Liberty and Peace" (quoted in Jeffrey Weeks, *Sexuality and Its Discontents: Meanings, Myths and Modern Sexualities*, London, Routledge and Kegan Paul, 1985, p. 71).

built by prisoners in the Nazi work camps, the labor required to quarry, trans-
port, and place the blocks for those bridges resulted in thousands of deaths.

The enactment of the inquest conducted by a Gestapo doctor, which concludes with the stunned young man signing a prepared confession, is performed
in an understated and cinematically spare style that is consistently used in the
tape. Instead of exploiting the conventional television techniques that render
rhetorical constructions invisible (the fast-paced editing, multiple camera angles,
and portentious music demonstrated in *Bright Eyes*'s opening sequence and then
abandoned), Marshall prolongs shots and silences, intercuts printed texts, and
frustrates identification by not revealing off-screen speakers and by casting the
same actors in different roles. For example, the actor who plays the condemned
gay man and the former concentration camp inmate in this second part of the
tape also played the modern doctor in the opening sequence and the nineteenth-
century physician-author immediately following. In the tape's third part, he will
play first a television talk-show host, then an undercover cop in a vignette
demonstrating British police practices used to entrap gay men for soliciting.[14]

The effect of these devices is that Marshall's analysis of the conflation of
truth with photographic imagery is extended to television's own forms of veristic
representation. At the beginning of the tape's third section, broadcast journalism's role in shaping perceptions of AIDS is underscored in a sketch in which a
TV crew prepares for an interview with a man with AIDS. A belligerent audio
technician afraid of "catching" AIDS refuses to place a microphone around the
neck of the talk-show guest, who realizes that his only option is to speak to the
interviewer on an off-stage telephone — in other words, to be invisible. Although
enacted according to the rules of realist drama, the characters and their situation
seem too exaggerated to be credible. But Marshall anticipates this response and
answers it with a close-up of a newspaper item about just such an event that
occurred on a TV program called *A.M. San Francisco*.

Bright Eyes's third and final part consists mostly of a series of interviews with
people whose work involves AIDS — John Weber, a doctor and AIDS researcher; Richard Wells, a nursing advisor who coauthored guidelines for the
care of people with AIDS; Tony Whitehead, chairperson of the Terrence Hig-
gins Trust, Britain's first AIDS education and service organization — as well as
Nick Billingham of the Campaign for Homosexual Equality, and Linda Semple,
manager of Gay's the Word bookstore in London. Never cross-cut, this sequence
of interviews moves from Weber's calm commentary on misunderstandings
about AIDS to broader, though related cultural and political issues discussed by
Billingham and Semple. Each speaker is shot from a single angle and edited
sparingly. Though an interviewer's voice occasionally intercedes, the interviewer

---

14.   This is a device Marshall rigorously employs in his earlier tapes that deal with characterization
and the construction of representations, such as *The Love Show* and *A Question of Three Sets of
Characteristics*, both 1980.

himself never appears. The absence of cut-aways is somewhat unconventional, but otherwise this section of the tape conforms to recognizable television documentary form, or so it would seem if this material were divorced from everything that precedes it. But what these people say — together with the speech by People with AIDS Coalition cofounder Michael Callen at the tape's conclusion — has everything to do with what has come before. When Semple describes a raid by British customs officials on her bookstore and the subsequent confiscation of all imported materials, including those on AIDS, the interviewer asks, "Do you know what will happen to the confiscated books?" "They'll be burned," she replies, "Books that are confiscated are always burned."

The discussions with all six subjects abound with current examples of the relationship between forms of representation and ideas of deviance examined earlier. Weber, Wells, and Whitehead all confirm the influence of the mass media on public responses to AIDS, citing instances in which sensationalizing reports in the media created waves of paranoia and resulted in surges of telephone inquiries from people who believed, incorrectly, that they had contracted AIDS and therefore suffered morbid anxieties. Whitehead notes that, to the mass media, a gay person with AIDS is "not a story," and that gay people are seen as the cause or perpetrators of AIDS, whereas straight people with AIDS are frequently portrayed as innocent victims.

Callen's statement, a recitation of his testimony before a New York State legislative committee in 1983, serves as a counterpoint to the representations of disease in the first section of the tape. His passionate, detailed, and well-argued description of the experiences of PWAs ends with an eloquent (though now outdated) account of knowledge about AIDS and the responsibilities of medical and government institutions, not only in preventing AIDS but toward those who have been diagnosed with AIDS and ARC. Here, at last, a man with AIDS speaks for himself. But even here speech and image are not presented as unmediated, transparent truth. Although his address was originally conceived for a public forum, Callen appears in *Bright Eyes* against the background of an unpopulated, bucolic London garden. The scene is not constructed to feign spontaneity, and no effort is made to disguise the fact that Callen is reading a text. The camera remains fixed, and the edits are few, although at each edit the camera moves several steps closer. The emotional strength of Callen's testimony consists not in pathos but in his direct, careful, unapologetic language and delivery, which contradicts all concepts of an object of medical curiosity or a pitiable victim of disease.

*

> *I went to see this National Health psychia-*
> *trist. . . . I was quite taken aback when he*
> *said something which didn't seem to have*
> *anything to do with me whatsoever, which*
> *was, "When you are older you will start*
> *hanging around public toilets. Do you want*
> *this?" I was totally shocked. I thought,*
> *"What's he talking about? He's nuts."*
>
> —*Bright Eyes*, Part One

I've strayed from the subject of fear—specifically, homophobia and its relationship to disease. This is in part because fear is *not* invoked in *Bright Eyes*. On the contrary, analysis of the pathology of fear and its manipulation are fundamental to the tape. Instead of counseling the imagined audience to correct irrational fears by following the advice of designated experts—the favored "solution" in the mass media's approach to AIDS—*Bright Eyes* encourages a recognition of fear's results—hatred of and discrimination against those classified as abnormal and therefore degenerate or dangerous or both—and the complicity of systems of expertise in establishing the authority of such categories in the first place.

Having reviewed the structure of Marshall's analysis of representations of disease and deviance, I want now to retrace my steps in order to discuss the less overt emotional content of the tape, which contradicts and exposes the insidious and oppressive links between mechanisms of identification and the narrative gambit of provoking anxiety and then providing psychic satisfaction through its resolution. For example, by thwarting identification with actors and thus abjuring a central tactic of emotional manipulation, Marshall dissociates the language of anxiety from the personal attributes and actions of characters and shows it to exist instead on the plane of political relations. The final scene of Part One, in which the speech quoted above appears, makes this clear.

The sequence of pictures of "abnormal" individuals—Ellis's "criminals" juxtaposed with the *Sunday People* photos of Ramsaur—immediately precedes an obviously contrived interview with a man whose face is obscured in shadow, the sort of disguise used in television interviews to conceal the identities of informants or criminals fearful of discovery. An apparently middle-aged man tells about coming out when he was eighteen years old—of an early memory of his mother's denigrating comment about a gay man in a TV drama, his father's dismay when his son tells him he loves a man, his visit to a psychiatrist who offers to cure him, and his recognition that he doesn't want to be cured because he is happy. He recalls telling the psychiatrist that he made the decision to refuse treatment because he understood, "The problem's not mine; it's my father's." In the annals of gay social history, similar accounts have often been reproduced as stories of courage in the face of oppressive scientific attitudes toward homosexuality, which often condoned torture in the name of therapy (the man accurately notes that the prescribed treatment for homosexuality twenty years ago was electric shock "therapy"). The scene works as an addendum to the cross-cutting of nineteenth-century taxonomies of unnatural bodies with present-day depictions of sick homosexuals. The ambiguous lighting not only invokes television styles used to ensure anonymity, but also suggests a correlation with other texts in the tape, especially one spoken as a commentary on a nineteenth-century painting, Sir Luke Fildes's *The Doctor*:

> A Victorian country doctor sits in the darkness of a worker's cottage trying to get a picture of a sick child's condition. . . . Night has begun to fall and he has angled the shade of the oil lamp to see more clearly. Light and dark, doctors and disease. The beam of lamplight pierces the darkness of the cottage, and the doctor's gaze pierces the darkness of her illness. . . . Someone else, possibly the child's father, is also watching from a dark corner, but, unlike the sick child, this person is not the object of medical surveillance, and so the beam of lamplight is not angled in his direction and he barely becomes a picture.

"Light and dark, doctors and disease." This elliptical sentence establishes the axes along which the discourse of homosexuality travels. Occurring at the approximate center of the tape's first part, the sentence refers to an earlier observation concerning the mass media's reportage on gay subjects. This activity, Marshall notes, often entails a visit to a "shadowy back street bar" and is couched in expressions such as the "smoky gloom" of such hideaways, emblematic of the "twilight world" of gay culture. Such reports are reminiscent of those written by explorers of foreign lands, addressed to readers of the same class, race, and culture as the writer—in this case, those who have never frequented gay bars. Analogously, the man hovering in the shadows of the Fildes canvas, outside the doctor's lamplight, remains mysterious and vaguely ominous.

The light/dark dichotomy is recapitulated in the opening scene of Part Two, which consists of a parody of nineteenth-century empiricist prose, earnestly but ironically recited by a black actor. Appearing among the potted palms and stuffed peacocks of a room decorated in the Orientalist style, speaking in a deadpan manner that downplays the text's racist overtones, the actor outlines the scientific excuse for imperialism: the "classification and categorization of all that is unknown," bringing "the light of scientific knowledge . . . to play upon the twilight world of nature and the exotic species which inhabit its dark corners."

In the sequence prior to the interview with the obscured gay man, there is a short interlude consisting of a few uncaptioned portraits of men. A voice-over considers the effects of being designated an object of "the light of scientific knowledge," or, alternately, of voluntarily emerging from the shadows:

> Every image of a gay man is in danger of becoming two pictures of a homosexual. When his image is just a depiction of a man, then he remains an individual. When he is identified as a homosexual, then he becomes a member of an exotic species and a case history of a pathological sickness.

The half-lit face of the gay man recounting his own history similarly presents two pictures, but not the same two: a picture of an unidentified man — neither exotic specimen nor visible case history — and the shadowy figure that troubles the image of heterosexual normality by refusing to "become a picture." But he also becomes a nearly literal representation of those "denizens of the twilight world of homosexuality," thereby placing himself on the negative side of the hierarchical terms of Enlightenment ideology — associations of light with order and dark with chaos, light with civilization and dark with nature. His ambiguous presence and the content of the interview represent a complex of historical conditions and relations. He is a man who was able to follow his own desires despite his parents' disapproval, but he did so within a set of predetermined social coordinates that relegate him to a shadowy existence. Nevertheless, he raises the question of who is really "nuts" — the "pervert," the doctor offering a "cure," or the father — and thus his story carries radical social meaning.

The positivist equation of visibility — pictures — with truth is disrupted by this man's refusal to accept an identity defined as abnormal, as is the assertion of the political neutrality of representations. Magnus Hirshfeld assembled his photographic archive in the same positivist spirit as Cesare Lombroso and Havelock Ellis, collecting photographic records to establish the visibility — and thus the viability — of a social group, what Hirshfeld called an intermediate or third sex. Although it was not his belief in rational science that made him a target of the Nazis, but rather his untiring political organizing on behalf of full civil rights for gay men and lesbians (as well as for all women and for illegitimate children), Hirshfeld misunderstood the ideological malleability of representations, their uses in systems of thought, systems of social ordering. It is that malleability of meaning that Marshall makes evident.

A detail of the concluding interviews in the third part of the tape, where Marshall appears to abandon the complex constructions of the previous sections, also implies a subtle but important comparison involving the ideological function of images. Each speaker is captioned, labeled with superimposed words indicating each one's name and occupation and/or place of work. These bits of information appear to be nothing more than the standard means of identification used in television or film documentaries, but here they must also be considered in relation to the labels applied to the only other captioned pictures in the tape: the photographed deviants: "a moral imbecile," "an hysteric," "an intermediate type," and the "group of perverts." The labels accompanying these photographs indicate their subjects' status as unsocialized, abnormal people whose bodies are

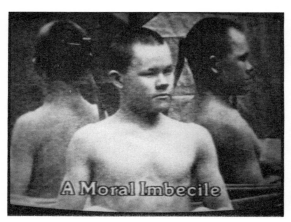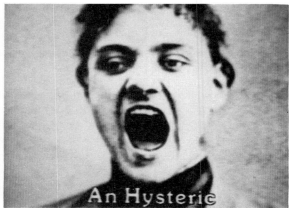

Stuart Marshall. Bright Eyes, *Part I. 1984.*

made to exhibit symptoms of degeneracy. The textual information provided about the people who speak in "Part Three" is, by contrast, specific to each subject; the categories of identification are associated with social integration.

The nameless and practically faceless gay man at the end of Part One serves as a kind of mediator between these two groups. His speech indicates his understanding of his father's homophobia and his doctor's normalizing mission. But his anonymity bespeaks the impossibility, if he is *seen* as representative, of escaping the tyranny of being classified as a homosexual.[15] By the time Weber, Wells, and the others appear, Marshall has reversed the question of identity, away from abnormal, perhaps exotic, and disruptive sexual identities toward the self-identification of gay men and lesbians who understand the mechanisms of oppressive power and work to defeat them. Callen's speech extends this contradiction to people with AIDS, refuting the stereotype of AIDS "victim" Kenny Ramsaur, the grotesque product of insidious viruses and unnatural sexual practices, whose portrait is meant to serve as an icon of moral decay.

When the reigning ideology is subjected to scrutiny, as it is in *Bright Eyes*, the emotional constructions that it engenders and feeds upon lose their force. The photos of Kenny Ramsaur, for example, inspire neither horror nor pity, nor

15.   Similarly, Adrienne Rich objects to the word *lesbianism*, because, she writes, it "has a clinical and limiting ring." See her influential essay "Compulsory Heterosexuality and Lesbian Existence," *Signs*, vol. 5, no. 4 (1980). Gay male writers such as Simon Watney have similarly insisted on the word *gay* rather than *homosexual* in order to counteract the oppressive medical connotations of the latter term.

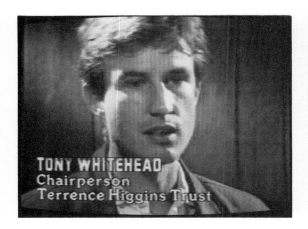 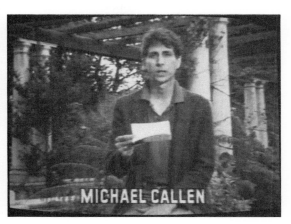

Stuart Marshall. Bright Eyes, *Part III. 1984.*

can they any longer be seen as proof of this man's inherent decadence. They signify instead only a rhetorical ploy devised by *Sunday People*'s editors. Probably naively, these media workers follow the dictates of scientific theology, taking pictures to "reveal . . . truth" about "sick homosexuals," in the tradition of the scientific objectivity that they claim to uphold. For science, and for those who subscribe to its power, AIDS represents social chaos that only rationalization can put in order. But those systems of rationalization are already in place, complete with their mania for classification and categorization and their ideological utility for opportunistic politicians, as well as for the mass media that makes those politicians authoritative public figures.

I do not wish to prescribe *Bright Eyes*, or any single work or action, as *the* sobering antidote to the effects of the institutions and instruments of social control. Nor will the tape be found "inspirational" in the sense of those works that attempt to counter stereotypes with stories of heroic role models. But the means Marshall employs to expose the relationships between the mass media, scientific systems of classification, and definitions of pathology suggest an important direction for sexual politics, a politics articulated in *Bright Eyes* by various representatives of gay institutions. These are gay men and lesbians who have initiated programs for AIDS education and advocacy for PWAs, who guarantee the availability of literature on gay subjects, and who promote political awareness about and organize resistance to official discrimination and antigay violence. Their participation in *Bright Eyes*, separately and collectively, does not constitute a plea for social acceptance, but rather proposes an outspoken, unequivocal assertion of the processes of self-identification that Marshall recognizes and represents. As their various contributions demonstrate, these identities are neither abstract, absolute, nor limited to individual integrity, but shaped through active engagement in social relations. Just as AIDS has sanctioned expressions of homophobia and revived supposedly outmoded methods for controlling sexuality, the conflation of AIDS with homosexuality has clarified political positions for many gay men and lesbians. And just as AIDS has confirmed and even escalated the hostility of the mass media toward lesbians and gay men, an extended critique of the mass media has become central to gay political work. *Bright Eyes* is a part of that work.

AMBER HOLLIBAUGH,
MITCHELL KARP,
and KATY TAYLOR

interviewed by DOUGLAS CRIMP

The AIDS Discrimination Unit of the New York City Commission on Human Rights was established in 1983 to document and respond to complaints of AIDS-related discrimination. It now has a full-time staff of sixteen, aided by several interns. In addition to handling individual complaints of discrimination through advocacy and litigation, the commission initiates complaints in cases of widespread systemic discrimination, issues reports on varying forms of discrimination, produces educational materials on AIDS and AIDS-related discrimination, and trains other agencies and groups to respond to discrimination issues. The Human Rights Law of New York City prohibits discrimination in areas of housing, employment, and public accommodation on the basis of an individual's handicap or disability. Thus the commission accepts complaints from and offers assistance to:

— People with AIDS
— People with ARC (AIDS-Related Complex)
— Those who have tested HIV antibody positive
— Members of groups perceived to be at risk for AIDS
— Family members, coworkers, lovers, and/or friends of someone in the above categories who believe they have been discriminated against because of their association with this individual.

*

Crimp: How did the AIDS Discrimination Unit come to be formed?

Taylor: The first AIDS-related complaint came to the Human Rights Commission in mid-'83. The case was that of an Hispanic grandmother unable to find a funeral home to bury her daughter, who had died of AIDS. Keith O'Connor, a gay man who had worked at the commission for many years and was at the time director of the unit dealing with patterns of discrimination, simply helped to find a funeral home willing to provide burial services.

It had already become obvious in 1983 that AIDS-related discrimination was a very real problem. Groups such as the Lambda Legal Defense Fund were raising the issue from outside the commission, and Keith was pushing from inside to get the commission to take an active role in responding to the backlash unleashed by AIDS. The administration was supportive, but as usual there was a problem of money and staff, so Keith simply handled the AIDS-related cases on top of all the other work he was doing. When Keith hired me, I found myself with a caseload that was almost entirely AIDS-related. In those days we did a lot of what I call "cowboy advocacy"—like the Wild West, it was all new territory, there were no rules, so you figured it out as you went along. For example, if someone called and said, "I can't find a place that will bury my child," you couldn't say, "Come in and file a complaint and we'll do an investigation and take it to a hearing."

The administration of the commission realized right away that our usual process wouldn't work, so the AIDS Discrimination Unit was set up to expedite these problems. It was decided to use advocacy, up-front problem-solving, as the first form of intervention. But documentation has also been a crucial aspect of our approach. Since there has been so much confusion about, and denial of, the impact of discrimination, it was necessary to prove that widespread discrimination existed both against people with AIDS and people associated with them— caretakers, family members, friends, coworkers—or people perceived to be members of groups at higher risk of HIV infection, such as gay men. From the beginning we knew that the hardest hit communities were where we had to start building our networks. At that time AIDS was still seen largely as a "gay disease," but our caseload reflected the actual diversity of people struck by the disease, and by discrimination.

There was an interesting development that came about because of our early work. Because the commission was visibly dealing with AIDS, we got a lot of calls from healthy gay men and lesbians who were encountering both antigay and AIDS-related discrimination—being fired from their jobs, thrown out of their homes, called "queers" and "AIDS carriers"—simply because they were gay or, as is also the case, because they were *perceived* to be gay. At that time there was no protection against discrimination based on sexual orientation (except for an executive order protecting city employees), but we could sometimes take on these problems as perceived disability cases. Ironically AIDS, an illness mistaken as gay-related, became the basis for finally affording gay people some civil rights protection.

At the same time, we received a steady stream of old-fashioned, garden-variety sexual-orientation discrimination reports, about which there was nothing we could formally do. Wherever possible we tried to help out, and at the very least we could document those incidents. We knew that AIDS had triggered an antigay backlash, so we began a Lesbian and Gay Discrimination Documentation Project. Over a two-year period we received nearly 500 complaints, and this documented discrimination was instrumental in finally getting the gay rights law passed in 1986.

Crimp: As I understand it, people with AIDS in New York City are legally protected from discrimination on the basis of disability and, where applicable, sexual orientation. But how do these laws protect people who are neither disabled nor gay, but are simply *perceived* to have AIDS.

Karp: Courts in other states have ruled that even though a statute might not use the words "perceived disability," the law would be rendered meaningless if it could only be applied to people who were actually disabled. What the law attempts to rectify is differential treatment based on someone else's assumptions. The disability laws here go back to the '70s, so we already had jurisdiction; the question was only whether or not AIDS would be treated as a disability. We decided at the commission to take a very broad view of the law. Last year, in a case involving a teacher with tuberculosis, the US Supreme Court held that a contagious disease could be construed as a physical disability as that term is defined in law. AIDS, of course, is not contagious but infectious, which makes it even more obvious that it should be construed as a disability.

Hollibaugh: Because there is such terror about transmission, and because there's a crisis of information about AIDS, discrimination based on misperception is one of the major problems we deal with.

Karp: The media continues to refer to the "AIDS test" and the "AIDS virus," so how can people be expected to make the distinction between AIDS and HIV seropositivity? In our job we have to deal with the ripple effect of constant misstatements in the media and by public officials.

A telling thing has happened with AIDS discrimination. We've taken complaints against funeral homes for years on the basis of racial and religious discrimination, and it was automatically assumed that we should handle those complaints. But when we took an AIDS-related complaint against a funeral home, suddenly our jurisdiction was challenged.

Crimp: Hasn't accurate AIDS information—in spite of continuing misinformation—begun to have an effect?

Karp: In some respects it definitely has. Over the past year, we've had calls from lawyers for employers, personnel directors, and union presidents, saying they want to anticipate problems and develop AIDS policies. So there's work being done to educate people, to formulate rational policies before problems arise. But this exists side by side with the most blatant displays of ignorance. And as the number of sick people continues to climb, the social impact is reaching further and further into previously untouched areas.

Hollibaugh: Mitchell and I do a lot of public speaking on AIDS, and much of mine is about transmission. I find that people have very wild fantasies about how you can come into contact with the virus. What I think this reflects is, first, extreme distrust of the government—"Why should we trust the government on this one when we know they lie to us about other things?" And second, it takes time for people really to learn about transmission. Education is a process; it's not a single brochure, a single PTA meeting with health officials. Our work consists of repeating this information in as many believable forms as possible, and allowing people to work through their resistance, work out their fears, not only of transmission, but of illness generally, of drugs, of sex, of death. Most people are extremely isolated in their attempts to deal with this crisis. No one in our culture has faced an epidemic of this sort. And epidemics have not previously been attached to such forbidden kinds of behavior as gay sexuality and IV drug use.

Crimp: Obviously education is the best means of fighting discrimination, but it hadn't occurred to me that this would be such a major focus of the unit. I had assumed you were mostly involved with narrow legal issues. What is your mandate?

Karp: Our mandate under the Human Rights Code is to prevent and eliminate discrimination, and we don't take a passive approach. For example, we sued a number of funeral homes for discrimination, hoping to use it as an educational tool for the funeral industry, and indeed we wound up speaking to 200 funeral-home directors about the issue. We also do large mailings. We sent out thousands of copies of our report *AIDS and People of Color: The Discriminatory Impact*, which condensed what had been only anecdotal information into an authoritative document that could be cited by others. We also ask to be invited to speak to large groups, especially those involved in policy planning. We work in conjunction with the AIDS Education Unit of the City Health Department. They do basic transmission education, and Amber, Katy, and I discuss the social ramifications of the epidemic, trying to put the social questions on an equal footing with medical questions.

Taylor: For most people, human rights are an afterthought, and that's what we want to change. Our position is that not only is there no conflict between public health and civil rights, but effective public health policy *depends* on civil rights. If you look at diseases in the US such as malaria and small pox, which have been virtually eliminated, as against sexually transmitted diseases, which are currently on the increase, you can see that social stigma undermines, even confounds, our best public health efforts.

Crimp: What are some of the discrimination issues that affect specific constituencies?

Karp: At the outset it should be said that currently fifty-five percent of people with AIDS in New York City are people of color, and the majority of requests for intervention by the unit come from blacks and Hispanics. But not surprisingly, the people comfortable with using the *formal* process, with using the legal system, are primarily white and middle-class. People who come to us with cases of employment discrimination, for example, are often those who have prior expectations of fair treatment. People in marginal kinds of employment — undocumented workers, let's say — are already so used to being treated prejudicially that AIDS-related discrimination doesn't feel very different to them. But in public accommodations cases, all types of people come to us. In fact, the poorer you are, the more likely you are to be subjected to economic discrimination in these areas: "If you want this person buried, you'll need a glass cover — $500 — and a steel coffin — $1,500." When you don't have money for a taxi, you have to rely on ambulances, which either won't come or, when they do come, the paramedics arrive fully outfitted in space suits, which alerts the entire neighborhood to the fact that you have AIDS. Or, a landlord with no particular bias about AIDS can use AIDS or HIV positivity as an opportunity to vacate a rent-controlled apartment.

Taylor: We've always recognized that the people we most wanted to reach were the most disenfranchised, people for whom government had long been the enemy — gay people, Haitians . . . And that shaped our initial focus on systemic discrimination, on agency-initiated complaints, which have the widest ameliorative effect on discrimination generally and thus reach people who would never come to a human rights agency.

Crimp: When you speak of systemic discrimination, I assume you're speaking of, let's say, industry-wide discrimination in the insurance business. But truly systemic discrimination is not simply the desire of the insurance companies to discriminate against people with AIDS or people perceived to be at risk for AIDS, but is entirely endemic to the system of medical insurance that exists in the US, or to our health care system. Because these are private, profit-making industries, there are built-in inequities according to income. Is there any way that you can address such discrimination?

Hollibaugh: All of us are well aware of contradictions. We're not naive about how deep discrimination runs in this society. But we feel that at least the contradictions can be mediated and that we can be involved in changing the attitudes that keep the systems as they are. In fact, AIDS provides an avenue toward addressing precisely these problems. AIDS has given many people insight into what really goes on in our society. For instance, gay men were not, for the most part, involved in attempts to change the health care system ten years ago; today they are.

Karp: Unfortunately, much of the history of the gay movement has involved a denial of disenfranchisement or an attempt to sneak in the back door to become enfranchised. But AIDS has shown us that gay men are entirely disenfranchised.

Hollibaugh: If you know that different communities are affected differently by oppression, and want to address the contradictions while not making those communities compete with one another, AIDS provides a mechanism. And if you don't address the contradictions in your approach to AIDS, your work will be irrelevant.

The fact that we're a part of the New York City Commission on Human Rights lends a credibility to our work that most activists or people working within disenfranchised communities don't have. There is a disproportionate amount of attention paid to what we say, as opposed to what is said by the Minority Task Force on AIDS, for example, even though what we say is often identical. But our report on AIDS and people of color can be used as supporting evidence when, let's say, Suki Ports (formerly of the Minority Task Force on AIDS) testifies at a state hearing. We try to help empower people working within the communities to continue doing their work.

Karp: The commission can take some pride in having been among the groups that put pressure on the City Health Department to remove Haitians from the list of so-called risk groups, which was followed by a decision by the Centers for Disease Control to do the same. The commission recognized the absurdity of and harm caused by this risk-group classification. In 1984, when the impact of AIDS on the Haitian community was so devastating — with physical assaults, boycotting of businesses, and so on — Katy spoke about the issue on Haitian radio.

Taylor: The radio program was done with Joe Placide, a Haitian-American who works for the commission, and Lola Poisson, who was the head of the Haitian Coalition on AIDS at the time. We were on Fritz Marshall's show, called "Moments Créole," to which virtually the entire Haitian community tunes in on Sunday afternoons. Our problem, however, was that you cannot simply walk into the Haitian community and talk about AIDS. In a Haitian context AIDS looks very different from the way it does in a gay context, or a hemophiliac context. To begin with, there's *profound* distrust. So our strategy was to approach it as a "Know Your Rights" series. Many Haitians don't know they have civil rights, even if they're naturalized, or that they have some protections even if they're not here legally. AIDS was just a part of a wider discussion. We began with housing, which is a primary concern in the community, and then health care, and so on, and through these other issues were able to discuss AIDS. We were flooded with calls after the programs, which alerted us both to the extent of the problems the Haitian community faces and the increased level of discrimination against that community, with AIDS as the excuse.

Karp: But locating AIDS discrimination within a nexus of other issues, such as housing and health care, is also consistent with our efforts to show the ways in which this new form of discrimination intersects with other biases that preceded the disease, biases based on class, race, gender, and so on. Our report on AIDS and people of color is an example of these efforts.

Taylor: At the time the report was completed, very few people were talking about AIDS and race. And government officials generally tend to be wary of issues that are seen as new or sensitive. In addition, there was still a lot of denial in the minority communities, a resistance to confronting the AIDS crisis. Several white people reviewing the report worried that even talking about the issue might be racist. But basically this is just a reflection of what racism does: it confuses white people, makes them overly cautious and fearful, so they can't determine what must be done, even if it's obvious.

Karp: All of us in this unit come out of community activism, so instead of being threatened or frightened by the AIDS community, we can be an effective liaison with it. One of the things we've tried to do is to validate people with AIDS as the *real experts*.

Crimp: I think it would be helpful to discuss some details of specific instances of discrimination against people with AIDS or those perceived to be at risk.

Karp: There are three different actual situations that I'd like to mention. The first concerns a nurse who was planning to have a child and who is married to a man with some past homosexual experience. Public health pronouncements insist that any woman who has had any risk of exposure should have an HIV antibody test when contemplating pregnancy. So this woman, in response to the public education campaign, went to the office of occupational health in her hospital and inquired about the test. She was told that the hospital performs the test and that the results would have no bearing upon her employment. She was also given a document outlining the confidentiality provisions issued by the City Department of Health. Believing this, she took the test, which determined that she was seropositive. Confidentiality was immediately broken, the hospital administrators were informed, and they decided as a matter of general policy that no staff member who is HIV antibody positive would be permitted to work in an operating room, emergency room, or intensive care unit. They therefore offered the nurse, who worked in intensive care, either a transfer to another unit or one month's severance pay. The nurse refused both options, which the hospital construed as a voluntary resignation, and they terminated her employment.

I think the hospital's real concern in this case was that it might be accused of being the source of transmission to a patient who might, at some point in the future, test positive. But what is the real likelihood of such a transmission? All hospital personnel use infection control guidelines in invasive procedures. Nevertheless, the hospital responded to *anticipated irrational fear* instead of education and denied the nurse her rights. The same hospital does not test its staff routinely, nor should it. So the nurse could have gone to an anonymous testing site, and this incident would not have occurred. Instead she followed the rules and was fired for her trouble.

The second case I want to mention involves an IV drug user who sought admission to a drug treatment center. The center said that as a condition of admission it was necessary to take an HIV antibody test. The person tested positive and was refused admission, probably because the center considered it a waste of resources to treat someone they assumed would die within a short time anyway. Public health officials say, "Get treatment, stop using drugs," yet when people pay attention and go for treatment, they're subjected to tests and denied treatment, and they risk having their test results leak out, which can further stigmatize them, cost them their jobs, their homes, and so on.

The third case came to us just yesterday. A woman arrested for prostitution was beaten up by a cop, whom she bit during the struggle. Although no one knew whether or not she was HIV antibody positive, she was charged with attempted murder. This charge was subsequently reduced to second-degree assault, to which the prostitute pleaded guilty, agreeing to accept a felony on her record in exchange for a six-month probation. At the time of sentencing, the judge was seen privately talking to the police officer and the officer's PBA representative, after which the DA's office was convinced that, as a condition of probation, she must take three HIV antibody tests over a period of time, with the results given to the cop. Now, the whole point of probation is that it will supposedly aid in rehabilitation. So unless you argue that knowing her HIV antibody status would help "rehabilitate" this woman, there can be no justification for the tests, and this is especially the case because the test results are intended for the cop, not for her. In addition, the judge, the DA, and everyone else involved are lending their authority to the unsubstantiated notion that biting is a means of transmission. In fact the only person at risk in such a case is the one who bites, not the one who is bitten. But of course no one is worried about the prostitute's health. Prostitutes are only thought of as "vectors" to the heterosexual population.

Crimp: Obviously cases of discrimination against people whose activities are criminalized—prostitutes, IV drug users, even gay people in some states—are more intractable. How are you able to deal with them?

Karp: We have no jurisdiction in the criminal justice system. We're limited to housing, employment, and public accommodations, so we can't make a formal complaint in such a case as the one I just described. But given our broad mandate to eliminate discrimination, we consider educating the legal and judicial community part of our function.

Crimp: But can't someone test the legality of demanding an HIV test as a condition of probation?

Taylor: Legal Aid is going to challenge it. The ACLU has challenged the mandatory testing law in Georgia. I'm not sure how many states have mandatory testing laws for prostitutes, but Nevada has already tested all of the prostitutes in legal brothels. Over 4,500 tests were conducted on 500 women, and *not one* was seropositive. Needless to say this fact did not make the front page of the *New York Times.* But, after all, the results are not so surprising. Most professionals take care of themselves. Prostitutes routinely used condoms long before AIDS. They're much more knowledgeable than most people about sexually transmitted diseases. Even according to the US Department of Health, prostitution is connected with only three to five percent of sexually transmitted diseases in the US.

   Very cogent objections to testing prostitutes have been raised. Money is not a mode of transmission. It is not prostitutes, but sexually active females, some of whom are sex workers, who could be said to belong to a "risk group"—a term that is misleading in any case; there's no such thing as a risk group, there are only risk behaviors or risk factors. Thus far, the only remotely scientific study of this group is that done by Project AWARE (Association for Women's AIDS Research and Education) in San Francisco, working with COYOTE (Call Off Your Old Tired Ethics), also based in San Francisco. In any case, every US study has found that if you separate out IV drug users and their sexual partners, the rate of HIV positivity among sex workers is comparable to that of other sexually active women, which is to say, very low.

Crimp: Does anyone remember that there are also *male* prostitutes? Has anyone done a study of them?

Taylor: There are some underway now. In New York, programs for runaway and "throw away" youth, such as the Hetrick-Martin Institute (formerly the Institute for the Protection of Lesbian and Gay Youth) and the Street Work Project, focus on the problems of hustlers, but this work is only now beginning.

Crimp: What disturbs me concerning hustlers is that, like female prostitutes, they are thought of only as "carriers" or "vectors," not as themselves at risk and very much in need of information and education so that they can protect themselves.

But this raises for me the question of another, equally deadly form of discrimination. The Helms Amendment, which outlaws AIDS education that directly or indirectly encourages homosexuality, effectively prevents gay people from getting the information they need in order to stay alive. Do we have any legal recourse?

Karp: The Helms Amendment only pertains to federal expenditures; it doesn't preclude the states' educating gay people. The situation is analogous to that of federal laws on abortion funding. The federal government claims that it is not denying the right of abortion by declining to fund abortions. There could be no clearer example of discrimination based on sex, class, and race, given who needs abortions and who can afford to pay for them. But challenges to the government's position have been unsuccessful.

Crimp: And another type of probable discrimination: I don't know precisely how patients are chosen for drug protocols at the officially designated ATEUs (AIDS Treatment Evaluation Units), but it's my assumption that they are not by and large drawn from minority communities.

Taylor: This issue has been raised in relation not only to race but also to gender. But there is some recognition, at least in New York, that this could be a potential problem, and people in minority communities have been very much on top of the situation with their demands. One of the first places where this type of concern arose was in prisons. Because of experimentation on prisoners in the past, legislation exists to prevent use of experimental drugs in prison. This became a problem with AZT, which is an experimental AIDS treatment, so the regulations had to be bent in order to get AZT to prisoners with AIDS. Dr. Robert Cohen, who is concerned about these issues and used to be directly involved with prison health care, is the doctor in charge of AIDS at the Health and Hospital Corporation. He sees to it that city clinics, such as Kings County Hospital, make AZT available. But clearly the fact that the drug costs $800 per month for each patient makes money a central issue.

Hollibaugh: I find that New York is better in this regard than most places I've visited. For example, in San Francisco, even very progressive white gay men still think of AIDS as mostly affecting only their own community, while at the same time minority AIDS organizations, many of whose members are gay, work in isolation from all the activity in the Castro district. Within a week there last summer, I was in touch with a very large number of AIDS organizations that did not know about one another. Of course, the shape of the epidemic in New York is such that you cannot refuse to notice affected communities other than your own. You have to include all of these other communities within your analysis of the situation or you'll lose your credibility. Grass-roots AIDS work in the city is surprisingly integrated, and that's one reason that we've had the successes we've had, in spite of funding problems. Beyond that, it's a question of who had the most legitimacy and power in the first place. It's no accident that members of ACT UP (AIDS Coalition to Unleash Power), most of whom are young white gay men, are the ones that can risk sitting down in the street and getting arrested. They, too, are very aware of other affected communities, and they don't agitate only for themselves. Even if it's a fairly homogeneous group of people, they don't have a one-dimensional analysis of the situation; they're concerned with prisoners' issues, prostitutes' issues, and so on. To give another example, in spite of their name, the Gay Men's Health Crisis says that from thirty to thirty-five percent of its current caseload is not gay men. At the same time it's not an accusation to say that different people have their own needs and priorities. That's why we try to hire in the unit to reflect the various affected communities.

Taylor: The integration of the various communities' concerns also reflects the players in New York. Most respected people in leadership positions in the AIDS community have worked to keep the context accurate. Jonathan Mann, who is in charge of the AIDS program for the World Health Organization, has said that from a global perspective, the countries dealing best with the AIDS crisis are not necessarily the richest, but rather those with the best leadership.

Crimp: I've read in some of your material that you are not pressing for specific legislation on AIDS discrimination, but that it's more practical to use anti-discrimination legislation already on the books. But would it in fact be useful to you to have such specific legislation?

Taylor: In general there's a tendency to try to deal with a particular problem with a neat package solution. So if AIDS is the problem there will be an AIDS-specific solution — AIDS-specific policies, AIDS-specific legislation, AIDS-specific facilities. Although tidy, this is ultimately a liberal approach, an approach that fails to see the overall context of the problem. It also tends to propagate stigma. When AIDS appeared, the funeral industry found itself with very few regulations on bio-hazardous conditions, so they established guidelines for AIDS. When funeral homes then refused to handle AIDS deaths, we pointed out that they should be handled just like other infectious diseases, like hepatitis, for example; their reply was that AIDS was different because they had a long list of regulations about it. Regarding stigma, I think that we are at the point now where you're either part of the problem or part of the solution. If you're not actively deconstructing stigma you're part of the construction of it. So wherever possible, everyone has to consider whether what they do will increase or decrease stigmatization. In the short run it might be necessary — given the overwhelming stigma and the magnitude of the problem — to have some separate facilities or programs, primarily to *protect* people with AIDS. But in the long run, it is deadly.

In addition, approaching specific problems with specific solutions reflects bad planning. The people who really understand this are those from the poorest communities. They've seen the hot issues come and go — the war on poverty, the war on crime, the war on drugs — overwhelming problems approached with short-term solutions. And then the communities are left with clinics or treatment centers that are no longer funded. People dealing with AIDS know that the response to it has to be embedded — "mainstreamed" — in the affected communities, because we cannot afford for these programs and services to dry up.

Karp: We shouldn't mislead you. Of course it would be helpful to have legislative action underscoring that AIDS and HIV antibody positivity should be protected, like any physical disability. But we know the political climate we're operating in and the amount of resources that would be required to get such legislation. And if it were defeated it would be debilitating.

Crimp: Can you tell me about *The Second Epidemic*, the unit's project for a broadcast video on AIDS-related discrimination?

Hollibaugh: The Second Epidemic will hopefully put discrimination squarely on the agenda. Part of the message is that this is not a cold legal issue or even a civil rights issue. It is something that determines how people will face this crisis. We are working within a cataclysmic situation that necessitates changing community attitudes, changing government policies . . . maybe it necessitates revolution. Discrimination has to be understood this broadly.

I'm focusing on some of the cases that have come through the unit, narrating them as vignettes, and shaping the narration within a broader context in which discrimination is shown to be a parallel epidemic. Whether or not we are able to eradicate discrimination will determine whether or not we are able to eradicate AIDS, because oppression and the effects of oppression are what prevent people from being able to protect themselves, or to take care of themselves if they're infected.

Taylor: We've found that the discrimination component of the AIDS epidemic has eluded many people, including those who should know better, like public health officials. In the beginning I thought we could just mention the problem and everyone would understand, but that hasn't been the case. So I knew we had to come up with something that was both detailed and accessible enough to convince people of the seriousness of the problem and help them identify the issues.

Hollibaugh: My job is not only to produce educational material, but to get it out to the communities. Until now, working as a video producer had always meant that I had to relinquish my role as an activist: I could tell wonderful stories but I

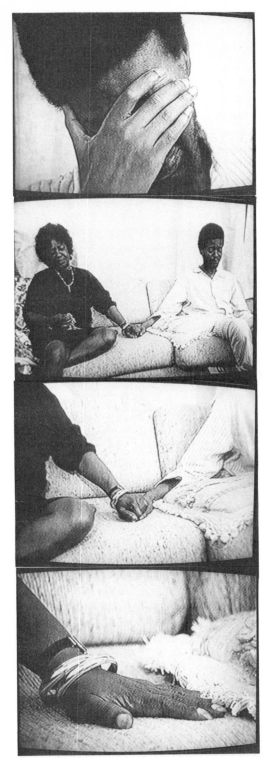

Amber Hollibaugh. The Second Epidemic. *1987–88.*

Cliff Gilchrist [who went blind through neglect while in the hospital]: "My eyesight started getting dim, so I pressed the call button in the bathroom, which didn't work. So I yelled for the nurse and told her I could not see. I couldn't find the buzzer. I yelled, I screamed, I tried to make a phone call. It was a push-button phone so I couldn't quite get it right. I was panicking. . . . I yelled out my phone number, asking, 'Somebody, please call my number. Give 'em your name and I'll pay you to get them.' But nobody came. I finally just screamed myself to sleep."

Charlotte Gilchrist [Cliff's mother]: "I made no secret that I would complain until somebody listened. I didn't care where I had to go. I didn't care how far I had to go. You see, it didn't matter to me. Somebody, somehow was gonna get the message that I wasn't gonna stop until something was done. Because people are suffering enough. AIDS is enough. You don't need to add bullshit to it, neglect, stupidity, fear. . . ."

Cliff: I was ready to die, but I was not going to let them kill me. And that's what it seemed like; they were just trying to bump me off. I was called a troublemaker many times because I asked for things I felt I was entitled to.

couldn't take them back into the communities from which they'd emerged and build on the work. But as a producer/educator it's part of my job to take the material I produce into the communities and see if it works.

Crimp: How will you distribute the video?

Hollibaugh: It will definitely air on WNYC, the local public television station, and I'm negotiating with PBS to have it aired nationally. But broadcast television is only one possible form of distribution. I want to maintain control of distribution to community organizations. I'm investigating a distribution network now, determining which communities are reached by which progressive distributors, which communities can use the materials, and so forth. Our work can also be integrated into programs set up by the Department of Health, so that when they show educational materials on transmission, they can also use ours on discrimination.

My eventual goal is to make a whole series of documentaries. After this general one, I hope to make others shaped around particular aspects of discrimination — blue-collar workplace issues, for example. Although there is a lot of information about AIDS in the workplace, the workplace in question always seems to be white-collar. You might learn that you won't get AIDS by sitting at the same computer terminal with someone who's infected, but what about the janitor who cleans up in the hospital? What about industrial settings where there can be serious accidents? These working people's fears are not being addressed, nor is there money available to help address them.

In addition, I intend to make a video about women and children with AIDS; I'm considering a video-novella in Spanish; and I want to make a video about successes, to show alternatives to discrimination. I want to say, "You don't have to respond as they did in Arcadia, Florida. You *could* respond as they did in Swansee, Massachusetts." Here was a virtually identical situation — a small, working-class town that found out about a hemophiliac schoolboy with AIDS. But in this case the school principal, the police chief, and the public health nurse educated themselves about AIDS and then helped educate the townspeople, with the result that the townspeople formed a committee to support the boy and his family through their ordeal. When the boy died, the people held a candlelight procession through the town.

Taylor: We hope to have the first tape subtitled in Spanish and captioned in ASL (American sign language). There was a large increase in the number of people born deaf between 1962 and '64, when there was a rubella outbreak in New York City. Many of these young adults are from poor and minority neighborhoods, where the disease was most widespread. Despite the fact that IV drug use and sexual activity, both straight and gay, are as much issues for this population as for anyone else, little information is reaching them.

Hollibaugh: There are special problems involved in making these documentaries. There are many women with AIDS, for example, who don't feel that they can afford to be public about it, especially if they have children. So if I find a woman who is willing to participate, I have to get there right away with a film crew, because I don't know how long she'll be in good enough health to do it. And there are other difficulties beyond that of finding people who can afford to go public. When I made the documentary entitled *Gay Greenwich Village*, I had similar problems finding people who could afford to show their faces, even though, being gay myself, I had no trouble getting access to gay people. But people with AIDS and their caretakers are constantly confronted with media of the most disgusting sort. I walk into the community following the producers that have just ripped these people off—exposed them, used their names, not protected them as they'd promised, edited their statements in misleading ways. I then have to go in and say, "I'm different. I won't do that to you." There's a very difficult balance between the importance of hearing directly from the people most affected by AIDS and the vulnerability of those very people, especially when exposed to the invasiveness of a camera.

Given these problems, what gives me confidence is the support I have from the unit. Everyone here is involved in the project, and it's grown significantly beyond what I had initially thought could be done. There hasn't yet been a documentary on AIDS-related discrimination, and it's urgently needed, not just here in New York, but in Wichita, in Bakersfield, everywhere. That's why it's important to make this for broadcast. All kinds of people watch TV, and they don't have to be able to read to understand what they see there. I'm planning to use computer animation and to do a faster-paced edit than is normally used for documentary, because most people find documentaries boring.

Crimp: Do you have the funding you need?

Hollibaugh: Yes, right now we do. If our current funding continues, we'll be in good shape. But you never know. Even though I'm on staff, the video budget is year-by-year, so I could be in the middle of a project and be unable to finish it, if I were to lose my budget. But something other than funding has made this project possible. Everyone that I've ever approached about it has cooperated. Everyone living with AIDS or working with AIDS knows how important this is, and that opens everything up.

Karp: Our unit has benefited from the interest and support of community-based AIDS organizations, who formed an alliance and put together an AIDS funding agenda that was backed by some elected officials, notably Manhattan Borough President David Dinkins. We're the largest unit of this type in the country, and New York City is one of very few cities that has this kind of program.

Taylor: Almost from the beginning, we've acted as a resource for places around the country—and even outside the country. I've consulted with the governments of Japan, Australia, the Netherlands, which is not exactly typical for your garden-variety civil servant. But this shows that the work we do here has ramifications far beyond the solution of individual cases brought to our attention. This is particularly true regarding systemic discrimination. Over the years we have tackled many areas—ambulances, dentists, and so on—but the response of the funeral industry is the best example. For years the Bureau of Funeral Directing wouldn't even return my phone calls. So, after all our efforts at education and persuasion failed, we filed formal complaints, and they immediately called to say, "Let's work this out." At the time, we were working with Gay Men's Health Crisis, whose initial survey of funeral homes turned up only a handful that they could recommend. Shortly after their survey was completed, we filed our complaints, and after six months they conducted a follow-up survey and found close to 200 that they could recommend.

Hollibaugh: Another thing I want to accomplish with *The Second Epidemic* is to publicize the AIDS resources that already exist. For example, I plan to use footage from a Spanish-language AIDS education tape in soap opera format that was made in San Francisco. Seeing this, people doing AIDS work will know that such a tape exists when they're looking for something that will reach Hispanics. People will also learn that the AIDS Discrimination Unit exists as a resource, and my hope is that after this tape is aired on WNYC more people will seek us out.

Karp: We want people to know that AIDS-related discrimination is illegal in New York City, that people with AIDS have rights. That's the bottom line. One of our biggest hurdles is getting people to identify discrimination. There's so much internalized oppression. People's coping mechanisms are such that they've learned to go on with their lives in spite of being subjected to discrimination. We're asking people to stop, to see it for what it is. We want to empower everyone as an activist fighting AIDS-related discrimination.

MAX NAVARRE

In the media, everyone's a victim: of fire, of cancer, of mugging, of rape, of AIDS. In the world of reportage, no one is doing well. Victims sell newspapers. Does anyone consider the impact of this cult of the victim? Does anyone realize the power of the message "You are helpless, there is no hope for you"?

As a person with AIDS, I can attest to the sense of diminishment at seeing and hearing myself constantly referred to as an AIDS victim, an AIDS sufferer, an AIDS case—as anything but what I am, a person with AIDS. I am a person with a condition. I am not that condition.

AIDS is so confusing and frightening. Apart from the devastating physical effects of AIDS, fear of AIDS can undo even the most confident and self-loving among us. Those who have it, those who think they have it, those who expect to get it, those who are terrified by the sound of the word—all are overly susceptible to any opinion or point of view that sounds authoritative.

I recently met a man who had been diagnosed with ARC. He was not ill at the time, nor had he had any opportunistic infections. He did not have AIDS. His symptoms were quite mild. Essentially, all he had was a lowered T-cell count, not necessarily significant in and of itself, but in the current diagnostic fashion, enough to warrant treatment with AZT. Here's how it goes: take someone with a lowered T-cell count who is asymptomatic, or who shows only mild symptoms, and treat him with AZT, known to be highly toxic, which might, at the very least, nauseate him, or, at worst, damage and suppress the bone marrow enough to cause severe anemia, not to mention liver damage—all in the name of suppressing a virus that might not even be the "cause" of AIDS.

My conversation with this man went something like this:

"How do you feel?"

"I feel good, but I'm sick."

"What do you mean?"

"My T-cells are down. I'm taking AZT. I must be sick."

"Why are you taking AZT?"

"My doctor told me to."

"Did you ask him why?"

"Because I'm sick."

"But you're not sick. You said you feel well."

"I do, but that doesn't mean I'm not sick."

I could not convince this man that being sick means you don't feel well. I couldn't make him listen to his body instead of his lab reports.

This is not uncommon. People are so frightened that it's as if they have to be sick even if they're not. After two and a half years of living with AIDS, I've come to realize that when I'm sick, I'm sick, and when I'm well, I treasure my health. Even so, I'm not immune to the reinforcement of hopelessness that surrounds me.

That reinforcement causes despair, and I believe that despair kills people with AIDS as much as any of AIDS's physical manifestations. If we could truly believe in the possibility of *living* with AIDS, I think that survival figures would be higher.

To survive, you have to overcome the fear factor on a daily basis. How can you go forward when the only apparent future is chronic illness and death? Where is the motivation to move on in life? Where is the security a future offers? Work becomes difficult or impossible, friends disappear, family and loved ones grieve in your presence. You're cruelly written off even when you're relatively well and still quite capable of living life from one day to the next, just like everybody else.

But, of course, everybody else isn't up against AIDS. It takes an enormous amount of personal power to sustain hope. And hope is one of the greatest healers. I know that sounds simplistic, but I also know too many people with AIDS living full and productive lives far longer than they're expected to not to believe it. The shared trait in those people is the belief that they are *entitled* to live, work, and function. In short: self-empowerment.

In 1983, the National Association of People with AIDS was formed at the second AIDS Forum in Denver. Attending the conference from all parts of the US was a very diverse group of PWAs whose unifying goal was to assert—for the public and especially for themselves—that people with AIDS have the right and the responsibility actively to determine their own experience with AIDS.

In spite of the opinions of so-called experts, the statistics, and the history of physician-patient relationships, these stubborn people insisted that they were not passive victims. They seized the opportunity of the meeting to draw up what became known as the Denver Principles (see pp. 148–149). This extraordinary document announced the birth of self-empowerment for PWAs.

Because AIDS is so often perceived as a moral problem instead of a health crisis, and because of the connection between AIDS and gay men, AIDS has from the beginning been a political issue, tied to the long and bitter struggle for gay and lesbian rights. The movement of self-empowerment for PWAs has its origins in this grass-roots struggle; the Denver Principles are its manifesto.

The creation of this document set the stage for a new kind of interaction between doctor and patient, between service provider and recipient. Of course, there have always been patients who have challenged their illnesses and questioned medical authority, but never before had patients, as a group, affirmed their right to be exceptional.

PWAs were saying no—no, we will not be characterized as victims; no, we will not be experimented upon without our complete understanding and approval; no, we will not be medicated without explanation; no, we will not go out with a whimper.

On paper, it looked great. In practice, convincing the public and ourselves that people with AIDS can participate in life, even prosper, has been an uphill struggle. The facts are all too clear: people suffer terribly, and we're dying by the thousands. But I'm not talking about not dying; I don't deny the reality that sooner or later most people with AIDS die; it would be foolish not to address death. I'm talking about the business of living, of making choices, of *not* being passive, helpless, dependent, the storm-tossed object of the ministrations of the kindly well. These are the pejorative connotations of *victim* that PWAs find unacceptable.

The point is to see AIDS, when it happens to you, less as a defeat and more as an opportunity for creative life management. That might seem glib, but, given the choice between what the *New York Times* recently called "a shattered life" and seeing AIDS as a chance to live life fully on a daily basis, it doesn't take much to realize which view is the more helpful. Taking the bull by the horns is a means of escaping the sentimental soap opera that the media has created around the experience of having AIDS.

In 1985, a group of five or six of us formed the PWA Coalition in New York. It was our initial intention to create a support system for ourselves and others in the health crisis. In two years we've grown and expanded enormously. We offer monthly public forums at which PWAs can meet and ask questions of doctors, researchers, and holistic practitioners. We provide meals three afternoons a week, offering an opportunity for people to gather for a lunch that they might otherwise—because of physical weakness or financial difficulty—be unable to enjoy. We host monthly "singles' teas" so that people diagnosed with AIDS or ARC can meet with others without having to explain or clarify their health status. We have ongoing support groups for Spanish-speaking PWAs, for women with AIDS, for people with ARC, and for mothers of PWAs. We appear before the press as publicly identified PWAs; we respond to publications and public figures that refer to us in ways that we consider diminishing; and we serve on the boards of other service-providing organizations—all in the belief that our experience offers something unique, *real* expertise about AIDS. Our two most consuming projects are the Community Research Initiative and our monthly magazine, the *PWA Coalition Newsline*.

Out of frustration with FDA foot-dragging on promising drugs for the treatment of AIDS and AIDS-related illnesses, the PWA Coalition developed the

Community Research Initiative (CRI) to study these drugs in a community setting. Backed by a powerful and influential Institutional Review Board, utilizing the facilities of local physicians, and maintaining FDA-quality research, CRI seeks to achieve two goals: to give people access to the study of promising drugs that would otherwise be unavailable to them, and to prod the FDA into processing drugs that they might not otherwise explore.

The initiation of drug research by people with AIDS and the expansion of existing drug protocols to reach a greater number of PWAs at the community level is such a revolutionary concept that many obstacles stand in its way. Funding is, of course, the major stumbling block. But we have nevertheless recently begun an expanded study of Aerosol Pentamadine as a prophylaxis for *Pneumocystis carinii* pneumonia, as well as a study of Erythropoietin's potential for counteracting anemia resulting from AZT or as a direct symptom of AIDS. Also in the works is a major study of Ampligen, sponsored by Dupont, its manufacturer. Other treatments that are under consideration for study by CRI are Antabuse, DHPG, Methionine Enkephalin, and egg lipids.

Our monthly magazine, the *Newsline,* was initiated by Michael Callen, its original editor, working with the other founding members of the coalition. It began publication in June 1985 as sixteen typed pages of information and suggestions, surreptitiously photocopied at someone's office and distributed by hand to doctors' offices and gay bookstores. Today the *Newsline* receives and prints letters, news, and features from PWAs and their friends all over the world. With a circulation of 11,000, it is read in hospitals, hospices, private homes, offices, and correctional facilities everywhere. The *Newsline* serves as the best available forum for sharing opinions, experiences, strength, and hope for PWAs. As its current editor, I am gratified to know that people with AIDS have a magazine that not only keeps them informed, but makes them feel united with others with similar experiences. AIDS is very isolating, particularly for people living in small or disenfranchised communities. Many people are forced by their illness to leave cities such as New York and San Francisco and go back to their hometowns to be cared for by family — "going home to die," as the *New York Times* so callously put it.

What kind of information do those people normally get? What kind of care? Thanks to the miserliness and homophobia of our federal government, there are very few support systems available to the people who need them most: those living in rural areas, the impoverished, the incarcerated. The *Newsline* reaches some of these people (it is free to PWAs), and all of them have an opportunity to speak out, to let other PWAs know about their situations, simply by writing in.

Hope must be constantly reinforced, taking action constantly encouraged. It's enough to be up against a baffling and inexorable disease without having to be undermined at every turn in the effort to continue living as well and as long as possible. We're up against a lot. PWAC has lost most of its original board members. Whenever a friend dies, it's a big setback. Whenever there's an illness among us, sadness sets in. Loss and fear haunt us. But we continue to fight.

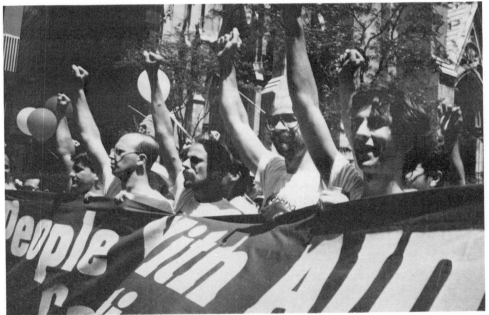

Photo: Jane Rosett

The following statements, articles, letters, and photographs are selected from issues one (June 1985) through twenty-eight (November 1987) of the PWA Coalition News-line, *and from* Surviving and Thriving with AIDS: Hints for the Newly Diag-nosed, *edited by Michael Callen and published by the People with AIDS Coalition in 1987. In some cases this material is excerpted; deletions are indicated by ellipsis points. While giving an impression of the self-representation of PWAs, these items do not encompass the full range of material published by the* Newsline, *which also prints announcements of events, services, and studies; a resource directory; treatment informa-tion, including alternative healing possibilities; news briefs; and memorials. — ed.*

Founding Statement of People with AIDS/ARC (The Denver Principles)

We condemn attempts to label us as "victims," which implies defeat, and we are only occasionally "patients," which implies passivity, helplessness, and dependence upon the care of others. We are "people with AIDS."

We recommend that health care professionals:
1. Who are gay, come out, especially to their patients who have AIDS.
2. Always clearly identify and discuss the theory they favor as to the cause of AIDS, since this bias affects the treatment and advice they give.
3. Get in touch with their feelings (fears, anxieties, hopes, etc.) about AIDS, and not simply deal with AIDS intellectually.
4. Take a thorough personal inventory and identify and examine their own agendas around AIDS.
5. Treat people with AIDS as whole people and address psychosocial issues as well as biophysical ones.
6. Address the question of sexuality in people with AIDS specifically, sensitively, and with information about gay male sexuality in general and the sexuality of people with AIDS in particular.

We recommend that all people:
1. Support us in our struggle against those who would fire us from our jobs, evict us from our homes, refuse to touch us, separate us from our loved ones, our community, or our peers, since there is no evidence that AIDS can be spread by casual social contact.
2. Do not scapegoat people with AIDS, blame us for the epidemic, or generalize about our lifestyles.

We recommend that people with AIDS:
1. *Form* caucuses to choose their own representatives, to deal with the media, to choose their own agenda, and to plan their own strategies.
2. Be involved at every level of AIDS decision-making and specifically serve on the boards of directors of provider organizations.
3. Be included in all AIDS forums with equal credibility as other participants, to share their own experiences and knowledge.
4. Substitute low risk sexual behaviors for those that could endanger themselves or their partners, and we feel that people with AIDS have an ethical responsibility to inform their potential sexual partners of their health status.

People with AIDS have the right:

1. To as full and satisfying sexual and emotional lives as anyone else.

2. To quality medical treatment and quality social service provision, without discrimination of any form, including sexual orientation, gender, diagnosis, economic status, age, or race.

3. To full explanations of all medical procedures and risks, to choose or refuse their treatment modalities, to refuse to participate in research without jeopardizing their treatment, and to make informed decisions about their lives.

4. To privacy, to confidentiality of medical records, to human respect, and to choose who their significant others are.

5. To die and to *live* in dignity.

> (*Newsline*, no. 1, June 1985,
> and *Surviving and Thriving with
> AIDS,* 1987)

Mr. John Vinocur
Metropolitan Editor
New York Times

Dear Mr. Vinocur:

I am writing regarding the news obituary of Kenneth Meeks which appeared in today's *New York Times*.

We protest the *Times*'s not listing Ken's surviving life-mate of over ten years, Mr. Jack Steinhebel. Upon calling your office, I spoke to "Fred," who told me that it was the policy of the *Times* "not to include lovers" as survivors. That policy is totally inappropriate in that it lacks sensitivity and basic respect. "Fred" also informed me that in his "six years at the *Times* and with hundreds of phone calls the policy had not changed" and that we should "not expect it to change in the future." How sad.

We were also disappointed that the article failed to mention Ken Meeks's involvement with the People with AIDS Coalition as cofounder and former president.

Finally the labeling of People with AIDS as "victims" in Ken's obit was incorrect and more so in light of Ken's extensive work to end such practices. We are greatly disappointed by such journalism.

Sincerely,
Michael Hirsh
Executive Director, PWA Coalition

Reply to Michael Hirsch:

No slurs were intended, insofar as I can determine, but I can well understand your feelings about Kenneth Meeks's obituary. We are reviewing our obituary conventions regarding mention of intimates other than blood relatives and spouses. I cannot predict what we will decide to do, but think you have contributed to consciousness-raising.

As for the word "victims," I cannot agree that it is pejorative. Along with most of society, we have long written about "stroke victims," "heart attack victims," and "cancer victims." The logic is equally applicable to AIDS, and I am uncomfortable about drying idiom [sic] for any cause, no matter how meritorious.

Sincerely,
Alan M. Siegel
News Editor
New York Times

(Newsline, no. 18, December 1986)

Media Watch
(And It's *Still Ticking*)

MICHAEL CALLEN

Have you noticed? Everywhere you turn, people seem to talk of nothing but the asshole. In newspapers and magazines, on TV and radio, we are now regularly treated to the bizarre spectacle of the mayor and the governor and ass-orted newscasters wrapping their untrained lips around the words *anal intercourse*. Even the constipated *New York Times* finally broke down and printed "anal intercourse."

One distressing presumption that runs throughout this asshole coverage is that anal intercourse and male homosexuality are synonymous. When will someone point out that heterosexuals can *and do* engage in anal intercourse? . . .

I was in a government office building last week when I discovered two young, presumably straight men behind a counter passing around a xerox and giggling. In disbelief, I asked for a copy (reproduced below), which they provided.

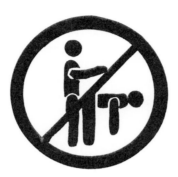

I am appalled by the sentiment that all one has to do to wipe out AIDS is eliminate anal intercourse. (Childbirth has often been fatal to women, but no one has seriously suggested that the way to reduce or eliminate maternal mortality is to eliminate vaginal intercourse.)

But I fear that many in the gay community share the simplistic notion that anal sex per se is a death-defying act. What is going on here?

Consider GMHC's "trick card" (which is based on guidelines formulated by NY Physicians for Human Rights). Check out Point 3: "Try to avoid anal sex." The only difference between this GMHC/NYPHR view and Governor Cuomo's is that Cuomo is willing to go to greater lengths to ensure that gay men "avoid anal sex." Aside from the sex negativity, the worst thing about this anti-anal-sex message is that it discourages the use of condoms: if condoms are protective, why "avoid anal sex"? . . .

As AIDS researcher Joe Sonnabend eloquently stated in a recent *Native* interview: "One should take an aggressive view. The rectum is a sexual organ, and it deserves the respect that a penis gets and a vagina gets. Anal intercourse is a central sexual activity, and it should be supported, it should be celebrated."

. . . Simply put, those who enjoy getting fucked should not be made to feel stupid or irresponsible. Instead, they should be provided with the information necessary to make what they enjoy safe(r)! And that means the *aggressive* encouragement of condom use!

(*Newsline*, no. 7, December 1985)

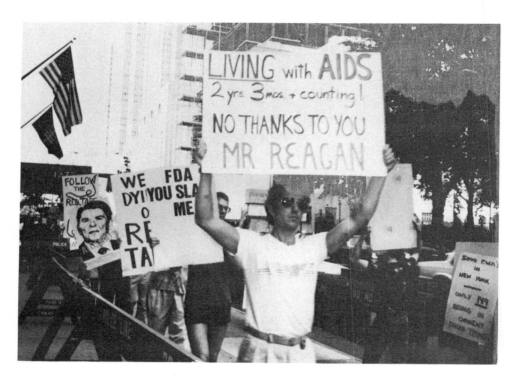

ACT UP demonstration at Memorial Sloan-Kettering Hospital, one of New York City's officially designated AIDS Treatment Evaluation Units, July 21, 1987.

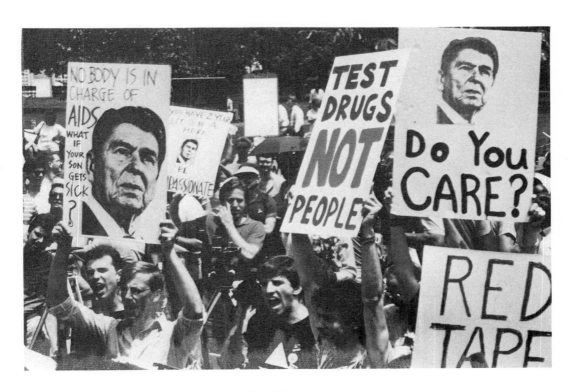

Demonstration by AIDS activists in front of the White House at the time of the Third International Conference on AIDS, June 1, 1987.

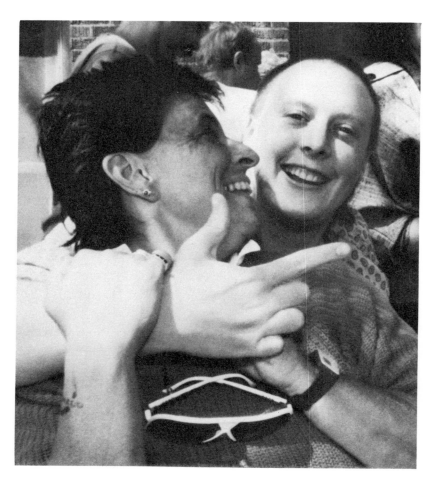

Carol LaFavor and Allyson Hunter, two lesbian PWAs,
at the National Association of People with AIDS
Conference held in Dallas, 1987.

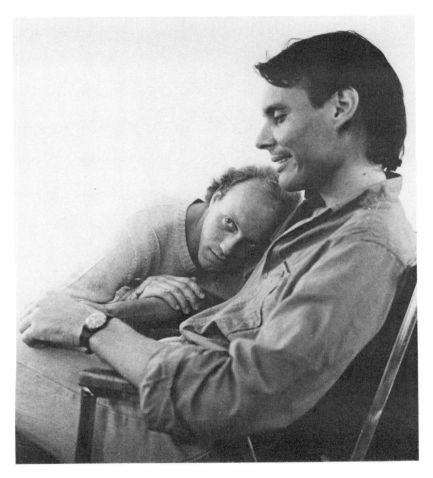

Joseph Foulon (right), board member of PWA Coalition and National Association of People with AIDS, with his lover Mark Senak, 1986. Foulon died in June 1987.

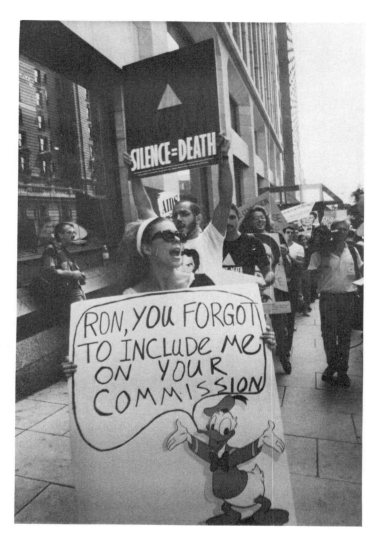

ACT UP demonstration at the first meeting of the
Presidential Commission on the HIV Epidemic,
Washington, D.C., September 9, 1987.

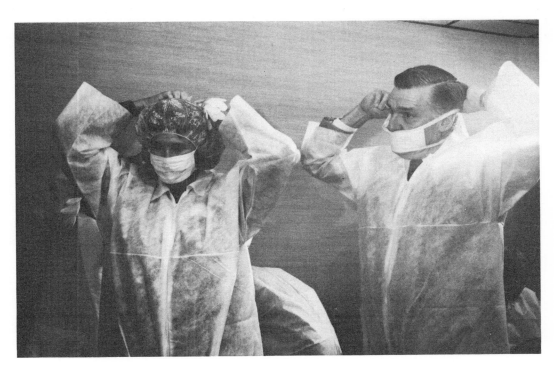

Presidential Commission members Theresa Crenshaw
and Admiral James Watkins gown up for a tour of the
HIV lab at Mt. Sinai Medical Center in Miami, 1987.

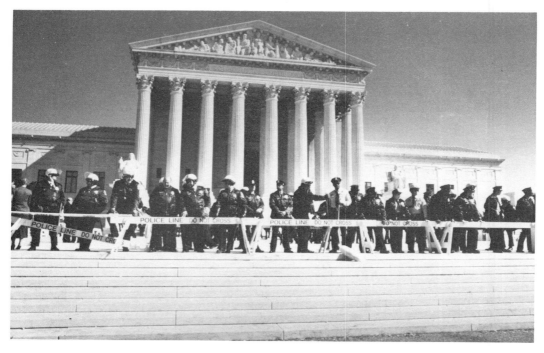

*Police stand in readiness for civil disobedience by
lesbians and gays to protest the Supreme Court's* Bowers
v. Hardwick *decision upholding anti-sodomy laws,
October 13, 1987.*

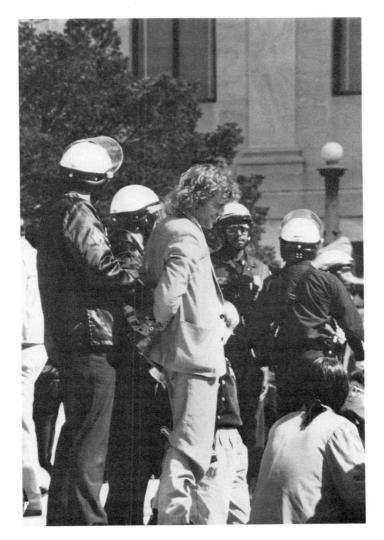

Michael Hardwick, plaintiff in Bowers v. Hardwick, *arrested in civil disobedience action.*

A Patient's Bill of Rights

1. The right to expect a full and complete diagnosis and prognosis in terms understandable to a non-medically trained patient.

2. The right to a full explanation of all recommended medical procedures and the risks involved.

3. The right to refuse specific treatments without jeopardizing the relationship between the patient and the health care professional.

4. The right to be released from institutional in-patient care upon request.

5. The right to refuse to participate in research-oriented treatment or studies without jeopardizing the treatment relationship between the health care professional and the patient.

6. The right to patient anonymity, privacy, and confidentiality.

7. The right to quality medical treatment and quality social services without discrimination based on sex, sexual orientation, economic status, diagnosis, race, or religious, political, or other beliefs.

8. The right to informed choices at the time of admission for medical care, so that the patient can continue his or her choice of the use of extraordinary measures to prolong life or to discontinue treatment that the patient feels no longer provides a quality of life worth living.

9. The right to accept dying without guilt of failure or a judgment that this decision is somehow wrong.

10. The right to the choice of "immediate family member" status for those the patient may designate.

(Newsline, no. 7, December 1985)

Statement of Prisoners in the AIDS Ward on Rikers Island

The following is a statement issued by PWAs incarcerated in the isolated AIDS ward on Rikers Island. It was issued in support of ACT UP's April 15, 1987, demonstration at the US General Post Office in New York City.

We, the undersigned (as well as those who could not sign), would like to communicate with you on this evening as you gather in the memory of those who have died. We would like to add our protest to yours as you stand before the post office and raise your voices against the lack of spending for AIDS research.

There is no doubt that the system is not providing us with proper medical care. Although we are in the hospital building, we have been relegated to the top floor, where the roof leaks whenever it rains, and the old windows do not keep out the cold winds that come off the river. We do not have hospital beds or reside in a hospital unit. Each AIDS unit is a regular cell unit. When one inmate complained about the large amount of pigeon shit that collects on the sills and blows in through the cracks in the window, even after writing to the grievance department, he was given a window scraper and told to do it himself.

I'm sure that you are all witness to the lack of concern that our society has shown in the face of this crisis. Up here and behind bars, that society has shown what it is truly capable of. Only your continual voice can make a difference. The horror stories that any one of us could tell are all possible out there if people forget, if people do not speak out. Currently a lot of us are waiting for court dates, which continually get postponed. The courts figure that, if we die first, they will not have to worry about us. Your presence, today and everyday, can prove them wrong.

We just wanted to take this opportunity to join our voice with yours, to reach out to our brothers and sisters on the outside who have the freedom to protest and get involved. We want you to know that we are with you in spirit. Please, do not stop raising your voices. Gay or straight, black or white, man or woman, we are all in this together and must unite. If we do this now, then maybe, God willing, we will walk away from this crisis, with our lives and our dignity.

(*Newsline*, no. 23, May 1987)

Remarks of Michael Callen,
American Public Health Association
Annual Meeting, Las Vegas, Nevada, 1986

In the fall of '84, I found myself tethered to an IV pole in room 557 of a building named after a homophobic — reputedly homosexual — Catholic cardinal in a hospital named after a Catholic saint. That week, the *current* Catholic archbishop was demonstrating his peculiar concept of Christian charity by opposing — with much fanfare — a mayoral executive order that offered limited protection from discrimination in employment, housing, and public accommodation to lesbians and gay men.

That day, a *Village Voice* headline screamed from every newsstand that what it referred to as the "AIDS virus" had been "found in the saliva of two patients."

My breakfast grew cold outside my room on the floor where it had been left. As I rang for the nurse, a middle-aged black man, wearing a surgical gown, gloves, and a mask, skittered nervously across my room (keeping close to the far wall). He flipped a switch that turned on the rental TV and fled.

I paused to consider whether the tableau I formed might well be the quintessential image of an urban gay man in the Reagan '80s: sick, shunned, frightened, and frightening, and largely unprotected by either law or popular opinion. There in the largest gay ghetto on the East Coast, I found myself dependent on the kindness of some very strange strangers.

*

. . . For me and my fellow members of the People with AIDS Coalition, AIDS is about living daily with the very real possibility that tomorrow—or maybe the day after tomorrow—we may be dead.

AIDS is about bedpans and respirators. It's about loss of control—control of one's bowels and bladder, one's arms and legs, one's life. Sometimes the loss is sudden; sometimes its tortuously gradual. It's about the *anticipation* of pain as well as actual pain. It's about swelling and horrible disfigurement, the fear of dementia. It is horror.

AIDS is the moment-to-moment management of uncertainty. It's a roller coaster ride without a seat belt. Once this ride begins, there is never a moment when the rush of events that swirl around you stops long enough for you to get your bearings. AIDS is like motion sickness, except you realize that you'll never stop moving; one way or another, you'll be dealing with AIDS for the rest of your life.

It's like standing in the middle of the New York stock exchange at midday: buzzers and lights flashing, everyone yelling, a million opinions, a momentum.

Some of us who've seen too many friends die—who've had to remove too many lives from our Roladexes—talk about "the look" and "the smell" that characterize the terminal stage of AIDS. Although "the look" varies from person to person, it's essentially the look of someone who has just seen clearly—perhaps for the first time—the image and imminence of his own death. The eyes are sunken with resignation and wasting, yet wide open with terror; vacant yet certain. It is a look I've only seen elsewhere in gruesome photos from the holocaust.

"The smell" is like slightly rotten oranges moldering on the street in a cardboard box on a hot summer day—sprayed with Lysol. It is the smell of death.

*

. . . What I've just tried to describe is the experience of *dying* from AIDS. And certainly the experience of AIDS for a great many of those diagnosed is the experience of dying. But if I can challenge one assumption about AIDS in this speech, it is the assumption that everyone dies from AIDS—that AIDS is an automatic death sentence—that AIDS has a 100 percent mortality rate.

There are a handful of us—estimated variously at ten to eighteen percent —who happen to be quite alive more than three years after our diagnoses and who intend to be alive for many more years. *The unthinking repetition of the notion that everyone dies from AIDS denies both the reality of—but more importantly the possibility of—our survival.*

I want to expose the tautology behind the definition of AIDS. When most people use the word *AIDS*—as in CDC-defined AIDS or full-blown AIDS—they mean the terminal stage in a spectrum of illnesses. If you're only going to count as frank AIDS those cases that are terminal, then by definition the mortality rate is going to be 100 percent. Death from AIDS will become a self-fulfilling prophecy, because anyone who doesn't have the good sense to die will be demoted from the fraternity—if they're not dead within three years, maybe they never *really* had AIDS.

What I'd like to shake from the definition of AIDS is the sense of hopelessness that seems to have been built in. It is my own perception that the disease is changing—people are living longer, seem to be somehow less sick. Perhaps AIDS is becoming less virulent. Or possibly we have a better handle on it now—earlier diagnosis of opportunistic complications, more accurate treatment regimens for specific infections. I suspect that one reason the mortality rate for AIDS was so high in the early days was the rush to aggressive chemotherapy. Most of my friends from the early days seemed to have died from their treatments, not the diseases they were being treated for.

. . . We must begin to make room for survival, to admit it as a possibility. I know it may be painful. The one consolation of believing that AIDS is 100 percent fatal is the comfort of some certainty about a disease for which so little is certain. If AIDS is truly 100 percent fatal, then those caring for us know how the roller coaster ride is going to end. They can humor us in our protestations of survival and hand us Kubler-Ross and ration out their emotional strength, certain that however draining, however horrible it is to watch the progression of AIDS, the end is inevitable. Admitting the possibility of survival will require that others around us suffer the disappointment of our hopes along with us in a new way. It's a tall order, I know, but it's time to begin admitting hope into the AIDS picture.

*

. . . It is a principle of the PWA movement that when one speaks as a PWA or PWArc, it is useful briefly to state what one's own medical history has been. . . .

In the spring of '81, when the CDC made its first report, I was sick: fevers, night sweats, thrush, weight loss, diarrhea, and malaise. The standard tests showed nothing conclusive. As it happened, my doctor was Joe Sonnabend, a microbiologist of international repute who had left the research world to go into private practice. He initiated some of the earliest AIDS research using samples provided by me and other patients from his practice. As a result Dr. Sonnabend was able to tell me as early as December 1981 that I had almost no T-helper cells left and that other blood parameters indicated that I was dangerously immuno-suppressed. My results, he warned me, were identical to those of his patients who had—or were soon to develop—PCP and KS. . . .

If there had been such a term, I would, in early 1982, have been diagnosed with ARC (AIDS-Related Complex). At the time, the very namelessness of the condition compounded the terror.

I continued to lose weight, to sleep twelve or fourteen hours, to vomit up my food. And I had bloody diarrhea eight to ten times a day. In June of 1982, I collapsed in my home from dehydration and was taken to the emergency room with a 104-degree fever by Dr. Sonnabend's physician's assistant.

During that first hospitalization—the first in a series—they finally diag-nosed my problem as cryptosporidiosis, a parasite that, in the . . . words of the hospital doctor, had been "previously found only in livestock." Cryptosporidiosis (which we PWAs refer to as crypto) is one of the diseases that qualifies one for an official diagnosis of AIDS. . . . As far as I and my doctors (and, incidentally, my insurance company) were concerned, as of June 1982 I had AIDS, CDC-defined AIDS, full-blown AIDS, frank AIDS—call it what you will.

But the clinical reality of AIDS is actually a lot more complicated than it seems on paper. There is clearly a range of illnesses. There are some people who have, say, a few lesions, who don't otherwise look or feel sick. There are people with AIDS-related conditions for whom it is an effort to get out of bed in the morning and who are in and out of hospitals all the time.

In my own case, there has been some debate—much of it painful to me—about whether I "really" have AIDS or whether I "only" have ARC. I remember one AIDS conference where three doctors got into a shouting match over my diagnosis.

Dr. A suggested that if all I've had is crypto, if I hadn't "yet" had PCP or KS, then as far as *he* was concerned, I didn't *really* have AIDS. He suggested the novel notion that I was "on the cusp between ARC and AIDS" (I thought this was an interesting mix of astrology and epidemiology).

Dr. B pointed out that I *was* AIDS, but only by a technicality (an interesting mix of sports and epidemiology, the sport of epidemiology, if you will). Since the CDC lists crypto in humans as one of the diseases indicative of immunodeficiency that qualifies one for a diagnosis of AIDS, since I was in a risk group, and since I had all other immunologic parameters indicative of AIDS, then, he said, it *had to be admitted* that I met the *technical* definition of AIDS.

Dr. C pointed out that the debate, in addition to being offensive, was Talmudic (the religion of epidemiology?). What, he asked, are we debating? At least a thousand individuals are believed to have died from ARC. These are people whose immunologic parameters match those of people with AIDS, but who have died from diseases that happen not to be on the CDC's arbitrary list. Does it mean much that they are therefore disqualified from a diagnosis of AIDS? . . .

As my own story illustrates, *AIDS* is a slippery term that is often sloppily used. From the standpoint of emotional anguish, having AIDS-Related Complex, lymphadenopathy, being antibody positive, or, for that matter, being a member of a so-called high risk group, differs from the experience of having CDC-defined AIDS mostly as a matter of degree.

The stigma attached to the so-called lesser forms of AIDS is essentially the same as for strict, CDC-defined AIDS. Those in the "general population" who are afraid of AIDS don't bother to make distinctions between AIDS, ARC, and lymphadenopathy. . . . The parents of a gay man who has flown home to announce that he has been diagnosed with AIDS-Related Complex won't hear much beyond the word *AIDS*. . . .

Much anxiety is caused by the fact that there really isn't a very good definition of ARC. . . . There are some doctors for whom the definition of ARC is a gay man with a cold, doctors who diagnose *Pneumocystis* over the phone. There are others who steadfastly withhold the diagnosis of ARC because they believe the term to be too vague. . . .

*

Finally, the stigma of AIDS often extends to *healthy* members of so-called high risk groups. In many unfortunate ways, the stigma I have suffered as a gay man *with AIDS* has been an exaggeration of the stigma I have suffered as a gay man. The imagery and language of *sickness*—mental, moral, and medical—link the perception of AIDS and gay maleness.

Growing up in Ohio during the '60s, the overwhelming message that I absorbed about my then-secret sexual desires was that I was "sick." Coming out as a gay man was for me a process of refuting the stigma of sickness and undoing all that damage in order to get on with the business of living and loving. But because AIDS imagery often resonates uncomfortably with the language of sickness historically associated with gayness, because in many circles gay maleness and AIDS are now synonymous, most discussion about AIDS implicitly if not explicitly communicates messages about gayness as well. I no doubt belabor the obvious when I state that the aggressive marketing of AIDS as a conflation of gay male sex, disease, and death is having a subtle but corrosive impact on many gay men's self-perceptions.

Today, gay men are often presumed guilty of AIDS until proven innocent. A gay male friend of mine was recently hospitalized with a herniated disk. Although otherwise completely healthy, blood precaution signs—the same as those used for AIDS—were put up outside his room. As a result, he now must continually confront the rumor that he has AIDS and is merely denying it.

   . . . AIDS has undoubtedly made being gay more difficult for many gay men; but it has also had the effect of making some gay men fight harder to convince themselves and the world that gayness is something to be proud of. As the success of the AIDS service organizations demonstrates, AIDS has encouraged some to come out who might never have done so under any other circumstances. And the sight of people mobilizing to take care of those in their community who are sick is a legitimate cause for pride. . . .

*

I'll end by saying that I'm a skeptic. If I believed everything I was told, if I believed that tiresome boilerplate that AIDS is "100 percent fatal," then I'd probably be dead by now. . . . If I didn't arm myself with information, with diverse views, I would be unable to defend myself from the madness and gibberish that daily assault those of us who have acquired immune deficiency syndrome.

(Surviving and Thriving with AIDS, 1987)

An Open Letter to the Planning Committees of the Third International Conference on AIDS

THE INTERNATIONAL WORKING GROUP ON WOMEN AND AIDS

AIDS is a women's issue.

—In the US, women are proportionately the fastest growing group of people with AIDS.

—In NYC, AIDS is the primary cause of death for women 25–29 years old.

—In the US, 51% of all women with AIDS are black and 21% are Latina, although blacks make up only 18% of the total US population, and Latinos 11%.

—The number of children with AIDS is doubling every 8–9 months; over 90% of affected children under 5 years old are children of color.

—50% of people with AIDS in Africa and the Caribbean are women.

—In Western Europe, women comprise 9% of cases; in Africa, the male-to-female ratio is almost 1:1.

AIDS is a women's issue, with a particularly devastating and disproportionate impact on the lives of women who have the disease, who have family or who live in communities beset with the disease, and who care for the people who are sick with the manifestations of HIV infection.

Throughout the world, women are the caretakers of the family and of the sick. Women comprise about 90% of all the nurses, social workers, educators, home health aides, and health workers. Women are the most poorly paid of all health workers and frequently are recruited from the populations already most severely affected by HIV-related disease.

Throughout the world, the burden of unpaid health services has always fallen to wives, mothers, grandmothers, sisters, aunts, daughters, and women friends. Volunteerism is increasingly seen as the answer to the escalating costs of caring for those with AIDS and ARC, without regard for the enormous burden this illness already places on those communities with the least support and resources from the health care delivery system.

Furthermore, AIDS offers a paradigm for all of the critical issues which impact on women:

—Deeply ingrained societal racism and sexism.

—Inadequate quality and inaccessibility of health care, including outpatient, hospice, and respite care as well as more traditional facilities.

—Absence of decent affordable housing, particularly for female-headed households, the impoverished, and the working poor.

—Insufficient child-care facilities and support services for raising children.

—Unequal educational opportunities and illiteracy.

—Underemployment and low paying jobs which enforce dependency on social service agencies.

—Devaluation of female sexuality as an important element of health and a part of our life experience, which has been suppressed and distorted by cultural insensitivities and overt discrimination.

Of particular concern is the paternalistic and cavalier disregard for the reproductive rights of women at highest risk for HIV infection. Because, historically, women of color have been repeatedly subject to forced sterilization and coerced family planning decisions, it is essential that all public health measures respect the dignity and autonomy of the pregnant woman. No meaningful reproductive options exist in the absence of adequate nutrition, prenatal and medical care, or without day care, education, and schooling for all children, including those born with disease or HIV positivity, and the availability of abortion on demand for women who choose it.

Women cannot be subject to compulsory, mandatory, "routine," or any other testing which is not entirely informed and voluntary. Testing mandates adequate counseling in a culturally sensitive manner using appropriate language. Anonymous testing and counseling must be available to women on request.

In this third international conference on AIDS, which has been a major forum for the discussion and definition of issues and problems involving AIDS, women are largely invisible except in two roles: as vectors for transmission either perinatally or (putatively) through prostitution. Even in those sessions that have focused on issues impacting on women's lives, for example heterosexual transmission, women are not adequately represented on the panels.

The International Women and AIDS Caucus insists that:

1. Women participate on the organizing, steering, and program committees for the international AIDS conferences in significant numbers.

2. A series of sessions on issues of concern to women be planned for the next international AIDS conferences.

3. Women's perspectives be represented in all sessions that address topics impacting on women and children.

4. Services be expanded to ensure accessibility to the conferences, including child care and sliding scale based on income, and travel subsidies.

We recognize that other affected groups have been similarly disenfranchised by the conference organizers and therefore support similar inclusion for all who have been excluded.

We believe that these recommendations carry the possibility of bringing us all closer to our mutual goal: victory over this devastating epidemic — the foremost public health challenge of our lifetime.

(*Newsline,* no. 25, July–August, 1987)

Needed (For Women and Children):

SUKI PORTS

AIDS is the major killer of women between the ages of twenty-five and thirty-four in New York City. In December of 1985, there were 487 women and 103 babies with AIDS. The majority were black, Hispanic, Asian, Native American, and "unknown other." Exactly two years later, in December 1987, the numbers in New York had risen to 1,364 women with AIDS and 231 pediatric cases — with the majority again being disproportionately from minority communities. AIDS occurs mainly among the poor, whose opportunities for obtaining comprehensive services during pregnancy or illness, at death, and for survivor children are slight. Appropriate housing, family case management, child care, and mental health support systems are even more limited, and AIDS has only exacerbated this situation.

Women are normally the care givers for the ill, so when they themselves become ill, who will care for them? There is no inclusive coordinated care system in place for them. We must not continue the patchwork, band-aid approach to AIDS care for women. Comprehensive extended support systems must be developed for families — whether traditional nuclear families, extended families, single sex couples and lovers with children, or the growing numbers of single parent families.

The fastest growing numbers of AIDS cases are among women, and, again, this means primarily minority women (eighty-four percent in New York City). While black and Hispanic women are disproportionately and increasingly affected by AIDS, the media insensitively and incorrectly tells us that the heterosexual spread of AIDS is not really a threat. How does a black or Hispanic woman feel when she hears this? Prostitutes, of course, continue to receive headlines, but only to be scapegoated as "vectors" of the disease, even though female-to-male transmission is considerably less common (or documented) than male-to-female transmission. Women have not achieved full equality in the job market, let alone in bed, and yet condom ads continue to place the necessity of protected sex on women.

While women have displayed incredible stamina, courage, and resourcefulness, AIDS has played a cruel trick upon their coping skills. Their strength is sapped caring for children, preparing meals, cleaning, shopping, and doing laundry—leaving little energy for personal care or the mother's additional duties of relating to schools, taking her children to the park or on special outings. Exhaustion is compounded by a sense of isolation. Among the factors that contribute to this additional impact of AIDS upon women are fear of eviction if neighbors find out that they or their children have AIDS, loss of support if the extended family finds out, loss of a lover or husband, "coping" if drugs are in any way involved, dismissal of their children from school if other parents or school board members find out. The low-income mother faced—alone—with these seemingly never-ending problems does not have recourse to, say, insurance-paid psychiatric counseling—a need that is of primary importance for anyone faced with HIV infection, both at the time of diagnosis and during the extended process of explaining such information to children, family, or friends.

Counseling, as an aid to coping and healing for those affected by AIDS, is generally frustrated by the limited availability of personnel who can relate to specific ethnic, racial, class, or language needs. The counselor must be able to deal effectively and with compassion with a broad range of psychosocial concerns, often including confronting a drug problem in whatever way it might be manifested. For adults, there is the need to face death and to make practical as well as emotional decisions about children. For children in a family affected by AIDS there are equally powerful and emotionally complex issues. One young nine-year-old recently stated, "When Mommy dies, it will be my fault." No counselor of the same ethnic background was immediately willing to visit the home of this young boy. AIDS often means that young people must come to an understanding of the illness and/or death of the person closest to them. It also means that they must comprehend why certain other parents might forbid their children to play with them, or why even a family member might shun them. And it means they have to face the fears they have now and, more frighteningly, an ultimate grief upon the death of a loved one, which they might have to bear alone or with little immediate or sustained empathy.

NEEDED: An appropriate means of dealing with death in a family, tailored to the needs of individual children of different ages. If we do not train people now, we will face—unprepared—thousands of children left behind by the deaths of their mothers, fathers, or both. This loss, this legacy of children left behind and unable to cope with their grief, will precipitate a crisis that we have yet to tackle in any nationwide or community-specific manner. We have an entire generation of physically well (or possibly potentially ill) children to plan for and protect.

—Originally diagnosed and hospitalized with tuberculosis, Jane, the grandmother of a three-year-old boy, was soon diagnosed with AIDS. Because there was no nursing home willing to care for her, she lived the next seven—and final—months of her life in a major urban hospital. Already overburdened with an average daily caseload of forty-five people with AIDS or other HIV-related illnesses, the hospital's infectious disease, psychiatric, and social support personnel interpreted Jane's early signs of AIDS-related dementia as nothing other than a grandmother's senility or lack of cooperativeness. Generally on alternate-level (as opposed to acute) care, Jane was resented by a staff forced to attend to her when they knew that what she really needed was a nursing care facility. Jane, in turn, resented their lack of attention. At some point during her hospitalization, her lower plate was lost, and its replacement was not a high priority on anyone's list but Jane's. Her once dry sense of humor and winsome smile contrasted sharply with the erratic and uncooperative behavior of this often cranky and complaining woman, whose facial appearance had now changed as much as her temperament. On one of my visits to another patient in her room I discovered that Jane and I were "twins"—sharing the same birth date and year. We compared stories of our "grands," and she always spoke of her sadness at missing out on seeing her grandson grow up. The little boy finally did see his grandmother . . . he was all dressed up in a gray suit and matching tie, shiny black shoes, and a look of puzzlement as he was walked past her open coffin.

NEEDED: A change in funding streams, which will provide, from the federal to the city level, housing for indigent seniors, including and especially those with AIDS. A little far-sightedness will ultimately result in fiscal soundness. The needs of senior citizens are the same as those of PWAs—ramps, handrails, elevators, doors with wheelchair and/or stretcher access, and spaces for group social activities including meals, family meetings, outpatient medical care, and private counseling. The housing required by both groups could be built into any rehabilitation of abandoned structures. Per diem costs would be far less than the toll now paid in actual dollars and in the demoralization of personnel, to say nothing of that of clients.

NEEDED: The funding necessary to enable care givers to get special training that would not only provide them with the most accurate and updated AIDS information to help them respond to PWAs' myriad questions, but take into account the extraordinary stress and strain of such a health care service by building-in adequate internal support and respite systems for all workers. AIDS care must not be static, lacking in compassion, or inadequate because of ignorance or overwork.

NEEDED: The ability to provide other than acute medical care for low-income PWAs, i.e., dental care, mental health counseling, and planning for legal and other business needs for both PWAs and their families.

NEEDED: Additional auxiliary personnel who have the time to consider and plan for the fulfillment of human needs. Jane, whose long life ended separated from family, and with the added indignity of not being able to eat well due to the lack of lower teeth, is but one painful example of an overburdened system's turning its back on the needs of individuals. Low-income communities cannot produce the same numbers of volunteers ("candy stripers") as the more affluent communities, which have both public and private hospitals within their boundaries.

—Mary was a tall, statuesque, thirty-one-year-old woman who became weak and thin almost before your eyes. Oral thrush made it difficult for her to talk and, consequently, difficult for her boyfriend to communicate with her. He eventually became discouraged by this, as well as by Mary's countless trips to the hospital's inpatient and outpatient clinics, and so he left her—which, needless to say, sent Mary into a deep depression. Only the stern intervention of a very caring infectious disease physician made the boyfriend see the vital role he played in both her physical and emotional health.

NEEDED: Time and funds for additional trained staff to participate in the education of family members—including lovers—and neighbors of PWAs. Where appropriate, family reconciliation needs to be nurtured.

—Betty, who had a teenage daughter, acted like a spoiled, manipulative adolescent herself. She frequently suffered from boredom, which caused her moods to swing dramatically from those of a crying, wily childlike person, who begged for cigarettes and specific candy or food, to a completely uncooperative patient whose abusive behavior was directed primarily at the overburdened nursing staff.

NEEDED: The availability of a TV in a social setting. This space might also serve as a place where some vocational or other training classes (i.e., writing skills or crafts) might be taught. Such an allotted space within an institution would allow patients who are sometimes in the hospital for long periods of time the opportunity to occupy themselves, while also providing them with valuable information that we mistakenly assume they get by osmosis. It could be the location for the dissemination of reading materials and information about AIDS, ranging from general home precautionary guidelines to practical nutrition recommendations. Nutrition information cannot be taken for granted within poor communities. AIDS care is completely out of step with the needs of people who must make their purchases on food stamps or whose ethnically oriented local grocery stores limit the availability of certain foods.

—Rosa, with five children from ages two to twenty, struggled with her religious upbringing and country of origin's traditions and finally decided it would be most responsible if she aborted her sixth child and had her tubes tied.

She did not count on the fact that this very difficult personal decision would be met by a three-week delay due to fear and unwillingness to deal with an HIV-infected woman on the part of a surgeon, a lab technician, and a nurse. After going through the humiliation of rejection by one medical staff person after another, she finally was scheduled for an overnight stay. We asked the appropriate city agency that child care be provided by a caretaker who was familiar to the children and who was willing to spend the night, although existing norms place children in temporary foster care. During the surgical procedure Rosa's uterus was perforated, thus requiring that a total hysterectomy be performed. She remained in pain many hours after returning to her room because no one had written orders for medication for this procedure. Given the lack of attention to Rosa's immediate health needs, it should come as no surprise that no one authorized the extension of the child care for the entire week now required for her hospitalization.

NEEDED: Coordination and sharing of information and training of all hospital personnel, particularly those who might come into contact with AIDS-related problems, and not only those in infectious disease units. Social services must be sufficiently organized and coordinated with medical personnel so that, for example, the infectious disease staff can alert general surgery (or others) when a particular patient might be hospitalized for a reason other than AIDS.

NEEDED: Child and family care based upon a Family Case Management system responsive to the needs of any member of a family in which there is a person with AIDS or HIV infection. This seemingly simple and commonsense need is not met because of existing rules for reimbursement, job definition, union work regulations, and scope of training. A major overhaul of child care and home care is long overdue, but AIDS-related needs have created a new crisis, and the gaps are glaring, as are the ramifications for affected families. In many cases the lowest-paid women are asked to provide the most support for difficult situations— without provisions for their own health, vacation, and other benefits.

—A mother with an income in the low twenty-thousand-dollar range has to quit work to take care of her child, who is HIV positive, because her income is too high to be eligible for free child care and too low to pay the going rates for private care. She cannot put her daughter in day care, as the child must be taken to a clinic weekly for medication and checkups. The mother's welfare payments do not cover her rent increase, the extra carfares needed to go to and from the hospital, extra pampers and special foods required by the child so as to avoid effects of diarrhea. As if it were not enough that this woman, who has never been on welfare, must face the emotional stress of a change in financial status and the painful realities of a child sick with a life-threatening disease (which might engender feelings of guilt and inadequacy on her part), she must also deal with the possibility of losing her home.

—Another mother is single and weak with AIDS. She qualifies for home care, but her children, who are healthy, might be sent to foster care because the adult-care worker is reporting that the mother neglects her children. Existing regulations do not require or even permit the home attendant assigned to an adult to feed the children the same food prepared for the mother. A duplication of workers is provided only after further reports of "neglect." This loving mother, who wishes to keep her family intact as long as possible, is faced with the "choice" of sending them to foster care or having neglect charges filed against her. The final result was that her children were placed in the home of strangers.

NEEDED: The development of a new definition of AIDS family care givers, with special training in AIDS care for any and all members of a "family." Perhaps the Peace Corps could serve as a model for a program that would draw people from a variety of backgrounds, including mothers whose children have grown up and left the nest, recent graduates with related academic interests who are undecided in career choice; these people might also include women who had been incarcerated and had received a special training certificate while institutionalized, or women on welfare who would be allowed to augment payments or who could get off welfare entirely, having been trained with skills for a new family health care career.

The foregoing examples of women who have experienced a multitude of problems with the onset of AIDS or HIV infection — either their own or that of a member of their family — represent but a glimpse of the multi-dimensional effects of AIDS upon women. But of what women are we speaking? For the most part, women who have lived difficult lives already: women who are (or were) drug users or who have been sexually involved with a drug user. They are also women who generally have low incomes, who have had little opportunity for higher education, and who have limited job opportunities. In the United States they are, for the most part, black and Hispanic. As a group of women at the Third International Conference on AIDS in June of 1987 stated, "AIDS offers a paradigm for all of the critical issues which impact upon women" (see pp. 166–168).

—A young black mother recently stated, with tears in her eyes, gripping the hand of her husband, "If it was not for Robert's support and being there, I would have committed suicide. When my baby was born she was beautiful. Now my baby is dying of AIDS."

—Lisette, when well enough to be ambulatory, helps older patients eat, combs their hair, acts as a nurse's aide and personal care giver, and is generally an outgoing spirit-picker-upper. But she has recently been depressed. She worries about her baby (age three) who is now seropositive, and her only healthy child (an adolescent), who just had an abortion. Lisette lost her husband, middle child, and a stepsister to AIDS. She has tried to commit suicide. Abused as a young girl, Lisette escaped from the world of school into a world of sex and drugs and became pregnant at sixteen. She cautions young women, "Learn more about life and yourself before trying to raise a family."

But we must ask: What are responsible adults doing to ensure that adolescents are getting specific AIDS prevention information? What is the prevailing knowledge among teenagers? What precautions are they taking?

In the December 1987 issue of *New Youth Connections, NYC,* the results of a survey from the previous month were printed in an article entitled "Thinking about AIDS." It is a sobering look at what teens believe in the city with the highest case incidence of AIDS in the world:

— Thirty-three percent think that you can only get AIDS by having sexual relations with a gay man.

— Sixty-eight percent of the sexually active readers who responded either never or only sometimes use a condom.

— Forty-two percent know people who shoot drugs.

While young people continue to shoot drugs, have unprotected sex, and get pregnant at the same alarming rates as before the advent of the AIDS epidemic, adults on school boards and boards of education are embroiled in emotional, diversionary controversies about sex education — how explicit to be about sex and drugs; whether methods of birth control, which are the only available artificial methods of preventing AIDS, should be discussed, displayed, or distributed.

If we are to ensure the well-being of our children, we must aggressively pursue the education, follow-up education, and, even more importantly, the follow-up counseling of adolescents, who are at the stage in life during which they are least receptive to adult intervention — when they are confronted with adulthood themselves, an adulthood that includes the challenge and excitement of sex and drugs.

If we are to ensure and encourage stable environments and compassionate care for PWAs, we must educate family members and communities to respond to those in need of care. Family case management is critical, but existing informal networks must also be encouraged. Only such steps will help kill the climate of fear about AIDS.

If we are to ensure that those already infected receive the best care, regardless of insurance coverage or class status, we must provide ongoing education to current care givers, create new sources of care givers, and provide respite and support for those providing care.

Because AIDS has disproportionately affected black and Hispanic women and children, future planning must involve the input of black and Hispanic women at the highest levels. We must base care and planning upon the most accurate knowledge and the most creative and promising guesses we can make, while also providing the compassion and coordination of services so lacking now. We must anticipate; we cannot luxuriate in testing the limits of women's endurance. Prevention, yes, and foresight based upon what is happening now. New policy issues will be arising in proportion to new situations, such as the lack of housing for adolescents with AIDS or HIV positivity. In New York City we must develop policy recommendations based upon large minority caseloads in a city torn apart by racism. While we may have the ability, the question is whether we have the will, the will to act immediately — to provide care and services for those already affected/infected and to inform and protect others from contracting this devastating disease.

CAROL LEIGH

"Deviants"

According to the figures of the National Task Force on Prostitution, there are from one to one and one-half million prostitutes in the US today. The average length of a prostitute's career is less than four years. In spite of the fact that nearly ten percent of the female population have worked as prostitutes, and many others have worked in other capacities in the sex business, sex workers are assumed to be a very small minority of the female population—the exception rather than one of the many rules regarding women's lives. Fear of stigma prevents this truth from coming out, as prostitutes remain closeted to their closest friends and families, even when they are in the midst of sex-business careers. Ex-prostitutes (and other women and men who have worked in the sex business) are often quick to disavow their histories, and as part of the process join in the censorship of those currently working. This cycle determines that there will be few advocates for the rights of sex workers.

Feminist debates within and among prostitutes' groups center on whether prostitution should be considered a forced or chosen profession. The women of WHISPER (Women Hurt in Systems of Prostitution Engaged in Revolt) focus on the exploitation, hypocrisy, and destructive socialization entailed in prostitution. COYOTE (Call Off Your Old Tired Ethics) emphasizes the range of prostitutes' experiences and works actively for prostitutes' rights. US Pros, concerned with women who work on the street, stresses economic analysis and also works for prostitutes' rights. But however prostitution is analyzed, as sex workers within the movement we must insist on the necessity of recognizing the contributions of prostitutes, both men and women, and accepting them as full and equal members of the community. We must work to dispel the myths that stigmatize us and divide us from one another and from other supposedly deviant communities. Especially in the midst of the AIDS epidemic, we must fight to protect everyone's right to engage in consensual sex. And we must fight against all those who would use this crisis as an excuse to legislate or otherwise limit sexuality.

The Crisis: A Personal History

In 1983, Priscilla Alexander and Margo St. James of COYOTE began warning me about a mysterious disease that was affecting gay men, and they insisted that I use condoms to protect my health. I did not respond immediately. I was trying to earn money to finance the production of a play I'd written. I had only five or six clients at the time, and they were not using condoms.

Prior to the epidemic, I'd been working as part of a network of call girls who shared a relatively elite clientele in San Francisco. We were a group of educated women using sex work to supplement careers in real estate, law, word processing, and the arts. Some of us had previously been teachers, others were paying for educations, and still others had begun as street prostitutes and worked their way up. Our clients were stockbrokers, bankers, lawyers, business executives, and middle management, white-collar workers, both single and married. In these circles, many men objected to the use of condoms, and in such a highly competitive milieu I found it too stressful to insist. Friends that worked outside of our network (in the street or in massage parlors) were extremely critical of the practices of call girls, who charged less and gave more time for the privilege of working in a system that provided a steady base of affluent, referred clients, and thus eliminated the risks of encountering strangers who could turn out to be police or rapists.

As time went on, COYOTE's warnings became more urgent. The news media began to be filled with horror stories about heterosexual transmission: "Prostitute Spreads AIDS" was a typically hysterical headline. I became terrified that I might have AIDS. Every cold seemed to portend a shameful death. Confronted by my mortality, I was overwhelmed with fear.

News of AIDS created an undercurrent of panic in our midst. We spoke for hours on the phone, as call girls do, discussing our fears and risks, vowing to abandon condom-phobic customers. Some of us began relying more on individual, wealthy clients. Others shifted their focus to family and schoolwork. Most of us were tested for exposure to HIV; none of us tested positive. Clients I'd been seeing for years left, vowing celibacy or monogamy. Business dropped off by twenty-five to fifty percent.

As the danger of AIDS to heterosexuals attracted more media attention, police stepped up the enforcement of laws against prostitution. Working girlfriends who had provided discreet services for many years began getting busted —after providing those services to a policeman. There is almost always a violation of rights in a prostitution bust, because enforcement of the law in victimless crimes requires entrapment. Often prostitutes' money and records are confiscated and disappear before court appearances. In most cities, police take condoms away from prostitutes during arrests; sometimes they simply punch holes in the condoms.

In January 1986, a law took effect in California making it a crime to *agree* to

take money for providing sexual services. Before, prostitutes were arrested—
theoretically—only for solicitation, for initiating the sexual contract. This new
law legalizes entrapment, in obvious violation of our civil rights. Police use this
law, together with new enforcement priorities, to arrest prostitutes who work
discreetly and privately, advertising in newspapers and sex-business journals. In
depositions taken at the 1987 Hookers' Convention, a large percentage of
women reported that police often engaged in sex with them as part of the arrest
procedure—obviously a form of rape.

Violations of our rights are nothing new to us. Some of us, survivors of
incest and child abuse, have weathered greater traumas using strategies of avoidance and compromise. The majority of prostitutes, like the majority of women in
general, are accustomed to seeing violations of our rights written into law. As
disenfranchised citizens, prostitutes are sometimes at the mercy of the violent
and exploitative men (and women) to whom we turn for protection from law
enforcement agencies. The situation is worse for poor women, especially blacks
and Hispanics, who are forced to work on the street because escort services and
massage parlors almost exclusively employ whites and Asians.

Five years after COYOTE's first warnings about AIDS, most of us are still
involved in the business, although we're earning less, working longer hours, and
having to supplement our incomes. It took me about a year to accept my
mortality, to resolve the fact that it is no shame to die. It took less time to
rearrange my priorities. I gave up my play, my apartment, and the clients that
still balked about using condoms, and I moved away from the city to escape the
media barrage. After leaving San Francisco I looked for opportunities to educate
other prostitutes about AIDS, and other AIDS activists about the violations of
prostitutes' rights.

Prostitutes as Educators

Since the onset of the AIDS epidemic, many prostitutes have been eager to
assume roles as safe sex educators. CAL-PEP (California Prostitutes Education
Project), a COYOTE offshoot, was recently awarded a $40,000 grant by the
California State Department of Health for the purpose of educating street prostitutes about safe sex and IV hygiene. In city- and state-funded programs such as
the Mid-city Consortium to Combat AIDS, in San Francisco, prostitutes and
ex-prostitutes in drug treatment centers and halfway houses assume key roles as
social workers providing much needed outreach to street communities. Prostitutes' rights organizations in some cities have organized support groups to discuss
a range of personal issues, including safe sex, IV hygiene, and HIV testing.

Prostitutes' rights advocates insist upon the necessity of consulting working
prostitutes on all matters that affect our situation, including treatment and
job-training programs. Policymaking must include outreach to the sex workers'
community.

Mandatory HIV Testing of Prostitutes

Legislation has been passed in some states, and is under consideration in many others, requiring mandatory HIV tests for anyone convicted of prostitution. Other legislation makes it a felony for prostitutes knowing they are HIV antibody positive to provide sexual services, even if their sexual practices are completely safe (e.g., manual stimulation). Such legislation scapegoats prostitutes because of our current status as outlaws and our traditional role as symbols of "immoral" sexual behavior. Violations of the rights of prostitutes as a means of allaying the unfounded fears of the "general public" is a diversionary tactic often devised by public officials who are perfectly aware of prostitutes' negligible impact on the spread of AIDS. The fear of "contamination" by prostitutes is not based in fact. Here are some of the real facts:

— According to the US Department of Health, prior to the AIDS epidemic prostitutes were involved in only three to five percent of cases of venereal disease in this country (in contrast, teenagers accounted for thirty-five percent). Current studies show that prostitutes practice safe sex with their clients.

— In a study conducted by AWARE (Association of Women's AIDS Research and Education) at San Francisco General Hospital, prostitutes showed no higher incidence of seropositive HIV test results than other women with three to five sexual partners per year. Seropositivity in prostitutes is confined to IV drug users, who comprise only ten percent of prostitutes. (Drug treatment programs must be designed to meet the needs of IV drug using prostitutes, and HIV tests must not be a prerequisite for eligibility. Livable income and job training alternatives must be provided for all those who want to stop working in the sex business. Special assistance must be provided to those exposed to HIV.)

— Mandatory testing and reporting of results will discourage participation in studies. Anonymity must be preserved to protect the rights of those choosing to be tested for their own information.

— Although mandatory testing purports to protect the clients of prostitutes (at the expense of prostitutes) by supposedly ensuring a "clean" pool of sex workers, test results do not necessarily indicate actual antibody status. Factors such as a possible six-month lapse time between infection and seroconversion, and the high numbers of false positives, limit the reliability of these tests. Mandatory testing can give clients a false sense of security and discourage safe sex practices.

— Many women are forced into prostitution by violence, both mental and physical. Mandatory testing and escalated charges are further forms of violence against these women and create greater dependence on abusive pimps. (Prostitutes must have the right to responsible management.)

— Only ten percent of those arrested in prostitution cases are clients. Laws against prostitution are therefore enforced in a discriminatory manner against women, particularly poor women of color. Although considerably less than half of all prostitutes in this country are women of color, they comprise eighty-five percent of those sentenced to prison for prostitution.

— Quarantining antibody positive prostitutes by charging them with felonies serves no purpose except to stigmatize and violate the civil rights of these people. Legislation already exists to cover any intentional infliction of bodily harm.

— Since sex is not defined in these new laws creating harsher sentences, those who engage in activities such as manual stimulation and fantasy-oriented sex can also be charged with felonies. This scapegoating legislation sets a precedent for criminalizing participation in erotic experiences for anyone who is HIV positive, even if practices are 100 percent safe.

AIDS is not a crime. We must defeat all legislation that violates the rights of those with AIDS and ARC, those testing HIV antibody positive, and those stigmatized as belonging to "high risk" categories. We must reclaim and protect the rights of gay people, prostitutes, prisoners, undocumented foreigners, mental health clients, IV drug users, hemophiliacs — all of whom are especially vulnerable during this epidemic. We are rarely allowed to speak for ourselves and we must therefore work toward self-empowerment and demand to be heard.

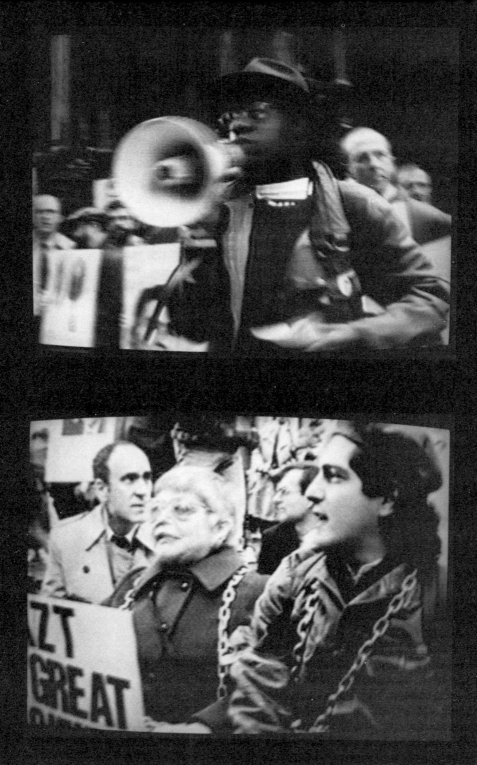

Testing the Limits: New York. 1987.

GREGG BORDOWITZ

As a twenty-three-year-old faggot, I get no affirmation from my culture. I see issues that affect my life—the issues raised by AIDS—being considered in ways that will probably end my life. For this reason I think that if there is to be a movement that will shift the discussion of AIDS away from the moralizing, punitive attitude that has characterized this country's policy, it will be built out of an emergent popular culture, one that affirms the lives of those affected. It will be a counterculture that will grow out of a broad-based mobilization to end the global epidemic.

There are already moves to contain this growing activism. Threats of mass mandatory HIV antibody testing and quarantine are written in banner headlines. Certain individuals and groups have already been subject to such assaults—within those institutions where surveillance is most easily enforced. This is not even to mention the discrimination people living with AIDS (PLWAs) have faced in all aspects of social life. The first targets of repression are, as always, the most disenfranchised. Thus, New York City's health commissioner Stephen Joseph has recently called for consideration of "mandatory AIDS testing [*sic*] for prostitutes and sex and drug offenders, as well as a heavy crackdown on all forms of prostitution."[1]

What purpose will enforced testing serve? Test results will establish much more than the extent to which a population has been exposed to a virus. Their

1.   Ronald Sullivan, "AIDS Test Is Weighed in Sex Cases," *New York Times*, November 21, 1987, p. B30.
On December 10, 1987, members of the Metropolitan Health Association, an affinity group of gay AIDS activists, staged a peaceful sit-in at the office of Health Commissioner Stephen Joseph to protest what MHA member David Harris called "Joseph's malign neglect of widespread explicit educational efforts to stem the course of AIDS in favor of punitive measures scapegoating the most vulnerable and disenfranchised members of society." Their list of demands included "an end to Dr. Joseph's flailing about on the AIDS issue. Long-term planning is needed today to prepare for an excess of 100,000 New Yorkers who will have AIDS and AIDS-related illnesses by 1991. There is no time for false posturing on testing in an attempt to appear tough on the problem, while doing far too little to create workable solutions." Eight MHA members were arrested after Joseph refused to state publicly that he would reconsider his position.

purpose is to identify an entire social group on the basis of the presence of antibodies. A whole new class of people will be designated as seropositives. The limits of the AIDS community will be established.

What is really being tested? The limits of control that can be exerted over our bodies. The limits of constraint that can be placed on our actions.

We are being tested. The Reagan Administration spends funds for costly, inefficient testing programs instead of for medical research, preventive education, and health care. This misuse of our tax dollars and neglect of our real needs tests the limits of our tolerance. It tests the limits of our will to fight back.

We in the communities affected by this epidemic will not stand for further intrusion into our already disempowered lives. Through direct action we will wrest control of the public discussion of AIDS. Through direct action we will make known the demands of the sick. Through direct action we will establish a national health care policy in the interests of people living with AIDS.

Drastic measures are being adopted. Activists are taking to the streets, making demands on their elected officials. Activists are providing alternative health care, educating their communities, researching alternative treatments. Activists are producing alternative media.

When circumstances require that drastic measures be adopted, independent media activists assume a central role. This role is twofold: to assist other activists in clarifying their positions and goals, and to represent those positions and goals to the world. Adopting the agenda of AIDS activists, media activists make armed propaganda.[2]

Video activists are everywhere met with the same challenges. We must call into question the established structures of the media. We must create new ways to make and distribute media. We must work toward participatory forms of representation that incorporate people into the communication process.

In the AIDS crisis, all of this must be done in order to facilitate moves toward the treatment and cure of AIDS and ARC, the distribution of preventive education materials, and the protection of civil rights. Video activists must clarify

---

2.   "The guerrilla expresses him or herself basically through armed activities, even if sometimes he or she uses other means of communication with people, like papers, pamphlets, radio messages, interference on radio and TV stations. . . . Armed propaganda takes on special importance . . . when it is a question of clarifying for the people, in periods when drastic measures must be adopted, positions whose goals are not sufficiently clear and which, thus, are difficult for the working-class mind to understand" (Actas Tupamaras, "Tactics of the Urban Guerrilla" [1971], quoted in Armand Mattelart, "For a Class and Group Analysis of Popular Communication Practices," in Seth Siegelaub and Armand Mattelart, eds., *Communication and Class Struggle, Liberation, Socialism,* New York, International General, 1983, vol. 2, p. 20). Although the above quotation evidences voluntarist tendencies of revolutionary media theory regarding the "working-class mind," it adequately describes the radical potential of alternative media in times of struggle.

A war is being fought over our bodies. Thus, through civil disobedience we will use our bodies as means of contention. Continuing government inaction necessitates militancy. Even armed resistance may become necessary in response to widespread mandatory testing and/or quarantine.

situations, render relations, picture possibilities for the emerging AIDS movement.

*

In the spring of 1987 the Testing the Limits Collective, comprised of lesbians, gays, and straights, formed to document emerging forms of activism arising out of people's responses to government inaction in the global AIDS epidemic. The founding members of the collective, Sandra Elgear, Robyn Hutt, Hilery Joy Kipnis, David Meieran, and myself, are all activists who view our documentary work as organizing work. The productive capacity and efficacy of the collective's project depends on establishing and maintaining links with protest-oriented groups and support organizations in the communities affected by AIDS.

Most of the members of the collective are participating members of ACT UP (AIDS Coalition to Unleash Power), "a diverse, nonpartisan group united in anger and committed to direct action to end the global AIDS epidemic." ACT UP's first action was staged on Wall Street in March 1987 to protest the unavailability of promising drug treatments and the announcement by Borroughs-Wellcome that they would charge each patient up to $13,000 per year for AZT. Immediately following the action, at which seventeen people were arrested, the Food and Drug Administration announced plans to cut two years off the drug approval process. Media attention began to focus on drug treatment issues, and film of ACT UP's Wall Street demonstration became stock footage in subsequent reporting.

After this initial demonstration, ACT UP grew to be a core group of over 200 people. It coordinated the following actions in 1987:

— April 15th: A demonstration at the Main Post Office in New York City protesting the lack of tax dollars earmarked for AIDS research.

— June 1st: ACT UP joined other national activist organizations in civil disobedience at the White House. Washington police wore yellow rubber gloves as they arrested sixty-four people. Later that day, ACT UP demonstrated at the Third International Conference on AIDS. The civil disobedience garnered extensive international media attention. The second demonstration forced many public officials to break their seven-year silence.

— June 30th: A rally and civil disobedience in Federal Plaza, New York City, to protest mandatory testing, immigration policy, and the negligence of the federal, state, and local governments. Thirty-three people were arrested.

— July 21st: A four-day, around-the-clock protest at Memorial Sloan-Kettering Hospital, one of the four AIDS Treatment Evaluation Units (ATEUs) in New York funded by the National Institutes of Health (NIH). ACT UP called for the NIH to conduct more clinical trials on promising drugs other than AZT and to increase the number of PLWAs in these trials. As a result of this demonstration, ACT UP established an ongoing dialogue with all four ATEUs in New York City.

— August 4th: ACT UP quickly mobilized 100 people to protest Northwest Orient Airlines for refusing passage to PLWAs. In response to the demonstration and to law suits brought in conjunction with the Lambda Legal Defense League and the National Gay Rights Advocates, Northwest issued a policy statement that PLWAs will now be permitted to fly on the airline.

— September 9th: A demonstration at the National Press Building in Washington, D.C., where the Presidential Commission on the HIV Epidemic was meeting for the first time. Several ACT UP members testified before the commission. In addition, ACT UP formed a subcommittee that continues to supply certain commission appointees with accurate and thorough information.

— September 22nd: ACT UP sponsored a community forum consisting of a twenty-member roundtable discussion about the possibilities for coordinated actions focused on issues of education, civil liberties, and health care.[3]

Through participation in ACT UP at every level of its process, the Testing the Limits Collective has been able to document each of these events, resulting in material that was, in effect, produced by the entire membership of ACT UP. As a member of both the video collective and the activist organization, it was important to me to be able to integrate my participation into a single practice. Thus, within ACT UP, I insisted that my work as a documentarian be recognized as itself a form of activism. Such recognition is hard-won. Activist groups generally consider only the dominant media, to which they have a fundamentally contradictory relationship: seeing it as the enemy and at the same time seeking legitimation from it. Discussions of the media are often bogged down in such petty issues as how to write a good press release or how to get the organization two minutes coverage on local news broadcasts.[4] An activist group that expends too much of its energy on the presentation of its image before the dominant media only gives the impression that it is more interested in publicity than in achieving its goals through direct action.

Within ACT UP, Testing the Limits had to earn its support. We were initially regarded as hobbyists, just as we are by the mainstream media: we cannot get press passes and the network musclemen physically cast us aside because we don't have broadcast-level equipment. One of our tasks was therefore to educate the group about the importance of alternative media. We had to introduce and reintroduce ourselves as independent documentarians within the group. We arranged screenings to show people what we were doing. We had constantly to announce our intentions and explain our activities.

3.   All information taken from an ACT UP pamphlet.
4.   See Dee Dee Halleck, "A Few Arguments for the Appropriation of Television," *High Performance*, no. 37 (1987), pp. 38–44.

Through this process, it became clear that the production of documentary overlaps with the efforts of political organizing. In order to tear down the structures that house the "public discussion" of AIDS, we have to build alternative structures, structures that can generate and foster an affirmative culture for people living with AIDS.

As a member of ACT UP's Outreach Committee, I worked with others to establish relations with other AIDS activist and support groups. Such networking had also become the focus of Testing the Limits's project while documenting a teach-in, hosted by the *Village Voice*, at which many community representatives and groups were present. The collective also independently interviewed these organizations' members, including Suki Ports of the Minority Task Force on AIDS, Mitchell Karp of the Human Rights Commission's AIDS Discrimination Unit, and Yolanda Serrano of ADAPT (Association for Drug Abuse Prevention and Treatment).

The collective's videotaping coincided with and contributed to the work of the Outreach Committee in seeking to build a coalition between groups. In coorganizing the ACT UP-sponsored community forum in September 1987, I was able to get the participation of many of the community representatives with whom the collective had already worked. The community forum then generated still more documentary material, which was edited by Jean Carlomusto, producer of Gay Men's Health Crisis's cable program *Living with AIDS,* into a half-hour show broadcast on the program the following week.

All the material the collective produced within the first three months after its formation was compiled into a six-minute tape. Entitled *Testing the Limits,* the tape is a fast-paced trailer that serves as a short catalogue of resistance to government policy.[5] It draws on the experiences of people from many communities affected by the AIDS crisis. Taped in various social spaces around New York, people are shown in meeting halls, churches, parks, homes, in the studio, at rallies, demonstrations, forums.

Testing the Limits is scripted to the song "Living in Wartime" written by Michael Callen, a person living with AIDS and founding member of the PWA Coalition, and performed by the group Low Life.

> This is the time for doubting,
> To stop and wonder why.
> This is the time for shouting
> I don't believe the lies.
> One way or another
> No one will be spared.

---

5. The pilot was first described as a "catalogue of resistance" by Mark Dion. The designation is appropriate because the pilot tape is an "index" to the kinds of direct action being taken as well as to the documentary material that constitutes the tape.

Call out to my brothers
Doesn't anybody care?

We are living,
We are living in wartime.[6]

This song was used as a vehicle to organize information and propel the viewer
through the material. "Living in Wartime" figures far more significantly in the
tape than merely as a sound track. Both lyrics and melody are used as a formal,
rhetorical structure that narrativizes the roughly compiled material within the
tape. The song functions to organize the dense arrangement of information,
shaping it into a work of propaganda. This tape is an attempt to use the music
television form—a commodity form—as a form of truly popular culture. We
appropriated some of the tropes of MTV to deploy them as agit-prop.

The six-minute tape was used effectively as a VCR organizing tool,
screened in galleries, at meetings, fundraisers, and on cable TV. It was also
screened at the lesbian and gay film festivals in San Francisco, Chicago, and New
York. In addition, it functioned as a pilot for the collective's future documentary
projects.

*

Testing the Limits, the pilot tape, would become a model for a twenty-eight
minute video called *Testing the Limits: New York*. Like the pilot, this tape is a
catalogue of resistance drawn from the nearly 100 hours of video the collective
had produced. The collective made the decision to edit the material according to
voice, as opposed to image. We wanted to listen to what people had to say about
themselves and their situations.

Statements by activists from many communities were roughly ordered according to three areas of concern in the AIDS crisis: civil liberties, education, and
health care. The script was divided into three sections according to these categories, recognizing that each of the categories would be triangulated around every
issue, within each section. The collective discussed the many varied points of view
expressed in the material and arrived at editing decisions through a loose consensus process. We arranged and rearranged clusters of material according to the
particular relation of each of the members to the issues. Our task was complicated, sometimes painful, as our decisions had to be mediated by the multiplicity
of social relations in play.

This collective process resulted in a number of awkward juxtapositions

---

6.   "Living in Wartime," music and lyrics by Michael Callen, performed by Low Life, © Tops and
Bottoms, Inc., BMI.

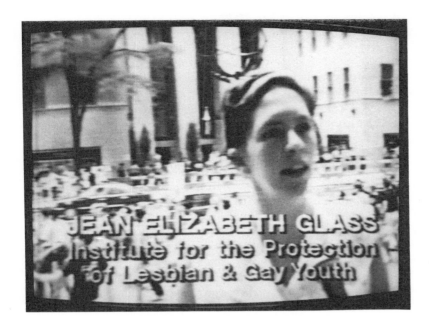

Testing the Limits: New York. 1987.

Jean Elizabeth Glass [a client of the Hetrick-Martin Institute, formerly the Institute for the Protection of Lesbian and Gay Youth]: "What's happening now in New York City is unthinkable: AIDS is now the leading cause of death for young men from the ages of eighteen to forty-four. Eighteen years old! That means they're contracting AIDS when? When they're fourteen? thirteen? fifteen? We're not educating these kids. AIDS is the leading cause of death in New York City in women twenty-six to thirty-seven. They caught it when? When they were eighteen? nineteen? They're not being educated. Obviously 'just say no' doesn't work for pregnancy. It doesn't work for veneral diseases like syphilis or gonorrhea. It's not going to work for AIDS.

One of the things that IPLGY does is tell kids the truth, and it's one of the few places that they get the truth. They're not getting it in the schools, they're not getting it in their homes, and they're not getting it on the street. At the institute, they at least have a shot to come in and ask very serious questions. Do I get AIDS if someone spits one me? Do I get AIDS if I have anal intercourse? Can I get AIDS from sucking my lover off? IPLGY uses terms that the kids understand. If you say 'anal intercourse,' they look at you like . . . 'what?' At least it's one place where you can come out and say 'fucking and sucking without a condom can give you AIDS.' The kids understand it and they respect it."

within the tape. One of the most jarring occurred in the section on education, in which a statement by Ruth Rodriguez of the Hispanic AIDS Forum was followed by a statement by Denise Ribble of the Community Health Project. Speaking in Spanish (subtitled in English), Rodriguez delivers an impassioned speech to members of her own community on issues of Latino representation and self-determination. Immediately following, Ribble describes the use of dental dams in lesbian safe sex practices. The conflict of the two segments involves more than the obvious. Rodriguez directly addresses the camera with a sense of rage. Then, relaxed in her clinical setting and clearly talking about something she enjoys, Ribble presents to the camera a piece of green latex, her "Christmas version" of the dental dam.

It is difficult to articulate what disturbed us about this juxtaposition. To my mind, we were confronted by our own internalized homophobia. We didn't think that a description of lesbian sexual practices should follow a statement about the cultural exclusion of the Latino community. We were afraid to risk offending the Latino community, assuming that that community would not view the issues as of equivalent importance.

This evidenced a historically specific discursive formation. For the sake of countering prevalent assumptions, such as "AIDS is a gay disease," many activists will deny that their sexual orientation is associated with their AIDS activism. This is counterbalanced by others who stress the problems the epidemic has posed for certain gay people to such an extent that they exclude recognition of the problems for anyone else. Regardless of intention, I think the collective, at times, recapitulated the homophobia exemplified by the former tendency. I think we experienced our own internalized AIDS-related homophobia. But there's no such thing as a thought crime. Editing occasioned a process that enabled us to work through some of the specular relations implicit in AIDS work. For me, each image that raised issues of sexuality was charged with questions about my own sexual orientation. Thus, I was forced to view issues of race, gender, and class as they figure in relation to gay sexual politics.

The juxtaposition between Ruth Rodriguez's statement and Denise Ribble's description did not seem to make sense at all, even though we had arrived at it through a reasoned process. In fact, what *does* make sense in the AIDS crisis would, in other circumstances, seem a non sequitur. The current situation involves a collision of issues that had existed before the epidemic. The response to the epidemic has thus enabled a number of groups to understand social injustices as systemic biases within society that affect all subaltern groups differently. For this reason, the experience of various issues by diverse groups must be rendered in terms of the common situation. Further, this compilation of experiences must be shown to result in a sense of shared goals.

In the end, we didn't retain the Rodriguez-Ribble juxtaposition. Other combinations of material seemed to approximate the historical conditions more accurately, according to the consensus of the collective. The entire section on

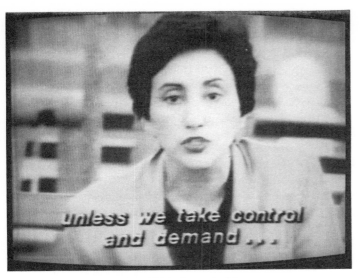

Ruth Rodriguez [Hispanic AIDS Forum]: "Our community needs education on the prevention of AIDS. That information has not reached us precisely because those who are in charge of protecting our rights, historically, have not done so and will not do so unless we take control and demand our rights for ourselves."

Denise Ribble [Community Health Project]: "For women, oral sex obviously constitutes a large part of what's going on. So we recommend dental dams. This is a dental dam. This is my Christmas version. A dental dam is a barrier between the virus and your body."

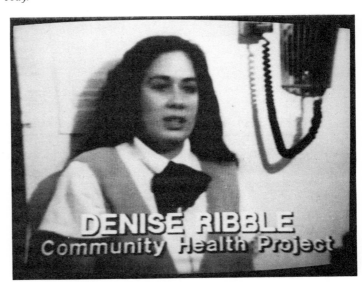

education became a collage in which issues of cultural sensitivity are formally anchored by Denise Ribble's safe sex instructions. These instructions are edited to intervene at regular intervals that determine the pace of what would otherwise seem arbitrary in the arrangement of material in the section. We arrived at this formal solution in view of our historical situation: experiences were grounded in a presentation of the principles of safe sex practices.

Editing decisions show the rough composition of issues that are the AIDS crisis, triangulated around civil liberties, education, and health care. This multiplicity is rendered — as voiced — by members of the affected communities. Concerns specific to each community are roughly juxtaposed. The single most important objective is to affirm the lives of people living with AIDS and the social relations these lives include. Finally, it is necessary to show courses of action that will bring about positive change. Protest and resistance must be militantly advocated.

Testing the Limits: New York is punctuated with powerful images of protest, explicitly intended to present direct action as the means to change. References to the print media and network television are occasionally introduced to situate the issues polemically in relation to the so-called public discussion of AIDS. The use of music serves a similar purpose, attempting to ground the tape in genuinely popular cultural production.

"Living in Wartime," the song used for the pilot, opened and closed the twenty-eight minute tape.

> They try to break our spirits.
> They try to keep us in our place.
> They do it to the women
> And the poor of every race.
> We face a common enemy,
> Bigotry and greed.
> But if we fight together
> We will find the strength we need.
>
> We are living,
> We are living in wartime.[7]

A section of the rap called "Respect Yourself," produced by the Philadelphia AIDS Task Force, was used in a transition between the section on civil liberties and that on education. The transition is a quick paced, diced selection of urban images contrasted with images of protest. Scripted with a simple theme of "movement" in mind, it is roughly edited to the rap beat.

---

7.   *Ibid.*

Be you a butcher, a baker, a candlestick maker,
AIDS don't care about the color of your skin.
You gotta keep your body strong.
Respect yourself and you will live long.[8]

The only other scored transition occurs between the sections on education and health care. A portion of the Romanovsky and Philips song "Homophobia" is played under a series of images about "touch." Shots of the Washington police wearing rubber gloves at a civil disobedience are paired with images of activists joining hands at the ACT UP civil disobedience at Federal Plaza in New York.

Now AIDS has claimed so many lives
And still there is no cure,
And if they don't spend more on research
It will keep on killing more.
Because it's called a gay disease
It's easy to ignore,
Which sounds a lot like blatant homophobia to me.[9]

Songs can succinctly render complex concerns in ways that are extremely accessible; music-making is central to building a popular culture. As we scripted sections of the tape to this music, it became clear that the collective's activity is part of an emerging cultural project.

*

The agenda of this project compels the video activist to organize the screening and distribution of material. People must be able to see themselves making history. People living with AIDS must be able to see themselves not as victims, but as self-empowered activists. In view of this agenda, distribution plans have to be fundamentally pragmatic: Generate as much material as possible. Show this material in as many forms and as many places as possible. Utilize every possible resource. Work by any means necessary.

The Testing the Limits collective has addressed issues of distribution by organizing its production as a self-generating process. The twenty-eight minute documentary is the "public image" for the work of the collective. As such, it is made to appeal to a wide audience. It has been screened in Los Angeles at the American Film Institute and in New York at both the New Museum of Contemporary Art and Global Village. Appropriate for broadcast, it is a means to

8.   "Respect Yourself," produced by Philadelphia Community Health Alternatives, Black and White Men Together, with the assistance of the US Conference of Mayors.
9.   "Homophobia," music and lyrics by Romanovsky and Philips, © 1985 Romanovsky and Philips. Thanks for their continuing commitment to lesbian and gay activism.

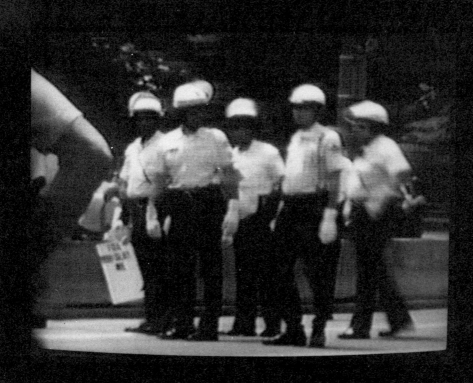

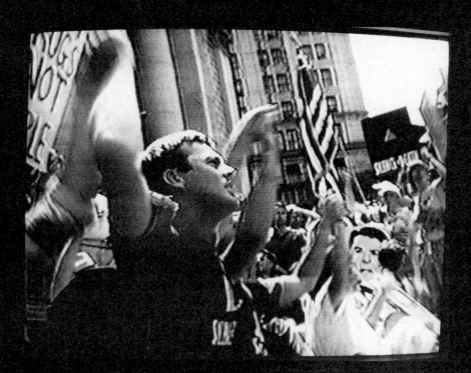

Testing the Limits: New York. 1987.

recognition and funding. More importantly, it provides an impetus to the community-based advocacy work in which the collective is engaged. Our material can be disseminated through local distribution, presented anywhere a screening is possible. The collective has a policy of sharing material with anyone in the movement. Aside from the local VCR circuit, material is fed to public access programs such as *Living with AIDS,* mentioned above, and *Out in the Eighties,* a gay cable TV show. It is possible to set up screenings anywhere. Some groups have organized screenings in parking lots, running tapes off the cigarette lighter of a station wagon, propping the TV on the tailgate.[10]

Imagine a screening. In a local community center a consumer VCR deck and a TV set sit on a table. Representatives from the various communities affected by AIDS sit in front of the TV. They watch a video composed of interviews with each of them. They see themselves pictured in relation to one another as they sit next to one another.

Consider this screening. It presents both means and ends for the video AIDS activist. The AIDS movement, like other radical movements, creates itself as it attempts to represent itself. Video puts into play the means of recognizing one's place within the movement in relation to that of others in the movement. Video has the potential to render the concerted efforts—as yet unimagined—between groups. The most significant challenge to the movement is coalition building, because the AIDS epidemic has engendered a community of people who cannot afford *not* to recognize themselves as a community and to act as one.

The AIDS epidemic has caused us to change our behavior. It has shaped our social relations as it has changed our views of ourselves. This became apparent to me recently, after coming out to my family. I realized that I had come out as a member of two disenfranchised groups. I am a member of the gay community and a member of the AIDS community. Furthermore, I am a gay member of the AIDS community, a community that some would establish by force, for no other end but containment, toward no other end but repression, with no other end but our deaths—a community that must, instead, establish *itself* in the face of this containment and repression. We must proudly identify ourselves as a coalition.

Picture a coalition of people refusing to be victims.

Picture a coalition of people distributing condoms and clean works.

Picture a coalition of people having safe sex and shooting up with clean works.

Picture a coalition of people staging a die-in in front of City Hall or the White House until massive funds for AIDS are released.

Picture a coalition of people getting arrested for blocking traffic during rush hour as they stand in the middle of Times Square kissing one another.

10.   See Halleck, p. 40.

Picture a coalition of people occupying abandoned buildings, demanding that they be made into hospices for people living with AIDS.

Picture a coalition of people chanting "Money for AIDS, not for war" as they surround and quarantine the Pentagon.

The government and the medical establishment denounce as "immoral" the people who get sick and the people they hope will get sick. They worry about themselves, their children, and the "innocent victims." They predict the kinds of people who get AIDS, the numbers of people infected, the numbers of deaths that will occur. But they are doing next to nothing to cure the sick and prevent the spread of AIDS.

People are asking, "If they won't do anything now, when will they?" "If they won't do anything for those who are sick now, for whom will they?"

Getting no answers, people are mobilizing.

Getting no answers, a movement is emerging.

Picture a coalition of people who *will* end this epidemic.

Is the Rectum a Grave?

LEO BERSANI

to the memory of Robert Hagopian

*These people have sex twenty to thirty times
a night. . . . A man comes along and goes
from anus to anus and in a single night will
act as a mosquito transferring infected cells
on his penis. When this is practised for a
year, with a man having three thousand
sexual intercourses, one can readily understand this massive epidemic that is currently
upon us.*

—Professor Opendra Narayan,
The Johns Hopkins Medical School

*I will leave you wondering, with me, why it
is that when a woman spreads her legs for a
camera, she is assumed to be exercising free
will.*

—Catherine A. MacKinnon

Le moi *est haïssable. . . .*

— Pascal

There is a big secret about sex: most people don't like it. I don't have any
statistics to back this up, and I doubt (although since Kinsey there has been no
shortage of polls on sexual behavior) that any poll has ever been taken in which
those polled were simply asked, "Do you like sex?" Nor am I suggesting the need
for any such poll, since people would probably answer the question as if they

were being asked, "Do you often feel the need to have sex?" and one of my aims will be to suggest why these are two wholly different questions. I am, however, interested in my rather irresponsibly announced findings of our nonexistent poll because they strike me as helping to make intelligible a broader spectrum of views about sex and sexuality than perhaps any other single hypothesis. In saying that most people don't like sex, I'm not arguing (nor, obviously, am I denying) that the most rigidly moralistic dicta about sex hide smoldering volcanoes of repressed sexual desire. When you make this argument, you divide people into two camps, and at the same time you let it be known to which camp you belong. There are, you intimate, those who can't face their sexual desires (or, correlatively, the relation between those desires and their views of sex), and those who know that such a relation exists and who are presumably unafraid of their own sexual impulses. Rather, I'm interested in something else, something both camps have in common, which may be a certain *aversion*, an aversion that is not the same thing as a repression and that can coexist quite comfortably with, say, the most enthusiastic endorsement of polysexuality with multiple sex partners.

The aversion I refer to comes in both benign and malignant forms. Malignant aversion has recently had an extraordinary opportunity both to express (and to expose) itself, and, tragically, to demonstrate its power. I'm thinking of course of responses to AIDS—more specifically, of how a public health crisis has been treated like an unprecedented sexual threat. The signs and sense of this extraordinary displacement are the subject of an excellent book just published by Simon Watney, aptly entitled *Policing Desire*.[1] Watney's premise is that "AIDS is not only a medical crisis on an unparalleled scale, it involves a crisis of representation itself, a crisis over the entire framing of knowledge about the human body and its capacities for sexual pleasure" (p. 9). *Policing Desire* is both a casebook of generally appalling examples of this crisis (taken largely from government policy concerning AIDS, as well as from press and television coverage, in England and America) and, most interestingly, an attempt to account for the mechanisms by which a spectacle of suffering and death has unleashed and even appeared to legitimize the impulse to murder.

There is, first of all, the by now familiar, more or less transparent, and ever-increasing evidence of the displacement that Watney studies. At the highest levels of officialdom, there have been the criminal delays in funding research and treatment, the obsession with testing instead of curing, the singularly unqualified members of Reagan's (belatedly constituted) AIDS commission,[2] and the general

1.   Simon Watney, *Policing Desire: Pornography, AIDS, and the Media*, Minneapolis, University of Minnesota Press, 1987. The present essay began as a review of this book; page references for all quotations from it are given in parentheses.
2.   Comparing the authority and efficiency of Reagan's AIDS commission to the presidential commission on the Space Shuttle accident, Philip M. Boffey wrote: "The staff and resources available to the AIDS commission are far smaller than that provided the Challenger commission. The Challenger panel had a staff of 49, including 15 investigators and several other professionals, operating

tendency to think of AIDS as an epidemic of the future rather than a catastrophe of the present. Furthermore, "hospital policies," according to a New York City doctor quoted by Watney, "have more to do with other patients' fears than a concern for the health of AIDS patients" (p. 38). Doctors have refused to operate on people known to be infected with the HIV virus, schools have forbidden children with AIDS to attend classes, and recently citizens of the idyllically named town of Arcadia, Florida, set fire to the house of a family with three hemophiliac children apparently infected with HIV. Television and the press continue to confuse AIDS with the HIV virus, to speak of AIDS as if it were a venereal disease, and consequently to suggest that one catches it by being promiscuous. The effectiveness of the media as an educating force in the fight against AIDS can be measured by the results of a poll cited by Watney in which 56.8 percent of *News of the World* readers came out "in favour of the idea that 'AIDS carriers' should be 'sterilised and given treatment to curb their sexual appetite', with a mere fifty-one percent in favour of the total recriminalisation of homosexuality" (p. 141). Anecdotally, there is, at a presumably high level of professional expertise, the description of gay male sex—which I quote as an epigraph to this essay—offered to viewers of a BBC *Horizon* program by one Opendra Narayan of the Johns Hopkins Medical School (background in veterinary medicine). A less colorfully expressed but equally lurid account of gay sex was given by Justice Richard Wallach of New York State Supreme Court in Manhattan when, in issuing the temporary restraining order that closed the New St. Marks Baths, he noted: "What a bathhouse like this sets up is the orgiastic behavior of multiple partners, one after the other, where in five minutes you can have five contacts."[3] Finally, the story that gave me the greatest morbid delight appeared in the London *Sun* under the headline "I'd Shoot My Son if He Had AIDS, Says Vicar!" accompanied by a photograph of a man holding a rifle at a boy at pointblank range. The son, apparently more attuned to his father's penchant for violence than the respectable reverend himself, candidly added, "Sometimes I think he would like to shoot me whether I had AIDS or not" (quoted pp. 94–95).

All of this is, as I say, familiar ground, and I mention these few disparate items more or less at random simply as a reminder of where our analytical inquiry starts, *and* to suggest that, given the nature of that starting point, analysis, while necessary, may also be an indefensible luxury. I share Watney's inter-

---

on a budget of about $3 million, exclusive of staff salaries. Moreover, the Challenger commission could virtually order NASA to perform tests and analyses at its bidding, thus vastly multiplying the resources at its disposal. In contrast, the AIDS commission currently has only six employees, although it may well appoint 10 to 15 in all, according to Dr. Mayberry, the former chairman. Its budget is projected at $950,000, exclusive of staff salaries. Although the AIDS commission has been promised cooperation by all Federal agencies, it is in no position to compel them to do its work" (*New York Times*, October 16, 1987, p. 10).

3.   "Court Orders Bath House in Village to Stay Shut," *New York Times*, December 28, 1985, p. 11.

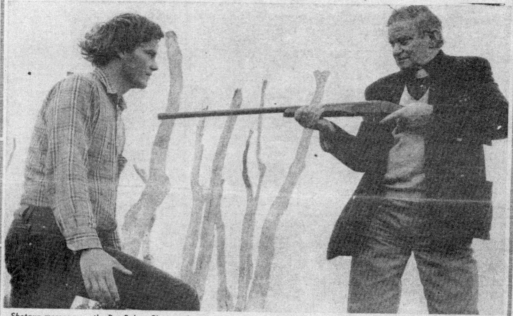

THE SUN, Monday.

I'D SHOOT MY SON IF HE HAD AIDS, SAYS VICAR!

Shotgun message . . . the Rev Robert Simpson demonstrates his point about AIDS with the help of son Chris

A VICAR vowed yesterday that he would take his teenage son to a mountain and shoot him if the boy had the deadly disease AIDS.

And to make his point, the Rev Robert Simpson climbed a hill behind his church and aimed a shotgun at his 18-year-old son Chris.

Mr Simpson, 64, said: "Chris would not get closer to me than six yards. He would be a dead man.

"Even though he is my own child I would pull the trigger.

"And that would go for the rest of my family as well as strangers."

Threat

"AIDS is so serious—there is no possible cure."

Bewildered Chris said: "I don't think I would like Dad to shoot me, but I know there is no chance with AIDS.

"Sometimes I think he would like to shoot me whether I had AIDS or not."

Another red hot Sun exclusive

He would pull trigger on rest of his family

BY JOHN LISNERS

But Mr Simpson, married with three other children, believes the disease is threatening Britain.

He said he would ban all practising homosexuals, who are most in danger of catching AIDS, from taking normal communion.

"I will not let anyone risk the health of my parishioners by allowing them to drink wine from the same chalice," he added at his home in Barnston, Humberside.

Mr Simpson said that in six years time, more than a million people in Britain would have AIDS. He went on:

● If it continues, it will be like the Black Plague. It could wipe out Britain. Family will be against family.

Nobody will trust anyone else and gun law will prevail.

But the fighting vicar says he has nothing against gays.

My criticism is of the unnatural acts they engage in."

Mr Simpson calls on the Government to repeal the law on homosexuality between consenting adults and prostitution — and to punish promiscuity.

● A TODDLER with AIDS has been banned from kindergarten in Sydney, Australia, after biting her best friend.

pretive interests, but it is also important to say that, morally, the only *necessary* response to all of this is rage. "AIDS," Watney writes, "is effectively being used as a pretext throughout the West to 'justify' calls for increasing legislation and regulation of those who are considered to be socially unacceptable" (p. 3). And the unacceptable ones in the AIDS crisis are, of course, male homosexuals and IV drug users (many of the latter, are, as we know, poor blacks and Hispanics). Is it unjust to suggest that *News of the World* readers and the gun-toting British vicar are representative examples of the "general public's" response to AIDS? Are there more decent heterosexuals around, heterosexuals who don't awaken a passionate yearning not to share the same planet with them? Of course there are, but — and this is particularly true of England and the United States — *power* is in the hands of those who give every sign of being able to sympathize more with the murderous "moral" fury of the good vicar than with the agony of a terminal KS patient. It was, after all, the Justice Department of the United States that issued a legal opinion stating that employers could fire employees with AIDS if they had so much as the suspicion that the virus could be spread to other workers, regardless of medical evidence. It was the American Secretary of Health and Human Services who recently urged Congress to defer action on a bill that would ban discrimination against people infected with HIV, and who also argued against the need for a federal law guaranteeing the confidentiality of HIV antibody test results.

To deliver such opinions and arguments is of course not the same thing as pointing a gun at your son's head, but since, as it has often been said, the failure to guarantee confidentiality will discourage people from taking the test and thereby make it more difficult to control the spread of the virus, the only conclusion we can draw is that Secretary Otis R. Bowen finds it more important to have the names of those who test positive than to slow the spread of AIDS into the sacrosanct "general public." To put this schematically: having the information necessary to lock up homosexuals in quarantine camps may be a higher priority in the family-oriented Reagan Administration than saving the heterosexual members of American families from AIDS. Such a priority suggests a far more serious and ambitious passion for violence than what are after all the rather banal, rather normal son-killing impulses of the Reverend Robert Simpson. At the very least, such things as the Justice Department's near recommendation that people with AIDS be thrown out of their jobs suggest that if Edwin Meese would not hold a gun to the head of a man with AIDS, he might not find the murder of a gay man with AIDS (or without AIDS?) intolerable or unbearable. And this is precisely what can be said of millions of fine Germans who never participated in the murder of Jews (and of homosexuals), but who *failed to find the idea of the holocaust unbearable*. That was the more than sufficient measure of their collaboration, the message they sent to their Führer even before the holocaust began but when the *idea* of it was around, was, as it were, being tested for acceptability during the '30s by less violent but nonetheless virulent manifestations of anti-Semitism, just as our leaders, by relegating the protection of people infected with HIV to local authorities, are telling those authorities that anything goes, that the federal government does not find the idea of camps—or perhaps worse—intolerable.

We can of course count on the more liberal press to editorialize against Meese's opinions and Bowen's urgings. We can, however, also count on that same press to give front-page coverage to the story of a presumably straight health worker testing positive for the HIV virus and—at least until recently—almost no coverage at all to complaints about the elephantine pace at which various drugs are being tested and approved for use against the virus. Try keeping up with AIDS research through TV and the press, and you'll remain fairly ignorant. You will, however, learn a great deal from the tube and from your daily newspaper about heterosexual anxieties. Instead of giving us sharp investigative reporting—on, say, *60 Minutes*—on research inefficiently divided among various uncoordinated and frequently competing private and public centers and agencies, or on the interests of pharmaceutical companies in helping to make available (or helping to keep unavailable) new antiviral treatments and in furthering or delaying the development of a vaccine,[4] TV treats us to nauseating processions of yuppie women announcing to the world that they will no longer put out for their yuppie boyfriends unless these boyfriends agree to use a condom. Thus hundreds of thousands of gay men and IV drug users, who have reason to think that they may be infected with HIV, or who know that they are (and who therefore live in daily terror that one of the familiar symptoms will show up), or who are already suffering from an AIDS-related illness, or who are dying from one of these illnesses, are asked to sympathize with all those yuppettes agonizing over whether they're going to risk losing a good fuck by taking the "unfeminine" initiative of interrupting the invading male in order to insist that

4.   On November 15, 1987—a month after I wrote this—*60 Minutes* did, in fact, devote a twenty-minute segment to AIDS. The report centered on Randy Shilts's recently published tale of responses and nonresponses—both in the government and in the gay community—to the AIDS crisis (*And the Band Played On*, New York, St. Martin's Press, 1987). The report presented a sympathetic view of Shilts's chronicle of the delayed and half-hearted efforts to deal with the epidemic, and also informed viewers that not a single official of the Reagan Administration would agree—or was authorized—to talk on *60 Minutes* on the politics of AIDS. However, nearly half of the segment—the first half—was devoted to the murderously naughty sexual habits of Gaetan Dugas, or "Patient Zero," the French-Canadian airline steward who, Shilts claims, was responsible for 40 of the first 200 cases of AIDS reported in the US. Thus the report was sensationalized from the very start with the most repugnant image of homosexuality imaginable: that of the irresponsible male tart who willfully spread the virus after he was diagnosed and warned of the dangers to others of his promiscuity. I won't go into—as of course *60 Minutes* (which provides the *best* political reporting on American network television) didn't go into—the phenomenon of Shilts himself as an overnight media star, and the relation between his stardom and his irreproachably respectable image, his longstanding willingness, indeed eagerness, to join the straights in being morally repelled by gay promiscuity. A good deal of his much admired "objectivity" as a reporter consists in his being as venomous toward those at an exceptionally high risk of becoming afflicted with AIDS (gay men) as toward the government officials who seem content to let them die.

he practice safe sex. In the face of all that, the shrillness of a Larry Kramer can seem like the simplest good sense. The danger of not exaggerating the hostility to homosexuality "legitimized" by AIDS is that, being "sensible," we may soon find ourselves in situations where exaggeration will be difficult, if not impossible. Kramer has recently said that "if AIDS does not spread out widely into the white non-drug-using heterosexual population, as it may or may not do, then the white non-drug-using population is going to hate us even more—for scaring them, for costing them a fucking fortune, for our 'lifestyle,' which they say caused this."[5] What a morbid, even horrendous, yet perhaps sensible suggestion: only when the "general public" is threatened can whatever the opposite of a general public is hope to get adequate attention and treatment.

Almost all the media coverage of AIDS has been aimed at the heterosexual groups now minimally at risk, as if the high-risk groups were not part of the audience. And in a sense, as Watney suggests, they're not. The media targets "an imaginary national family unit which is both white and heterosexual" (p. 43). This doesn't mean that most TV viewers in Europe and America are *not* white and heterosexual and part of a family. It does, however, mean, as Stuart Hall argues, that representation is very different from reflection: "It implies the active work of selecting and presenting, of structuring and shaping: not merely the transmitting of already-existing meaning, but the more active labour of *making things mean*" (quoted p. 124). TV doesn't make the family, but it makes the family *mean* in a certain way. That is, it makes an exceptionally sharp distinction between the family as a biological unit and as a cultural identity, and it does this by teaching us the attributes and attitudes by which people who thought they were already in a family actually only *begin to qualify* as belonging to a family. The great power of the media, and especially of television, is, as Watney writes, "its capacity to manufacture subjectivity itself" (p. 125), and in so doing to dictate the shape of an identity. The "general public" is at once an ideological construct and a moral prescription. Furthermore, the definition of the family *as an identity* is, inherently, an exclusionary process, and the cultural product has no obligation whatsoever to coincide exactly with its natural referent. Thus the family identity produced on American television is much more likely to include your dog than your homosexual brother or sister.

*

The peculiar exclusion of the principal sufferers in the AIDS crisis from the discourse about it has perhaps been felt most acutely by those gay men who, until recently, were able to feel that they could both be relatively open about their

---

5.   Quoted from a speech at a rally in Boston preceding a gay pride celebration; reprinted in, among other publications, the San Francisco lesbian and gay newspaper *Coming Up!*, vol. 8, no. 11 (August 1987), p. 8.

sexuality and still be thought of as belonging to the "general public," to the mainstream of American life. Until the late '60s and '70s, it was of course difficult to manage both these things at the same time. There is, I believe, something salutary in our having to discover the illusory nature of that harmonious adjustment. We now know, or should know, that "gay men," as Watney writes, "are officially regarded, in our entirety, as a disposable constituency" (p. 137). "In our entirety" is crucial. While it would of course be obscene to claim that the comfortable life of a successful gay white businessman or doctor is as oppressed as that of a poverty-stricken black mother in one of our ghettoes, it is also true that the power of blacks *as a group* in the United States is much greater than that of homosexuals. Paradoxically, as we have recently seen in the vote of conservative Democratic senators from the South against the Bork nomination to the Supreme Court, blacks, by their sheer number and their increasing participation in the vote, are no longer a disposable constituency in those very states that have the most illustrious record of racial discrimination. This obviously doesn't mean that blacks have made it in white America. In fact, some political attention to black interests has a certain tactical utility: it softens the blow and obscures the perception of a persistent indifference to the always flourishing economic oppression of blacks. Nowhere is that oppression more visible, less disguised, than in such great American cities as New York, Philadelphia, Boston, and Chicago, although it is typical of the American genius for politically displaced thought that when white liberal New Yorkers (and white liberal columnists such as Anthony Lewis) think of racial oppression, they probably always have images of South Africa in mind.[6] Yet, some blacks are needed in positions of prominence or power, which is not at all true for gay people. Straights can very easily portray gays on TV, while whites generally can't get away with passing for black and are much less effective than blacks as models in TV ads for fast-food chains targeted at the millions of blacks who don't have the money to eat anywhere else. The more greasy the product, the more likely some black models will be allowed to make money promoting it. Also, the country obviously needs a Civil Rights Commission, and it just as obviously has to have blacks on that commission, while there is clearly no immediate prospect for a federal commission to protect and promote gay ways of life. There is no longer a rationale for the oppression of blacks in America, while AIDS has made the oppression of gay men seem like a moral imperative.

In short, a few blacks will always be saved from the appalling fate of most blacks in America, whereas there is no political need to save or protect any homosexuals at all. The country's discovery that Rock Hudson was gay changed

6.   The black brothers and sisters on behalf of whom Berkeley students demonstrate in Sproul Plaza are always from Johannesburg, never from East Oakland, although signs posted on Oakland telephone poles and walls, which these same students have probably never seen, now announce— dare we have the optimism to say "ominously"?—"Oakland is South Africa."

nothing: nobody needs actors' votes (or even actors, for that matter) in the same way Southern senators need black votes to stay in power. In those very cities where white gay men could, at least for a few years, think of themselves as decidedly more white than black when it came to the distribution of privileges in America, cities where the increasingly effective ghettoization of blacks progresses unopposed, the gay men who have had as little trouble as their straight counterparts in accepting this demographic and economic segregation must now accept the fact that, unlike the underprivileged blacks all around them whom, like most other whites, they have developed a technique for not seeing, they—the gays—have no claims to power at all. Frequently on the side of power, but powerless; frequently affluent, but politically destitute; frequently articulate, but with *nothing but a moral argument*—not even recognized as a moral argument—to keep themselves in the protected white enclaves and out of the quarantine camps.

On the whole, gay men are no less socially ambitious, and, more often than we like to think, no less reactionary and racist than heterosexuals. To want sex with another man is not exactly a credential for political radicalism—a fact both recognized and denied by the gay liberation movement of the late '60s and early '70s. Recognized to the extent that gay liberation, as Jeffrey Weeks has put it, proposed "a radical separation . . . between homosexuality, which was about sexual preference, and 'gayness,' which was about a subversively political way of life."[7] And denied in that this very separation was proposed by homosexuals, who were thereby at least implicitly arguing for homosexuality itself as a privileged locus or point of departure for a political-sexual identity not "fixed" by, or in some way traceable to, a specific sexual orientation.[8] It is no secret that many homosexuals resisted, or were simply indifferent to, participation in "a subversively political way of life," to being, as it were, de-homosexualized in order to join what Watney describes as "a social identity defined not by notions of sexual 'essence', but in oppositional relation to the institutions and discourses of medicine, the law, education, housing and welfare policy, and so on" (p. 18). More precisely—and more to the point of an assumption that radical sex means or leads to radical politics—many gay men could, in the late '60s and early '70's, begin to feel comfortable about having "unusual" or radical ideas about what's OK in sex without modifying one bit their proud middle-class consciousness or even their racism. Men whose behavior at night at the San Francisco Cauldron or

7.   Jeffrey Weeks, *Sexuality and Its Discontents: Meanings, Myths and Modern Sexualities*, London, Boston, and Henley, Routledge & Kegan Paul, 1985, p. 198.
8.   Weeks has a good summary of that "neat ruse of history" by which the "intent of the early gay liberation movement . . . to disrupt fixed expectations that homosexuality was a peculiar condition or minority experience" was transformed, by less radical elements in the movement, into a fight for the legitimate claims of a newly recognized minority, "of what was now an almost 'ethnic' identity." Thus "the breakdown of roles, identities, and fixed expectations" was replaced by "the acceptance of homosexuality as a minority experience," an acceptance that "deliberately emphasizes the ghettoization of homosexual experience and by implication fails to interrogate the inevitability of heterosexuality" (*ibid.*, pp. 198–199).

the New York Mineshaft could win five-star approval from the (mostly straight) theoreticians of polysexuality had no problem being gay slumlords during the day and, in San Francisco for example, evicting from the Western Addition black families unable to pay the rents necessary to gentrify that neighborhood.

I don't mean that they *should* have had a problem about such combinations in their lives (although I obviously don't mean that they should have felt comfortable about being slumlords), but I do mean that there has been a lot of confusion about the real or potential political implications of homosexuality. Gay activists have tended to deduce those implications from the status of homosexuals as an oppressed minority rather than from what I think are (except perhaps in societies more physically repressive than ours has been) the more crucially operative continuities between political sympathies on the one hand and, on the other, fantasies connected with sexual pleasure. Thanks to a system of gliding emphases, gay activist rhetoric has even managed at times to suggest that a lust for other men's bodies is a by-product or a decision consequent upon political radicalism rather than a given point of departure for a whole range of political sympathies. While it is indisputably true that sexuality is always being politicized, the ways in which *having sex* politicizes are highly problematical. Right-wing politics can, for example, emerge quite easily from a sentimentalizing of the armed forces or of blue-collar workers, a sentimentalizing which can itself prolong and sublimate a marked sexual preference for sailors and telephone linemen.

In short, to put the matter polemically and even rather brutally, we have been telling a few lies — lies whose strategic value I fully understand, but which the AIDS crisis has rendered obsolescent. I do not, for example, find it helpful to suggest, as Dennis Altman has suggested, that gay baths created "a sort of Whitmanesque democracy, a desire to know and trust other men in a type of brotherhood far removed from the male bondage of rank, hierarchy, and competition that characterise much of the outside world."[9] Anyone who has ever spent one night in a gay bathhouse knows that it is (or was) one of the most ruthlessly ranked, hierarchized, and competitive environments imaginable. Your looks, muscles, hair distribution, size of cock, and shape of ass determined exactly how happy you were going to be during those few hours, and rejection, generally accompanied by two or three words at most, could be swift and brutal, with none of the civilizing hypocrisies with which we get rid of undesirables in the outside world. It has frequently been suggested in recent years that such things as the gay-macho style, the butch-fem lesbian couple, and gay and lesbian sadomasochism, far from expressing unqualified and uncontrollable complicities with a brutal and misogynous ideal of masculinity, or with the heterosexual couple permanently locked into a power structure of male sexual and social mastery

9.   Dennis Altman, *The Homosexualization of America, The Americanization of the Homosexual*, New York, St. Martins Press, 1982, pp. 79–80.

over female sexual and social passivity, or, finally, with fascism, are in fact subversive parodies of the very formations and behaviors they appear to ape. Such claims, which have been the subject of lively and often intelligent debate, are, it seems to me, totally aberrant, even though, in terms probably unacceptable to their defenders, they can also — indeed, must also — be supported.

First of all, a distinction has to be made between the possible effects of these styles on the heterosexual world that provides the models on which they are based, and their significance for the lesbians and gay men who perform them. A sloganesque approach won't help us here. Even Weeks, whose work I admire, speaks of "the rise of the macho-style amongst gay men in the 1970s . . . as another episode in the ongoing 'semiotic guerilla warfare' waged by sexual outsiders against the dominant order," and he approvingly quotes Richard Dyer's suggestion that "by taking the signs of masculinity and eroticizing them in a blatantly homosexual context, much mischief is done to the security with which 'men' are defined in society, and by which their power is secured."[10] These remarks deny what I take to be wholly nonsubversive intentions by conflating them with problematically subversive effects. It is difficult to know how "much mischief" can be done by a style that straight men see — if indeed they see it at all — from a car window as they drive down Folsom Street. Their security as males with power may very well not be threatened at all by that scarcely traumatic sight, because nothing forces them to see any relation between the gay-macho style and their image of their own masculinity (indeed, the very exaggerations of that style make such denials seem plausible). It may, however, be true that to the extent that the heterosexual male more or less secretly admires or identifies with motorcycle masculinity, its adoption by faggots creates, as Weeks and Dyer suggest, a painful (if passing) crisis of representation. The gay-macho style simultaneously invents the oxymoronic expression "leather queen" and denies its oxymoronic status; for the macho straight man, leather queen is intelligible, indeed tolerable, only *as* an oxymoron — which is of course to say that it must remain unintelligible. Leather and muscles are defiled by a sexually feminized body, although — and this is where I have trouble with Weeks's contention that the gay-macho style "gnaws at the roots of a male heterosexual identity"[11] — the macho male's rejection of his representation by the leather queen can also be accompanied by the secret satisfaction of knowing that the leather queen, for all his despicable blasphemy, at least *intends* to pay worshipful tribute to the style and behavior he defiles. The very real potential for subversive confusion in the joining of female sexuality (I'll return to this in a moment) and the signifiers of machismo is dissipated once the heterosexual recognizes in the gay-macho style a *yearning* toward machismo, a yearning that, very conveniently

10.   Weeks, p. 191.
11.   *Ibid.*

for the heterosexual, makes of the leather queen's forbidding armor and warlike manners a *per*version rather than a *sub*version of real maleness.

Indeed, if we now turn to the significance of the macho-style for gay men, it would, I think, be accurate to say that this style gives rise to two reactions, both of which indicate a profound respect for machismo itself. One is the classic put-down: the butch number swaggering into a bar in a leather get-up opens his mouth and sounds like a pansy, takes you home, where the first thing you notice is the complete works of Jane Austen, gets you into bed, and—well, you know the rest. In short, the mockery of gay machismo is almost exclusively an internal affair, and it is based on the dark suspicion that you may not be getting the real article. The other reaction is, quite simply, sexual excitement. And this brings us back to the question not of the reflection or expression of politics in sex, but rather of the extremely obscure process by which sexual pleasure *generates* politics.

If licking someone's leather boots turns you (and him) on, neither of you is making a statement subversive of macho masculinity. Parody is an erotic turn-off, and all gay men know this. Much campy talk is parodistic, and while that may be fun at a dinner party, if you're out to make someone you turn off the camp. Male gay camp is, however, largely a parody of women, which, obviously, raises some other questions. The gay male parody of a certain femininity, which, as others have argued, may itself be an elaborate social construct, is both a way of giving vent to the hostility toward women that probably afflicts every male (and which male heterosexuals have of course expressed in infinitely nastier and more effective ways) *and* could also paradoxically be thought of as helping to deconstruct that image for women themselves. A certain type of homosexual camp speaks the truth of that femininity as mindless, asexual, and hysterically bitchy, thereby provoking, it would seem to me, a violently antimimetic reaction in any female spectator. The gay male bitch desublimates and desexualizes a type of femininity glamorized by movie stars, whom he thus lovingly assassinates with his style, even though the campy parodist may himself be quite stimulated by the hateful impulses inevitably included in his performance. The gay-macho style, on the other hand, is intended to excite others sexually, and the only reason that it continues to be adopted is that it frequently succeeds in doing so. (If, especially in its more extreme leather forms, it is so often taken up by older men, it is precisely because they count on it to supplement their diminished sexual appeal.)

The dead seriousness of the gay commitment to machismo (by which I of course don't mean that all gays share, or share unambivalently, this commitment) means that gay men run the risk of idealizing and feeling inferior to certain representations of masculinity on the basis of which they are in fact judged and condemned. The logic of homosexual desire includes the potential for a loving identification with the gay man's enemies. And that is a fantasy-luxury that is at once inevitable and no longer permissible. Inevitable because a sexual desire for men can't be merely a kind of culturally neutral attraction to a Platonic Idea of the male body; the object of that desire necessarily includes a socially determined and socially pervasive definition of what it means to be a man. Arguments for the social construction of gender are by now familiar. But such arguments almost invariably have, for good political reasons, quite a different slant; they are didactically intended as demonstrations that the male and female identities proposed by a patriarchal and sexist culture are not to be taken for what they are proposed to be: ahistorical, essential, biologically determined identities. Without disagreeing with this argument, I want to make a different point, a point understandably less popular with those impatient to be freed of oppressive and degrading self-definitions. What I'm saying is that a gay man doesn't run the risk of loving his oppressor *only* in the ways in which blacks or Jews might more or less secretly collaborate with their oppressors — that is, as a consequence of the oppression, of that subtle corruption by which a slave can come to idolize power, to agree that he should be enslaved because he is enslaved, that he should be denied power because he doesn't have any. But blacks and Jews don't *become* blacks and Jews as a result of that internalization of an oppressive mentality, whereas that internalization is in part constitutive of male homosexual desire, which, like all sexual desire, combines and confuses impulses to appropriate and to identify with the object of desire. An authentic gay male political identity therefore implies a struggle not only against definitions of maleness and of homosexuality as they are reiterated and imposed in a heterosexist social discourse, but also against those very same definitions so seductively and so faithfully reflected by those (in large part culturally invented and elaborated) male bodies that we carry within us as permanently renewable sources of excitement.

*

There is, however, perhaps a way to explode this ideological body. I want to propose, instead of a denial of what I take to be important (if politically unpleasant) truths about male homosexual desire, an arduous representational discipline. The sexist power that defines maleness in most human cultures can easily survive social revolutions; what it perhaps cannot survive is a certain way of assuming, or taking on, that power. If, as Weeks puts it, gay men "gnaw at the roots of a male heterosexual identity," it is not because of the parodistic distance that they take from that identity, but rather because, from within their nearly mad identification with it, *they never cease to feel the appeal of its being violated.*

To understand this, it is perhaps necessary to accept the pain of embracing, at least provisionally, a homophobic representation of homosexuality. Let's return for a moment to the disturbed harmonies of Arcadia, Florida, and try to imagine what its citizens — especially those who set fire to the Rays' home — actually saw when they thought about or looked at the Rays' three boys. The persecuting of children or of heterosexuals with AIDS (or who have tested positive for HIV) is particularly striking in view of the popular description of such people as "innocent victims." It is as if gay men's "guilt" were the real agent of infection. And what is it, exactly, that they are guilty of? Everyone agrees that the crime is sexual, and Watney, along with others, defines it as the imagined or real promiscuity for which gay men are so famous. He analyzes a story about AIDS by the science correspondent of the *Observer* in which the "major argument, supported by 'AIDS experts in America,' [is] against 'casual sexual encounters.'" A London doctor does, in the course of the article, urge the use of condoms in such encounters, but "the main problem . . . is evidently 'promiscuity', with issues about the kinds of sex one has pushed firmly into the backgound" (p. 35). But the kinds of sex involved, in quite a different sense, may in fact be crucial to the argument. Since the promiscuity here is homosexual promiscuity, we may, I think, legitimately wonder if what is being done is not as important as how many times it is being done. Or, more exactly, the act being represented may itself be associated with insatiable desire, with unstoppable sex.

Before being more explicit about this, I should acknowledge that the argument I wish to make is a highly speculative one, based primarily on the exclusion of the evidence that supports it. An important lesson to be learned from a study of the representation of AIDS is that the messages most likely to reach their destination are messages already there. Or, to put this in other terms, representations of AIDS have to be X-rayed for their fantasmatic logic; they document the comparative irrelevance of information in communication. Thus the expert medical opinions about how the virus cannot be transmitted (information that the college-educated mayor of Arcadia and his college-educated wife have heard and refer to) is at once rationally discussed and occulted. SueEllen Smith, the Arcadia mayor's wife, makes the unobjectionable comment that "there are too many unanswered questions about this disease," only to conclude that "if you are intelligent and listen and read about AIDS you get scared when it involves your own children, because you realize all the assurances are not based on solid evidence." In strictly rational terms, this can of course be easily answered: there are indeed "many unanswered questions" about AIDS, but the assurances given by medical authorities that there is no risk of the HIV virus being transmitted through casual contact among schoolchildren is in fact based on "solid evidence." But what interests me most about the *New York Times* interview with the Smiths from which I am quoting (they are a genial, even disarming couple: "I know I must sound like a country jerk saying this," remarks Mr. Smith, who really never does sound like a country bumpkin) is the evidence that they have in fact received and thoroughly assimilated quite different messages about AIDS. The mayor said that "a lot of local people, including himself, believed that powerful interests, principally the national gay leaders, had pressured the Government into refraining from taking legitimate steps to help contain the spread of AIDS."[12] Let's ignore the charming illusion that "national gay leaders" are

12.   Jon Nordheimer, "To Neighbors of Shunned Family AIDS Fear Outweighs Sympathy," *New*

powerful enough to pressure the federal government into doing anything at all, and focus on the really extraordinary assumption that those belonging to the group hit most heavily by AIDS want nothing more intensely than to see it spread unchecked. In other words, those being killed are killers. Watney cites other versions of this idea of gay men as killers (their behavior is seen as the cause and source of AIDS), and he speaks of "a displaced desire to kill them all—the teeming deviant millions" (p. 82). Perhaps; but the presumed original desire to kill gays may itself be understandable only in terms of the fantasy for which it is offered as an explanation: homosexuals are killers. But what is it, exactly, that makes them killers?

The public discourse about homosexuals since the AIDS crisis began has a startling resemblance (which Watney notes in passing) to the representation of female prostitutes in the nineteenth century "as contaminated vessels, conveyancing 'female' venereal diseases to 'innocent' men" (pp. 33–34).[13] Some more light is retroactively thrown on those representations by the association of gay men's murderousness with what might be called the specific sexual heroics of their promiscuity. The accounts of Professor Narayan and Judge Wallach of gay men having sex twenty to thirty times a night, or once a minute, are much less descriptive of even the most promiscuous male sexuality than they are reminiscent of male fantasies about women's multiple orgasms. The Victorian representation of prostitutes may explicitly criminalize what is merely a consequence of a more profound or original guilt. Promiscuity is the social correlative of a sexuality physiologically grounded in the menacing phenomenon of the nonclimactic climax. Prostitutes publicize (indeed, sell) the inherent aptitude of women for uninterrupted sex. Conversely, the similarities between representations of female prostitutes and male homosexuals should help us to specify the exact form of sexual behavior being targeted, in representations of AIDS, as the criminal, fatal, and irresistibly repeated act. This is of course anal sex (with the potential for multiple orgasms having spread from the insertee to the insertor, who, in any case, may always switch roles and be the insertee for ten or fifteen of those thirty nightly encounters), and we must of course take into account the widespread confusion in heterosexual *and* homosexual men between fantasies of anal and vaginal sex. The realities of syphilis in the nineteenth century and of AIDS today "legitimate" a fantasy of female sexuality as intrinsically diseased; and promiscuity in this fantasy, far from merely increasing the risk of infection, is the *sign of infection*. Women and gay men spread their legs with an unquenchable appetite for destruction.[14] This is an image with extraordinary power; and if the good

---

York Times, August 31, 1987, p. A1.

13.   Charles Bernheimer's excellent study of the representation of prostitution in nineteenth-century France will be published by Harvard University Press in 1988.

14.   The fact that the rectum and the vagina, as far as the sexual transmission of the HIV virus is concerned, are privileged loci of infection is of course a major factor in this legitimizing process, but it hardly explains the fantasmatic force of the representations I have been discussing.

citizens of Arcadia, Florida, could chase from their midst an average, law-abiding family, it is, I would suggest, because in looking at three hemophiliac children they may have seen—that is, unconsciously represented—the infinitely more seductive and intolerable image of a grown man, legs high in the air, unable to refuse the suicidal ecstasy of being a woman.

But why "suicidal"? Recent studies have emphasized that even in societies in which, as John Boswell writes, "standards of beauty are often predicated on male archetypes" (he cites ancient Greece and the Muslim world) and, even more strikingly, in cultures that do not regard sexual relations between men as unnatural or sinful, the line is drawn at "passive" anal sex. In medieval Islam, for all its emphasis on homosexual eroticism, "the position of the 'insertee' is regarded as bizarre or even pathological," and while for the ancient Romans, "the distinction between roles approved for male citizens and others appears to center on the giving of seed (as opposed to the receiving of it) rather than on the more familiar modern active-passive division," to be anally penetrated was no less judged to be an "indecorous role for citizen males."[15] And in Volume II of *The History of Sexuality*, Michel Foucault has amply documented the acceptance (even glorification) *and* profound suspicion of homosexuality in ancient Greece. A general ethical polarity in Greek thought of self-domination and a helpless indulgence of appetites has, as one of its results, a structuring of sexual behavior in terms of activity and passivity, with a correlative rejection of the so-called passive role in sex. What the Athenians find hard to accept, Foucault writes, is the authority of a leader who as an adolescent was an "object of pleasure" for other men; there is a legal and moral incompatibility between sexual passivity and civic authority. The only "honorable" sexual behavior "consists in being active, in dominating, in penetrating, and in thereby exercising one's authority."[16]

In other words, the moral taboo on "passive" anal sex in ancient Athens is primarily formulated as a kind of hygienics of social power. *To be penetrated is to abdicate power.* I find it interesting that an almost identical argument—from, to be sure, a wholly different moral perspective—is being made today by certain feminists. In an interview published a few years ago in *Salmagundi*, Foucault said, "Men think that women can only experience pleasure in recognizing men as masters"[17]—a sentence one could easily take as coming from the pens of Catherine MacKinnon and Andrea Dworkin. These are unlikely bedfellows. In the same interview from which I have just quoted, Foucault more or less openly praises sado-masochistic practices for helping homosexual men (many of whom

15.   John Boswell, "Revolutions, Universals and Sexual Categories," *Salmagundi*, nos. 58–59 (Fall 1982–Winter 1983), pp. 107, 102, and 110. See also Boswell's *Christianity, Social Tolerance and Homosexuality*, Chicago, University of Chicago Press, 1980.
16.   Michel Foucault, *The Use of Pleasure*, trans. Robert Hurley, New York, Pantheon, 1985. This argument is made in chapter 4.
17.   "Sexual Choice, Sexual Act: An Interview with Michel Foucault," *Salmagundi*, nos. 58–59 (Fall 1982–Winter 1983), p. 21.

share heterosexual men's fear of losing their authority by "being under another man in the act of love") to "alleviate" the "problem" of feeling "that the passive role is in some way demeaning."[18] MacKinnon and Dworkin, on the other hand, are of course not interested in making women feel comfortable about lying under men, but in changing the distribution of power both signified and constituted by men's insistence on being on top. They have had quite a bit of bad press, but I think that they make some very important points, points that — rather unexpectedly — can help us to understand the homophobic rage unleashed by AIDS. MacKinnon, for example, argues convincingly against the liberal distinction between violence and sex in rape and pornography, a distinction that, in addition to denying what should be the obvious fact that violence *is* sex for the rapist, has helped to make pornography sound merely sexy, and therefore to protect it. If she and Dworkin use the word *violence* to describe pornography that would normally be classified as nonviolent (for example, porno films with no explicit sado-masochism or scenes of rape), it is because they define as violent the power relation that they see inscribed in the sex acts pornography represents. Pornography, MacKinnon writes, "eroticizes hierarchy"; it "makes inequality into sex, which makes it enjoyable, and into gender, which makes it seem natural." Not too differently from Foucault (except, of course, for the rhetorical escalation), MacKinnon speaks of "the male supremacist definition of female sexuality as lust for self-annihilation." Pornography "institutionalizes the sexuality of male supremacy, fusing the eroticization of dominance and submission with the social construction of male and female."[19] It has been argued that even if such descriptions of pornography are accurate, they exaggerate its importance: MacKinnon and Dworkin see pornography as playing a major role in constructing a social reality of which it is really only a marginal reflection. In a sense — and especially if we consider the size of the steady audience for hard-core pornography — this is true. But the objection is also something of a cop-out, because if it is agreed that pornography eroticizes — and thereby celebrates — the violence of inequality itself (and the inequality doesn't have to be enforced with whips to be violent: the denial to blacks of equal seating privileges on public busses was rightly seen as a form of racial violence), then legal pornography is legalized violence.

Not only that: MacKinnon and Dworkin are really making a claim for the realism of pornography. That is, whether or not we think of it as constitutive (rather than merely reflective) of an eroticizing of the violence of inequality, pornography would be the most accurate description and the most effective promotion of that inequality. Pornography can't be dismissed as less significant socially than other more pervasive expressions of gender inequality (such as the

18. *Ibid.*
19.   Catherine A. MacKinnon, *Feminism Unmodified: Discourses on Life and Law*, Cambridge, Massachusetts, and London, England, Harvard University Press, 1987, pp. 3 and 172.

abominable and innumerable TV ads in which, as part of a sales pitch for cough medicine and bran cereals, women are portrayed as slaves to the normal functioning of their men's bronchial tubes and large intestines), because only pornography tells us why the bran ad is effective: the slavishness of women is erotically thrilling. The ultimate logic of MacKinnon's and Dworkin's critique of pornography—and, however parodistic this may sound, I really don't mean it as a parody of their views—would be *the criminalization of sex itself until it has been reinvented*. For their most radical claim is not that pornography has a pernicious effect on otherwise nonpernicious sexual relations, but rather that so-called normal sexuality is already pornographic. "When violence against women is eroticized as it is in this culture," MacKinnon writes, "it is very difficult to say that there is a major distinction in the level of sex involved between being assaulted by a penis and being assaulted by a fist, especially when the perpetrator is a man."[20] Dworkin has taken this position to its logical extreme: the rejection of intercourse itself. If, as she argues, "there is a relationship between intercourse per se and the low-status of women," and if intercourse itself "is immune to reform," then there must be no more penetration. Dworkin announces: "In a world of male power—penile power—fucking is the essential sexual experience of power and potency and possession; fucking by mortal men, regular guys."[21] Almost everybody reading such sentences will find them crazy, although in a sense they merely develop the implicit *moral* logic of Foucault's more detached and therefore more respectable formulation: "Men think that women can only experience pleasure in recognizing men as masters." MacKinnon, Dworkin, and Foucault are all saying that a man lying on top of a woman assumes that what excites her is the idea of her body being invaded by a phallic master.

The argument against pornography remains, we could say, a liberal argument as long as it is assumed that pornography violates the natural conjunction of sex with tenderness and love. It becomes a much more disturbingly radical argument when the indictment against pornography is identified with an indictment against sex itself. This step is usually avoided by the positing of pornography's violence as either a sign of certain fantasies only marginally connected with an otherwise essentially healthy (caring, loving) form of human behavior, or the symptomatic by-product of social inequalities (more specifically, of the violence intrinsic to a phallocentric culture). In the first case, pornography can be defended as a therapeutic or at least cathartic outlet for those perhaps inescapable but happily marginal fantasies, and in the second case pornography becomes more or less irrelevant to a political struggle against more pervasive social structures of inequality (for once the latter are dismantled, their pornographic derivatives will have lost their raison d'être). MacKinnon and Dworkin, on the other hand, rightly assume the immense power of sexual images to orient our

20.   *Ibid.*, p. 92.
21.   Andrea Dworkin, *Intercourse*, New York, The Free Press, 1987, pp. 124, 137, 79.

imagination of how political power can and should be distributed and enjoyed, and, it seems to me, they just as rightly mistrust a certain intellectual sloppiness in the catharsis argument, a sloppiness that consists in avoiding the question of how a center of presumably wholesome sexuality ever produced those unsavory margins in the first place. Given the public discourse around the center of sexuality (a discourse obviously not unmotivated by a prescriptive ideology about sex), the margins may be the only place where the center becomes visible.

Furthermore, although their strategies and practical recommendations are unique, MacKinnon's and Dworkin's work could be inscribed within a more general enterprise, one which I will call the *redemptive reinvention of sex*. This enterprise cuts across the usual lines on the battlefield of sexual politics, and it includes not only the panicky denial of childhood sexuality, which is being "dignified" these days as a nearly psychotic anxiety about child abuse, but also the activities of such prominent lesbian proponents of S & M sex as Gayle Rubin and Pat Califia, neither of whom, to put it mildly, share the political agenda of MacKinnon and Dworkin. The immense body of contemporary discourse that argues for a radically revised imagination of the body's capacity for pleasure—a discursive project to which Foucault, Weeks, and Watney belong—has as its very condition of possibility a certain refusal of sex as we know it, and a frequently hidden agreement about sexuality as being, in its essence, less disturbing, less socially abrasive, less violent, more respectful of "personhood" than it has been in a male-dominated, phallocentric culture. The mystifications in gay activist discourse on gay male machismo belong to this enterprise; I will return to other signs of the gay participation in the redemptive sex project. For the moment, I want to argue, first of all, that MacKinnon and Dworkin have at least had the courage to be explicit about the profound *moral revulsion* with sex that inspires the entire project, whether its specific program be antipornography laws, a return to the arcadian mobilities of childhood polysexuality, the S & M battering of the body in order to multiply or redistribute its loci of pleasure, or, as we shall see, the comparatively anodine agenda (sponsored by Weeks and Watney) of sexual pluralism. Most of these programs have the slightly questionable virtue of being indubitably saner than Dworkin's lyrical tribute to the militant pastoralism of Joan of Arc's virginity, but the pastoral impulse lies behind them all. What bothers me about MacKinnon and Dworkin is not their analysis of sexuality, but rather the pastoralizing, redemptive intentions that support the analysis. That is—and this is the second, major point I wish to argue—they have given us the reasons why pornography must be multiplied and not abandoned, and, more profoundly, the reasons for defending, for cherishing the very sex they find so hateful. Their indictment of sex—their refusal to prettify it, to romanticize it, to maintain that fucking has anything to do with community or love—has had the immensely desirable effect of publicizing, of lucidly laying out for us, the inestimable value of sex as—at least in certain of its ineradicable aspects—anticommunal, antiegalitarian, antinurturing, antiloving.

Let's begin with some anatomical considerations. Human bodies are constructed in such a way that it is, or at least has been, almost impossible not to associate mastery and subordination with the experience of our most intense pleasures. This is first of all a question of positioning. If the penetration necessary (until recently . . .) for the reproduction of the species has most generally been accomplished by the man's getting on top of the woman, it is also true that being on top can never be just a question of a physical position—either for the person on top or for the one on the bottom. (And for the woman to get on top is just a way of letting her play the game of power for awhile, although—as the images of porn movies illustrate quite effectively—even on the bottom, the man can still concentrate his deceptively renounced aggressiveness in the thrusting movement of his penis.)[22] And, as this suggests, there is also, alas, the question of the penis. Unfortunately, the dismissal of penis envy as a male fantasy rather than a psychological truth about women doesn't really do anything to change the assumptions behind that fantasy. For the idea of penis envy describes how men feel about having one, and, as long as there are sexual relations between men and women, this can't help but be an important fact *for women*. In short, the social structures from which it is often said that the eroticizing of mastery and subordination derive are perhaps themselves derivations (and sublimations) of the indissociable nature of sexual pleasure and the exercise or loss of power. To say this is not to propose an "essentialist" view of sexuality. A reflection on the fantasmatic potential of the human body—the fantasies engendered by its sexual anatomy and the specific moves it makes in taking sexual pleasure—is not the same thing as an a priori, ideologically motivated, and prescriptive description of the essence of sexuality. Rather, I am saying that those effects of power which, as Foucault has argued, are inherent in the relational itself (they are immediately produced by "the divisions, inequalities and disequilibriums" inescapably present "in every relation from one point to another")[23] can perhaps most easily be exacerbated, and polarized into relations of mastery and subordination, in sex, and that this potential may be grounded in the shifting experience that every human being has of his or her body's capacity, or failure, to control and to manipulate the world beyond the self.

Needless to say, the ideological exploitations of this fantasmatic potential have a long and inglorious history. It is mainly a history of male power, and by now it has been richly documented by others. I want to approach this subject from a quite different angle, and to argue that a gravely dysfunctional aspect of what is, after all, the healthy pleasure we take in the operation of a coordinated

22.   The idea of intercourse without thrusting was proposed by Shere Hite in *The Hite Report*, New York, Macmillan, 1976. Hite envisaged "a mutual lying together in pleasure, penis-in-vagina, vagina-covering-penis, with female orgasm providing much of the stimulation necessary for male orgasm" (p. 141).
23.   Michel Foucault, *The History of Sexuality, vol. 1, An Introduction*, trans. Robert Hurley, New York, Vintage Books, 1980, pp. 93–94.

and strong physical organism is the temptation to deny the perhaps equally strong appeal of powerlessness, of the loss of control. Phallocentrism is exactly that: not primarily the denial of power to women (although it has obviously also led to that, everywhere and at all times), but above all the denial of the *value* of powerlessness in both men and women. I don't mean the value of gentleness, or nonaggressiveness, or even of passivity, but rather of a more radical disintegration and humiliation of the self. For there is finally, beyond the fantasies of bodily power and subordination that I have just discussed, a transgressing of that very polarity which, as Georges Bataille has proposed, may be the profound sense of both certain mystical experiences and of human sexuality. In making this suggestion I'm also thinking of Freud's somewhat reluctant speculation, especially in the *Three Essays on the Theory of Sexuality*, that sexual pleasure occurs whenever a certain threshold of intensity is reached, when the organization of the self is momentarily disturbed by sensations or affective processes somehow "beyond" those connected with psychic organization. Reluctant because, as I have argued elsewhere, this definition removes the sexual from the intersubjective, thereby depriving the teleological argument of the *Three Essays* of much of its weight. For on the one hand Freud outlines a normative sexual development that finds its natural goal in the post-Oedipal, genitally centered desire for someone of the opposite sex, while on the other hand he suggests not only the irrelevance of the object in sexuality but also, and even more radically, a shattering of the psychic structures themselves that are the precondition for the very establishment of a relation to others. In that curiously insistent, if intermittent, attempt to get at the "essence" of sexual pleasure—an attempt that punctuates and interrupts the more secure narrative outline of the history of desire in the *Three Essays*—Freud keeps returning to a line of speculation in which the opposition between pleasure and pain becomes irrelevant, in which the sexual emerges as the *jouissance* of exploded limits, as the ecstatic suffering into which the human organism momentarily plunges when it is "pressed" beyond a certain threshold of endurance. Sexuality, at least in the mode in which it is constituted, may be a tautology for masochism. In *The Freudian Body*, I proposed that this sexually constitutive masochism could even be thought of as an evolutionary conquest in the sense that it allows the infant to survive, indeed to find pleasure in, the painful and characteristically human period during which infants are shattered with stimuli for which they have not yet developed defensive or integrative ego structures. Masochism would be the psychical strategy that partially defeats a biologically dysfunctional process of maturation.[24] From this Freudian perspective, we might say that Bataille reformulates this self-shattering into the sexual as a kind of nonanecdotal self-debasement, as a masochism to which the melancholy of the

---

24.   See Leo Bersani, *The Freudian Body: Psychoanalysis and Art*, New York, Columbia University Press, 1986, chapter II, especially pp. 38–39.

post-Oedipal superego's moral masochism is wholly alien, and in which, so to speak, the self is exuberantly discarded.[25]

The relevance of these speculations to the present discussion should be clear: the self which the sexual shatters provides the basis on which sexuality is associated with power. It is possible to think of the sexual as, precisely, moving between a hyperbolic sense of self and a loss of all consciousness of self. But sex as self-hyperbole is perhaps a repression of sex as self-abolition. It inaccurately replicates self-shattering as self-swelling, as psychic tumescence. If, as these words suggest, men are especially apt to "choose" this version of sexual pleasure, because their sexual equipment appears to invite by analogy, or at least to facilitate, the phallicizing of the ego, neither sex has exclusive rights to the practice of sex as self-hyperbole. For it is perhaps primarily *the degeneration of the sexual into a relationship that condemns sexuality to becoming a struggle for power.* As soon as persons are posited, the war begins. It is the self that swells with excitement at the idea of being on top, the self that makes of the inevitable play of thrusts and relinquishments in sex an argument for the natural authority of one sex over the other.

*

Far from apologizing for their promiscuity as a failure to maintain a loving relationship, far from welcoming the return to monogamy as a beneficent consequence of the horror of AIDS,[26] gay men should ceaselessly lament the practical necessity, now, of such relationships, should resist being drawn into mimicking the unrelenting warfare between men and women, which nothing has ever changed. Even among the most critical historians of sexuality and the most angry activists, there has been a good deal of defensiveness about what it means to be gay. Thus for Jeffrey Weeks the most distinctive aspect of gay life is its "radical pluralism."[27] Gayle Rubin echoes and extends this idea by arguing for a "theoretical as well as a sexual pluralism."[28] Watney repeats this theme with, it is true, some important nuances. He sees that the "new gay identity was constructed

25.   Bataille called this experience "communication," in the sense that it breaks down the barriers that define individual organisms and keep them separate from one another. At the same time, however, like Freud he seems to be describing an experience in which the very terms of a communication are abolished. The term thus lends itself to a dangerous confusion if we allow it to keep any of its ordinary connotations.
26.   It might be pointed out that, unless you met your lover many, many years ago and neither you nor he has had sex with anyone else since then, monogamy is not that safe anyway. Unsafe sex a few times a week with someone carrying the HIV virus is undoubtedly like having unsafe sex with several HIV positive strangers over the same period of time.
27.   Weeks, p. 218.
28.   Gayle Rubin, "Thinking Sex: Notes for a Radical Theory of the Politics of Sexuality," in Carole Vance, ed., *Pleasure and Danger: Exploring Female Sexuality*, Boston, London, Melbourne, and Henley, Routledge & Kegan Paul, 1984, p. 309.

through multiple encounters, shifts of sexual identification, actings out, cultural reinforcements, and a plurality of opportunity (at least in large urban areas) for desublimating the inherited sexual guilt of a grotesquely homophobic society," and therefore laments the "wholesale de-sexualisation of gay culture and experience" encouraged by the AIDS crisis (p. 18). He nonetheless dilutes what I take to be the specific menace of gay sex for that "grotesquely homophobic society" by insisting on the assertion of "the diversity of human sexuality in *all* its variant forms" as "perhaps the most radical aspect of gay culture" (p. 25). *Diversity* is the key word in his discussions of homosexuality, which he defines as "a fluctuating field of sexual desires and behaviour" (p. 103); it maximizes "the mutual erotic possibilities of the body, and that is why it is taboo" (p. 127).[29]

Much of this derives of course from the rhetoric of sexual liberation in the '60s and '70s, a rhetoric that received its most prestigious intellectual justification from Foucault's call — especially in the first volume of his *History of Sexuality* —for a reinventing of the body as a surface of multiple sources of pleasure. Such calls, for all their redemptive appeal, are, however, unnecessarily and even dangerously tame. The argument for diversity has the strategic advantage of making gays seem like passionate defenders of one of the primary values of mainstream liberal culture, but to make that argument is, it seems to me, to be disingenuous about the relation between homosexual behavior and the revulsion it inspires. The revulsion, it turns out, is all a big mistake: what we're really up to is pluralism and diversity, and getting buggered is just one moment in the practice of those laudable humanistic virtues. Foucault could be especially perverse about all this: challenging, provoking, and yet, in spite of his radical intentions, somewhat appeasing in his emphases. Thus in the *Salmagundi* interview to which I have already referred, after announcing that he will not "make use of a position of authority while [he is] being interviewed to traffic in opinions," he delivers himself of the highly idiosyncratic opinions, first of all, that "for a homosexual, the best moment of love is likely to be when the lover leaves in the taxi" ("the homosexual imagination is for the most part concerned with reminiscing about the act rather than anticipating [or, presumably, enjoying] it") and, secondly, that the rituals of gay S & M are "the counterpart of the medieval courts where strict rules of proprietary courtship were defined."[30] The first opinion is somewhat embarrassing; the second has a certain campy appeal. Both turn our attention away from the body — from the acts in which it engages, from

29.   A frequently referred to study of gay men and women by the Institute for Sex Research founded by Alfred C. Kinsey concluded that "homosexual adults are a remarkably diverse group." See Alan P. Bell and Martin S. Weinberg, *Homosexualities: A Study of Diversity among Men and Women*, New York, Simon and Schuster, 1978, p. 217. One can hardly be unhappy with that conclusion in an "official" sociological study, but, needless to say, it tells us very little — and the tables about gay sexual preferences in the same study aren't much help here either — concerning fantasies of and about homosexuals.

30.   "Sexual Choice, Sexual Act," pp. 11, 20.

the pain it inflicts and begs for—and directs our attention to the romances of memory and the idealizations of the presexual, the courting imagination. That turning away from sex is then projected onto heterosexuals as an explanation for their hostility. "I think that what most bothers those who are not gay about gayness is the gay life-style, not sex acts themselves," and, "It is the prospect that gays will create as yet unforseen kinds of relationships that many people cannot tolerate."[31] But what is "*the* gay life-style"? Is there one? Was Foucault's life-style the same as Rock Hudson's? More importantly, can a nonrepresentable form of relationship really be more threatening than the representation of a particular sexual act—especially when the sexual act is associated with women but performed by men and, as I have suggested, has the terrifying appeal of a loss of the ego, of a self-debasement?

We have been studying examples of what might be called a frenzied epic of displacements in the discourse on sexuality and on AIDS. The government talks more about testing than it does about research and treatment; it is more interested in those who may eventually be threatened by AIDS than in those already stricken with it. There are hospitals in which concern for the safety of those patients who have not been exposed to HIV takes precedence over caring for those suffering from an AIDS-related disease. Attention is turned away from the kinds of sex people practice to a moralistic discourse about promiscuity. The impulse to kill gays comes out as a rage against gay killers deliberately spreading a deadly virus among the "general public." The temptation of incest has become a national obsession with child abuse by day-care workers and teachers. Among intellectuals, the penis has been sanitized and sublimated into the phallus as the originary signifier; the body is to be read as a language. (Such distancing techniques, for which intellectuals have a natural aptitude, are of course not only sexual: the national disgrace of economic discrimination against blacks is buried in the self-righteous call for sanctions against Pretoria.) The wild excitement of fascistic S & M becomes a parody of fascism; gay males' idolatry of the cock is "raised" to the political dignity of "semiotic guerrilla warfare." The phallocentrism of gay cruising becomes diversity and pluralism; representation is displaced from the concrete practice of fellatio and sodomy to the melancholy charms of erotic memories and the cerebral tensions of courtship. There has even been the displacement of displacement itself. While it is undeniably right to speak—as, among others, Foucault, Weeks, and MacKinnon have spoken—of the ideologically organizing force of sexuality, it is quite another thing to suggest—as these writers also suggest—that sexual inequalities are predominantly, perhaps exclusively, displaced social inequalities. Weeks, for example, speaks of erotic tensions as a displacement of politically enforced positions of power and subordination,[32]

---

31.   *Ibid.*, p. 22.
32.   See Weeks, p. 44.

as if the sexual—involving as it does the source and locus of every individual's original experience of power (and of powerlessness) in the world: the human body—could somehow be conceived of apart from all relations of power, were, so to speak, belatedly contaminated by power from elsewhere.

Displacement is endemic to sexuality. I have written, especially in *Baudelaire and Freud*, about the mobility of desire, arguing that sexual desire initiates, indeed can be recognized by, an agitated fantasmatic activity in which original (but, from the start, unlocatable) objects of desire get lost in the images they generate. Desire, by its very nature, turns us away from its objects. If I refer critically to what I take to be a certain refusal to speak frankly about gay sex, it is not because I believe either that gay sex is reducible to one form of sexual activity or that the sexual itself is a stable, easily observable, or easily definable function. Rather, I have been trying to account for the murderous representations of homosexuals unleashed and "legitimized" by AIDS, and in so doing I have been struck by what might be called the aversion-displacements characteristic of both those representations and the gay responses to them. Watney is acutely aware of the displacements operative in "cases of extreme verbal or physical violence towards lesbians and gay men and, by extension, the whole topic of AIDS"; he speaks, for example, of "displaced misogyny," of "a hatred of what is projected as 'passive' and therefore female, sanctioned by the subject's heterosexual drives" (p. 50). But, as I argued earlier, implicit in both the violence toward gay men (and toward women, both gay and straight) *and* the rethinking among gays (and among women) of what being gay (and what being a woman) means is a certain agreement about what sex should be. The pastoralizing project could be thought of as informing even the most oppressive demonstrations of power. If, for example, we assume that the oppression of women disguises a fearful male response to the seductiveness of an image of sexual powerlessness, then the most brutal machismo is really part of a domesticating, even sanitizing project. The ambition of performing sex as *only* power is a salvational project, one designed to preserve us from a nightmare of ontological obscenity, from the prospect of a breakdown of the human itself in sexual intensities, from a kind of selfless communication with "lower" orders of being. The panic about child abuse is the most transparent case of this compulsion to rewrite sex. Adult sexuality is split in two: at once redeemed by its retroactive metamorphosis into the purity of an asexual childhood, and yet preserved in its most sinister forms by being projected onto the image of the criminal seducer of children. "Purity" is crucial here: behind the brutalities against gays, against women, and, in the denial of their very nature and autonomy, against children lies the pastoralizing, the idealizing, the redemptive project I have been speaking of. More exactly, the brutality is identical to the idealization.

The participation of the powerless themselves in this project is particularly disheartening. Gays and women must of course fight the violence directed against them, and I am certainly not arguing for a complicity with misogynist and homophobic fantasies. I am, however, arguing against that form of complicity that consists in accepting, even finding new ways to defend, our culture's lies about sexuality. As if in secret agreement with the values that support misogynist images of female sexuality, women call for a permanent closing of the thighs in the name of chimerically nonviolent ideals of tenderness and nurturing; gays suddenly rediscover their lost bathhouses as laboratories of ethical liberalism, places where a culture's ill-practiced ideals of community and diversity are authentically put into practice. But what if we said, for example, not that it is wrong to think of so-called passive sex as "demeaning," but rather that *the value of sexuality itself is to demean the seriousness of efforts to redeem it?* "AIDS," Watney writes, "offers a new sign for the symbolic machinery of repression, making the rectum a grave" (p. 126). But if the rectum is the grave in which the masculine ideal (an ideal shared—differently—by men *and* women) of proud subjectivity is buried, then it should be celebrated for its very potential for death. Tragically, AIDS has literalized that potential as the certainty of biological death, and has therefore reinforced the heterosexual association of anal sex with a self-annihilation originally and primarily identified with the fantasmatic mystery of an insatiable, unstoppable female sexuality. It may, finally, be in the gay man's rectum that he demolishes his own perhaps otherwise uncontrollable identification with a murderous judgment against him.

That judgment, as I have been suggesting, is grounded in the sacrosanct value of selfhood, a value that accounts for human beings' extraordinary willingness to kill in order to protect the seriousness of their statements. The self is a practical convenience; promoted to the status of an ethical ideal, it is a sanction for violence.[33] If sexuality is socially dysfunctional in that it brings people together only to plunge them into a self-shattering and solipsistic *jouissance* that drives them apart, it could also be thought of as our primary hygienic practice of nonviolence. Gay men's "obsession" with sex, far from being denied, should be celebrated—not because of its communal virtues, not because of its subversive potential for parodies of machismo, not because it offers a model of genuine pluralism to a society that at once celebrates and punishes pluralism, but rather because it never stops re-presenting the internalized phallic male as an infinitely loved object of sacrifice. Male homosexuality advertises the risk of the sexual itself as the risk of self-dismissal, of *losing sight* of the self, and in so doing it proposes and dangerously represents *jouissance* as a mode of ascesis.

---

33.   This sentence could be rephrased, and elaborated, in Freudian terms, as the difference between the ego's function of "reality-testing" and the superego's moral violence (against the ego).

AIDS in the Two Berlins*

JOHN BORNEMAN

In September 1987 West German Chancellor Helmut Kohl welcomed the German Democratic Republic's Party Chairman Erich Honneker to Bonn for the first time, and with the full ceremony attendant upon a visiting head of state. Coming nearly forty years after the founding of today's German states, this symbolic acknowledgment of political reality offered hope for the end of a postwar history of mutual avoidance, denial, and sabotage. Remarkably enough, the very first point of the communiqué signed by the two leaders had nothing to do with international politics in the conventional sense of the term; rather it was an agreement to conduct joint research on AIDS. That the two competing regimes could agree on the need for basic scientific work in virology and immunology—while avoiding any discussion of their ideological differences regarding public health and other policies affecting AIDS—creates the illusion that everyone is united in the struggle against the epidemic. It also points to the polyvocality of AIDS, as scientific entity and cultural myth, as abstraction and experience.

AIDS geht alle an ("AIDS concerns us all"), the official education slogan of the West German AIDS-Hilfen, or AIDS Support Groups, has been adopted by West German Minister of Health Rita Süssmuth to inform the entire populace of West Berlin and West Germany of its proper relation to the public health crisis. In contrast, there is no AIDS slogan in the German Democratic Republic, despite the fact that official slogans are otherwise as abundant there as advertising jingles in America. Furthermore, according to Dr. Niels Sönnichsen, the GDR's leading "AIDS expert," AIDS by no means *geht alle an*. Rather, it primarily affects the "homosexual risk group," and East German educational efforts are therefore to be directed particularly to "young homosexuals."

The striking difference in these two approaches cannot be explained by appealing to the East-West ideological divide, nor can it be accounted for by

*   My thanks to Jim Steakley for an ongoing exchange of ideas and critical commentary, which substantially contributed to this essay. I also wish to thank Albert Eckart for a most informative interview on AIDS policy in West Berlin.

referring to "the facts" of AIDS, since these, too, are subject to dispute. One fact, however, is obvious: AIDS has had very dissimilar impacts on different national populations. Compare these June 1987 statistics for reported cases of AIDS and resultant deaths in three countries:[1]

	AIDS cases	Deaths
USA	36,058	20,849
West Germany	1,089	499
GDR	30	2

AIDS may indeed concern us all, but it affects us very differently depending on who and where we are, and this is obviously no mere matter of caseloads. The gravity of the situation in the United States, beginning in 1981, has marked the scenario in neither of the Germanies.[2] Indeed, the differences are often far greater between the United States and the Germanies than they are between the two Germanies themselves, and this is again no mere matter of caseloads. In the following examination of the relation of cultural style to AIDS in the two Germanies, I shall focus on the situation in Berlin, where I am living and conducting research—on both sides of the wall. Before detailing the differences between the two Berlins, however, I shall offer three explanations as to why the social and cultural construction of AIDS in the United States differs so significantly from that in Berlin.

First, all Berliners, socialist or capitalist, have health insurance. In neither system is health care dependent upon income, class, or employment status, or even upon citizenship. Health care in both Germanies is contingent solely upon legal residence. In the United States, community groups organized to deal with the impact of AIDS must often spend their resources on basic medical and home care for people living with AIDS, or on legal support for those subjected to discrimination within the health care system, as well as in public accommodations, housing, and the workplace. Instead of lobbying for national health care in the United States, the existence of which would entirely change the context in which AIDS is experienced, support groups struggle against all odds simply to provide basic human necessities on a person-by-person or group-by-group basis.

---

1.   The statistics for the US are taken from the Centers for Disease Control, Atlanta; those for West Germany from the German Ministry of Health; and those for the GDR from the World Health Organization. Of the thirty cases included in the June statistics for the GDR, twenty were foreigners and only ten GDR citizens. Dr. Sönnichsen reported in November 1987 that there were thirty-one citizens of the GDR infected with HIV, of which four were cases of frank AIDS. Two of these had died.
2.   The largest incidence of AIDS in West Germany is in the Frankfurt area, which not coincidentally also has the highest concentration of American soldiers. In the GDR, only one of the total reported HIV-positive men lived in Berlin, and two-thirds of the total were foreigners.

Secondly, all Berliners have greater job security than do Americans. Of course, there are major differences in labor organization in the two Berlins, and labor-management relations in West Berlin are increasingly coming to resemble those in the US. But it is still difficult to fire workers in West Berlin, and when dismissal does occur, workers are entitled to considerable state support. In all the West German court cases brought by individuals experiencing AIDS-related job discrimination, the rights of the worker have been upheld.[3]

In East Berlin it is nearly impossible for workers to be dismissed, and very easy to find other jobs when they are. Consequently, the fear of losing work and financial support plays a decidedly minor role in comparison with the situation in the West. In fact, the GDR's emphasis on societal inclusiveness and security can directly result in the protection of individuals infected with HIV. In the spring of 1987, for example, a small-town theater employee diagnosed with AIDS decided to move to Berlin, where medical care for HIV-related illnesses is better. Fully aware of his condition, the Deutsches Theater, one of the most renowned theaters in East Germany, offered to employ him on humanitarian grounds. Since there are so few cases of AIDS in the GDR, this example cannot be said to be representative of patterns of employment of people living with AIDS. But it illustrates a situation opposite to a trend in the US, where many gay men have moved from large cities—whose already inadequate health care facilities are further strained by growing numbers of AIDS patients—back to small towns and parental care. The decision to seek private, family health care is a matter of choice in the Germanies, a matter of dire necessity in the US.

The third major difference lies in the area of housing. There are diverse rental arrangements in West Berlin, some of which guarantee nearly absolute security; others only provide limited tenant's rights; most but not all apartments are rent controlled. But compared to the housing market in the United States, or for that matter in other West German cities, West Berlin is a renter's paradise. In East Berlin, as in the whole of the GDR, where some ninety percent of apartments are state owned, there can be neither major rent increases—many rents have not changed in fifty years—nor eviction, unless tenants are provided with another apartment. There are no reported cases of people with AIDS losing their apartments in East or West Berlin.[4]

Thus, the fundamental, systemic conditions of health care, job security, and housing in both Germanies provide a margin of protection for vulnerable individuals that is unimaginable in the United States. These systemic differences are

---

3. The conclusion to be drawn from this is not that Germans are less likely to discriminate than are Americans, but that individuals in both Germanies are better protected against AIDS-related discrimination than are US citizens. In 1983–84, the US-based McDonald's companies in West Germany attempted to restrict kitchen personnel suspected of having AIDS, but the company was subsequently forced to rescind the measures.

4. In contrast to this, New York City now has an estimated 400 homeless people with AIDS and is conservatively projected to have 900 three years from now.

further manifest in the ways people living with AIDS are represented. Americans testing positive for antibodies to HIV or diagnosed with AIDS are often called "AIDS victims." If they are children or have been infected through blood transfusions, they become "innocent victims," implying that all others are guilty —guilty of a reprehensible and immoderate "life-style." Nevertheless, all are expected to "marshall their defenses" and "fight for their lives." This reduction of all aspects of AIDS to personal guilt and responsibility is a distinctive feature of the American myth of the individual, helping to ensure that no critique of the system will occur.

Apart from a few scandal-mongering tabloid writers in West Berlin, Germans in both Berlins use similar terms when talking about AIDS. Those that test HIV-positive are called "carriers"—hardly a neutral term—or "positives." Those suffering from an AIDS-related illness are most often simply called "people sick with AIDS," and their illness is not seen as a question of personal guilt. West Berliners rarely portray specific individuals with AIDS, and even though gay men still comprise the vast majority of cases, the groups now most discussed in the West German media are babies, women, and drug addicts. Unlike Americans, Germans do not romanticize those who die of AIDS; the emphasis instead is on understanding how to live with danger, illness, and death.

*

Perhaps the most immediately striking difference between West and East Berlin in the cultural style of AIDS discussion is that of the relationship of public officials to local actors. The Federal Republic of Germany must provide the illusion of dialogue between elected officials and their constituents, while a monologue by officially sanctioned experts is the norm in the German Democratic Republic. Because of restrictive government controls on information production and consumption in the GDR, special effort is required for individuals to learn about the diverse research into and opinions about AIDS in the West.[5] This is mitigated somewhat by the fact that, outside of southern Saxony (the area around Dresden), nearly all East Germans receive television broadcasts from the West. For the past three years, West German TV and radio coverage of AIDS has included both hysterical reporting and relatively balanced, detailed information. Since all media is controlled in the East, there is no tabloid press to incite fear and prejudice, but neither is there an alternative press to provide information that deviates from the official. East Germans therefore ultimately rely on their own direct experiences, which have thus far been very limited.

5.   A member of Berliner AIDS-Hilfe, Sabine L., accepted an invitation from a gay discussion group in East Berlin to conduct discussions on safe sex. After several visits, she was discovered at the border carrying an exceptionally large number of condoms—West German condoms are apparently of superior quality to those in the GDR—and was denied a visa to visit the East. GDR border officials are evidently not interested in cooperating in AIDS education.

Despite official education efforts, gay men in the GDR appear to live as if AIDS existed only under capitalism, while heterosexuals act as if it affected only gay men. In either case, AIDS is seen as someone else's problem. The idea that AIDS is solely a problem of the West is repeated in the West itself, as is suggested by anecdotal accounts offered by former East Germans—both gay and straight. Once in the West, they find themselves eagerly sought after as marriage and sex partners, since they are assumed to be free of "Western sexual diseases."

Official discussion of AIDS in the GDR began in 1983, when the Ministry of Health established an advisory group of medical experts to analyze the development of AIDS in other countries. The group has since taken a number of steps to increase knowledge about AIDS and its prevention: publishing articles in daily newspapers and weekly and monthly magazines, distributing AIDS education brochures, delivering public lectures in youth clubs, introducing blood testing in various cities, and establishing an AIDS counseling center in Berlin. The educational materials are best characterized as factual and terse.

The first discussion of AIDS published in the GDR was an interview with Dr. Sönnichsen, director of the Dermatology Clinic of Berlin's Charité Hospital; it appeared in 1985 in the *Berliner Wochenpost*, a general interest weekly magazine.[6] In the interview, Sönnichsen described the first reports of an "AIDS illness" in 1981 in the US, the subsequent geographical spread of the syndrome, the isolation of the virus in 1984 by Robert Gallo in the US and Luc Montagnier in Paris, and the "special risk groups." He explained that of the two largest risk groups in Western countries, only homosexual men were of concern to him, since there is virtually no IV drug scene in the GDR. At the time of the interview, there were no "AIDS-related illnesses in our country" (the first reported case came in late 1986). Sönnichsen went on to outline the steps being taken in the GDR by the Ministry of Health to prepare for dealing with "people sick with AIDS." In a nonmoralizing manner, he explained what people could do to prevent AIDS: know the identity of your sex partners, avoid unsafe sex practices, use condoms.

In early 1986, the East German Ministry of Health issued brochures—targeted at men and women separately—entitled "What does it mean to have positive indications of the antibody against LAV/HTLV III [now called HIV]? Consequences for your health, your sex life, and your social contacts." The two-page pamphlet explains in easily understandable terms the significance of a positive antibody test, clarifies what must be done to prevent infecting others, and advises how to protect one's own health. People are instructed to establish stable relationships, to avoid exchanges of blood, plasma, or semen, and they are provided with guidelines for keeping the immune system intact. The brochure does not engage in the kind of guesswork—such as, "We do not know defini-

6.   "AIDS—eine neue Infektionskrankheit," *Berliner Wochenpost*, no. 40 (1985), p. 19.

tively if the virus can be spread through saliva"—that often characterizes the media and public statements in the West—guesswork that often leads people either to reject sex altogether and isolate themselves socially, or, since they lack the expertise to decide between competing forms of advice, to take no health precautions at all in their sexual contacts.[7]

Discussion of sexuality had been entirely absent from official publications of East Germany's ruling Socialist Unity Party before March 1987, when both *Neues Deutschland* and *Berliner Zeitung* published long articles on AIDS, including brief catalogues of safe sex practices. The information in these articles was primarily distilled from several panel discussions among medical experts held in February at the Charité Hospital. The degree of interest in the subject was evidenced by a huge turnout, even though publicity for the event was primarily word-of-mouth. Each discussion was attended by approximately 1,000 people, with equal numbers turned away for lack of seating. For the first panel, which I attended, about a third of the audience were women and nearly half were medical students, and the discussion was largely technical. When describing safe sex practices, one panelist resorted to English-language gay jargon: thus, one should avoid "rimming" and "fisting." Since there was no attempt to paraphrase these terms in German, presumably due to squeamishness, a considerable number of listeners were left in the dark as to which practices to avoid. In his presentation, Dr. Sönnichsen stressed that gay men were not to be asked to give up sex, but that they should reorient themselves to safer sex practices and to stable, monogamous relationships.[8]

The future development of AIDS in the GDR will depend to some extent on the testing of blood products, and as of January 1986 all blood banks had implemented state-of-the-art testing procedures. Authorities have remained silent as to whether or not any contaminated blood was found, but have claimed that the current blood supply is virus-free. By November '86, health authorities had issued a directive designed, through guarantees of anonymity, to encourage people to have their blood tested voluntarily. Such a directive represents a radical departure from standard policy in the GDR, where people are routinely required to show their official identification. In this instance, however, all district

---

7.   This range of reactions is clearly illustrated in recent articles in *Der Spiegel*, August 30 and September 7, 1987.

8.   Local GDR gay groups do not simply depend upon state and local medical authorities for information about AIDS; they also rely on Western media and Western friends. Since the signing of a new church-state agreement in 1978, the Protestant church in the GDR has played an essential supportive role for groups whose interests might be at odds with those of the state. In the case of gay self-help groups, the church offers space for meetings and publishes articles in church bulletins. A local Protestant parish in Jena was host in late November 1986 to a gathering of the leaders of "Working Groups for Homosexual Self-Help." The first inter-city gathering of this sort had taken place in Leipzig in 1984. At the Jena gathering, sixteen groups from fifteen cities were represented. Of three such groups in Berlin, one operates with state support; that group did not send a representative to the Jena meeting. The conference included discussion of AIDS and safer sex.

hospitals have been instructed *not* to record the names of those requesting that their blood samples be sent to the regionally designated physician responsible for HIV antibody tests.[9]

*

The West German AIDS education campaign began in 1983, three years earlier than that in East Germany. It was initiated, however, not at the government level, but locally, by self-help groups (the first one was in West Berlin) organized to provide information to the public. From the beginning, gay men were primarily responsible for the effort, although the West Berlin municipal government financed administrative costs. In 1985, after nearly two years of local financing, the Deutsche AIDS-Hilfe was reorganized into a national coordinating body for regional groups, with financing provided by the federal government. A privately financed, student-produced monthly entitled *Vor-sicht* ("Caution/Pre-view") "for all those who are concerned about AIDS or who should be concerned"—appeared in May 1986. West German education efforts also include informative pamphlets mailed to every West German household, extensive radio and TV coverage, major magazine series, educational comics, and a variety of public service announcements and commercials in cinemas. An early educational poster produced by the Berlin AIDS-Hilfe bore the motto *Sicher besser— Safer Sex* ("Safe is better—Safer Sex") and depicted two nude male torsos in an erotic embrace. Another poster, produced by the Federal Ministry of Health and Family Policy, features a handsome family of four saying, *Weil ich dich liebe: Gib AIDS keine Chance* ("Because I love you: Don't give AIDS a chance") and simultaneously admonishes the viewer: *Handeln Sie verantwortlich* ("Behave re-

9.   Guarantees of anonymity are, of course, a practical problem of HIV antibody testing in every country, and there have been reports of tests performed without consent or knowledge of the subjects in both Germanies. In September 1987, the West Berlin AIDS-Hilfe uncovered secret testing, in the West German city of Fulda, of ninety-three applicants for civil service employment, seven black Africans, and four applicants for political asylum (See "Heimliche AIDS-Test in Fulda," *Tageszeitung*, September 10, 1987, p. 4; and an earlier report, "AIDS-infiziert—Im Computer registriert," *Tageszeitung*, July 9, 1987, pp. 1–3). In the GDR, it is commonly assumed that the numerous black African students are routinely tested and, if found to be positive, deported. According to GDR officials, one million HIV antibody tests had been conducted as of March 1987 (Clara Roth, "Heimliche AIDS-Tests," *Tageszeitung*, March 14, 1987, p. 25). It is unclear whether or not all of these tests were performed on individuals giving consent.

       Outside of Bavaria (see footnote 11) there is no mandatory HIV antibody testing in West Germany. Although the GDR requires registration of individuals testing positive, failures to do so are not criminalized. In the Soviet Union, anyone who tests positive and then infects another individual is subject to from five to eight years imprisonment. Czechoslovakia has instituted mandatory HIV tests for anyone with a record of venereal disease. Anyone testing positive must sign a statement agreeing to have a reduced number of sexual partners and to have sex only with a condom. The policy mentions neither sexual orientation nor sexual practices. If the individual becomes sick after signing the agreement and is then discovered to have infected others, he or she is subject to a five-year jail term.

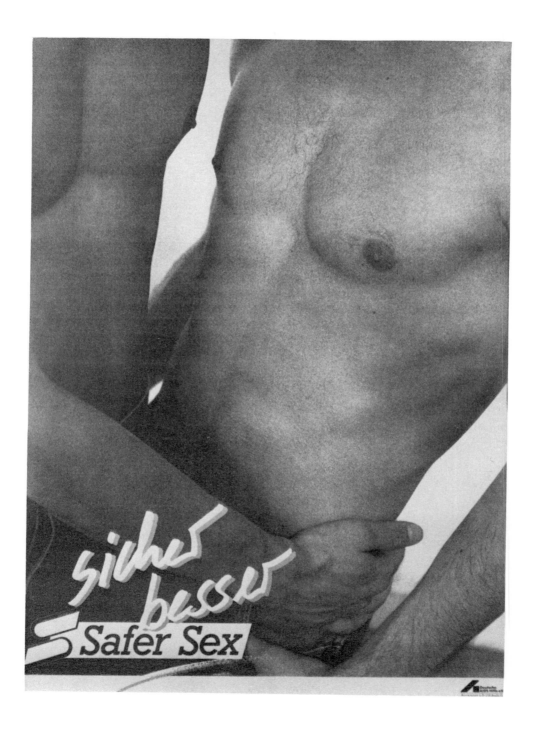

sponsibly"). The differences of message and target audience between the community-produced poster and that of the state could hardly be clearer.

Federal funds appropriated for AIDS education and research in West Germany (including West Berlin) amounted to seventeen million marks (about eight million dollars) in 1987, while the figure will increase to 180 million marks (nearly 100 million dollars) in 1988. Health Minister Süssmuth has set forth the following policy measures for the current fiscal year: the staffing of fifty social work agencies with personnel, psycho-social counseling for social workers, a project to aid infected mothers and children, AIDS counseling services in all 309

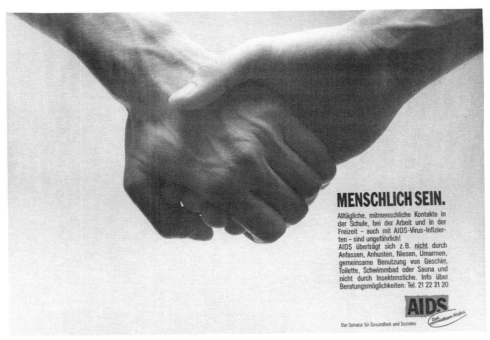

AIDS education poster produced by the Senator for Health and Human Services, Berlin. The text reads: BE HUMANE. Ordinary human contact at school, work, and play—even with those infected with the AIDS virus—is not dangerous! AIDS is not transmitted through, for example, touching, coughing, sneezing, hugging, or shared use of dishes, toilets, swimming pools, and saunas, or from insect bites.

AIDS education poster produced by the Berlin AIDS-Hilfe.

German AIDS-Hilfe. Safer Sex Comic 4, detail. 1985.

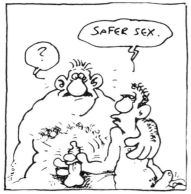

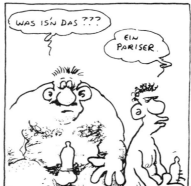

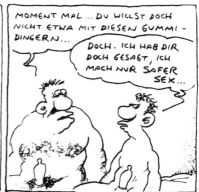

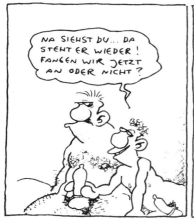

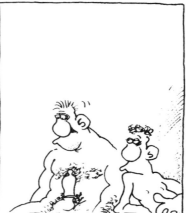

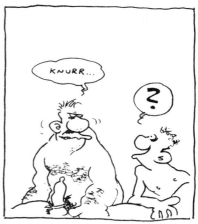

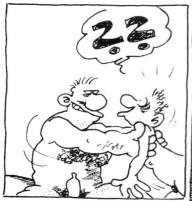

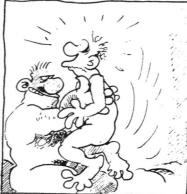

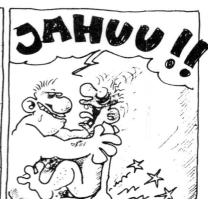

regional posts of the ministry, experimentation with new residential forms for those testing HIV positive and those who are sick, specific physicians' offices designated for AIDS research, clinics for documentation staffed with doctors and support personnel, and the continued financial support of already existing education and counseling facilities.[10] These measures were the first item on the agenda when the upper house of German Parliament began its session this past fall. Given that Süssmuth is a member of the ruling conservative Christian Democratic Union, her generally moderate policy recommendations and her resistance to the reactionary and repressive measures enacted in Franz Joseph Strauss's Bavaria came as considerable relief.[11] Largely because of her positions on AIDS, women's rights, and family policy, as well as her willingness to consult with the people most affected by these policies, Süssmuth has become one of the most popular political figures in West Germany.

*

Let us now turn to another dimension of the cultural construction of AIDS and compare the discursive style of the "free marketplace" of ideas in West Berlin with that of centralized planning in Berlin, GDR. Accounts of the etiology of AIDS, in which medical theories are thoroughly conflated with political ideology, are particularly revealing of symmetries and differences between the two systems.

East European theories, generally derived from those in the Soviet Union, assert direct connections between AIDS, drug abuse, sexual decadence, and Western capitalism. These explanations were given an entirely new twist in October 1986, when Dr. Jakob Segal, seventy-five-year-old emeritus professor of biology at Humboldt University in East Berlin, received a visit from two American diplomats "to question him about the AIDS virus." According to an account that promptly appeared in the West German weekly *Der Spiegel*, Segal declared afterward, "I'm sure they were from the CIA."[12] Following that visit, Segal undertook library research, then produced a manuscript detailing his contention that in the mid-'70s the US Army medical laboratory headquarters in Fort

10.   See Susanne Mayer, "Keine Kur nach Gauweilers Rezeption," *Die Zeit*, October 2, 1987, p. 5.
11.   At the hands of State Secretary Peter Gauweiler, AIDS policy in the Bavarian republic is directed toward the identification of perceived enemies, both internal and external. Public "health" measures there, which have not yet been fully enacted, include compulsory HIV testing of certain categories of foreigners seeking residence, prostitutes, drug users, prisoners, civil servants, and people found in gay bars during police raids. On November 16, in the Bavarian city of Nuremberg, a former US army cook with AIDS was convicted of attempting to inflict "grievous bodily harm" and sentenced to two years in prison for practicing unsafe sex. According to the *New York Times* (November 17, 1987, p. A5), "the law under which he was charged prohibits causing bodily harm with a weapon or 'dangerous treatment,' a clause normally reserved for poisons." The ex-soldier insisted all along that he had practiced safe sex. For an interview with Gauweiler about his AIDS policy, see "'Safer Sex ist nich sicher,'" *Der Spiegel*, May 25, 1987, pp. 25–32.
12.   Der Spiegel, November 10, 1986, p. 44.

Detrick, Maryland, had engaged in strange experiments with local prisoners: in exchange for their freedom, these prisoners had submitted to being infected with an assortment of viruses, one of which was the "AIDS virus," a genetically engineered combination, according to Segal, of the Maedi-Visna, known as the sheep virus, and HTLV-I, a retrovirus linked to human lymphoma.

Segal is not alone in advancing such a conspiracy theory. The Soviet newspapers *Trud* and *Literaturnaia gazeta* informed their readers several years ago that the virus was produced by the CIA and Pentagon in secret laboratories for use in biological warfare.[13] Similar theories are also propounded in the US, from such diverse positions as those of gay activist writer John Rechy and crypto-fascist Lyndon Larouche.[14] Of course, most establishment *scientists* in both Germanies (and in the Soviet Union) reject such theories, as do their counterparts in the US. The point here, however, is that conspiracy theories, including Segal's, linking AIDS with the CIA, have received considerable attention in West Germany, but have never once been published in the GDR.

The Segal story continued to receive West German press coverage into early 1987, when the West Berlin leftist daily *Tageszeitung* printed an entire series of articles on the Fort Detrick thesis. The series began with an interview with Professor Segal by Stefan Heym, a popular GDR writer living in East Berlin.[15] The article produced some resonance among certain anti-American West Berliners (the US has not, since the Vietnam War, regained the sympathy it enjoyed in Berlin during the Kennedy years). Consider the peculiarity of the situation: Two well-known, respected East Germans publish a theory propounding the notion that AIDS is caused by a man-made virus produced by American biological warfare researchers — but they do so in West Berlin. They are not permitted to publish their theory in newspapers in their own country, which is officially anti-American and especially vituperative about the CIA. It is impossible to give a verifiable explanation for this reticence, but one may surmise that in the GDR the politics of AIDS has remained the province of medical personnel rather than political propagandists. Meanwhile, in West Berlin, where 6,600 American "protection troops" and 30,000 support personnel reside, a widely read newspaper circulates a story that is virtually guaranteed to increase anti-American sentiment.

Coverage of the conspiracy theory of AIDS is only a variant of the Western press's tendency to sensationalize the AIDS crisis. The West's "free market-

13.   Complaints about this assertion were raised by Secretary of State George Shultz in an October 23 meeting with Mikhail Gorbachev in Moscow, after which *Isvestia* printed an official disavowal of the theory by Soviet scientists (see "Soviet Disavows Charges that U.S. Created AIDS," *New York Times*, November 5, 1987, p. A31).
14.   See also Robert Lederer, "Origin and Spread of AIDS: Is the West Responsible?" *Covert Action*, no. 28 (Summer 1987), pp. 43–54. Lederer relays, skeptically, the Segal thesis as well as other origin theories.
15.   "AIDS: Man-Made in the USA," *Tageszeitung*, February 18, 1987, pp. 11–13.

place" of ideas is, of course, not free; ideas are regulated by—precisely—the marketplace, leading, in the case of AIDS coverage, to the publication of whatever speculative theory or firsthand dramatic story will garner public attention. The majority of newspapers read in West Germany are controlled by Springer Verlag, which, like the Murdock chain in English-speaking countries, ensures its profits by pandering to existing prejudices—against gay people, for example.[16] By contrast, in the GDR press accounts of AIDS, public health officials stress their determination to prevent both widespread transmission of the virus and the "mass hysteria" they say is characteristic of the West. The East German media has handled the relationship between AIDS and homosexuality in such a way as to avoid any increase in homophobia; indeed, it appears that understanding of gay issues has increased. Homosexuality has been legal for consenting adults in the GDR since 1968, and public policy, while not actively encouraging or supporting gay people as a distinct group, has been generally oriented toward the toleration of homosexuality as a variant of human sexuality, with the goal of full and equal integration of gay people as "fellow citizens."[17]

Public attitudes and policy concerning minorities, including gay people, must be formulated in both Germanies against the background of a very particular history, that of the Nazi persecutions. Thus, the specter of concentration camps cannot fail to emerge in any suggestion of quarantining people with AIDS, especially insofar as it is now fully recognized that during the Third Reich homosexual prisoners, designated by the pink triangle, occupied the very bottom of the hierarchy in the camps. It is also understood that there was no need for massive propaganda campaigns—or indeed the creation of new laws—to bring public opinion in line with Nazi policy concerning homosexuals—a policy that included quarantine, sterilization, castration, and liquidation. Despite various attempts by politicians in both states (strongly supported in West Germany by the

---

16.   This treatment of AIDS in the Western press is condemned in an East German Protestant church publication, in which the author argues that hysterical reporting in Western capitalist countries has lead to the scapegoating of various minorities. He also suggests that one should speak not of AIDS deaths, but rather of deaths due to specific illnesses such as Kaposi's sarcoma or *Pneumocystis carinii* pneumonia. See Erhart Neubert, *Fallbeispiel AIDS: Eine sozialkritische Untersuchung*, Berlin, DDR, Theologische Studienabteilung beim Bund der Evangelischen Kirchen in der DDR, 1987.

17.   Medical "experts," such as Rainer Werner, in the first East German book entirely devoted to homosexuality (*Homosexualität: Herausforderung an Wissen und Toleranz*, Berlin, GDR, Ministry of Health, 1987), often insist that, unlike in the West, there is no separate gay culture in the GDR. This is patently false and reflects a combination of naiveté, ignorance, denial, and wishful thinking. As the experts maintain, government policy attempts to integrate homosexuals—labor shortages in the GDR make the possible loss of ten percent of their population unbearable. In pursuit of this goal, officials deny gay men and lesbians opportunities to build an autonomous culture. For a historical overview, see Jim Steakley, "Gays under Socialism: Male Homosexuality in the German Democratic Republic," *The Body Politic*, no. 29 (December 1976–January 1977), pp. 15–18. See also John Borneman, "Sexual Aufklärung and Sexual Practices in the German Democratic Republic," in *Homosexuality, Which Homosexuality?*, Amsterdam, Free University, International Conference on Gay and Lesbian Studies, 1987, Social Science vol. II, pp. 249–261.

Reagan Administration's ambassador Richard Burt) to escape the legacy of this shared past, history continues to resurface.

*

Just as the two German states have benefited from the earlier and proportionately greater experience of the United States with AIDS, Americans have much to learn from the Germanies. The clearest lesson concerns the systems of health care discussed above; it cannot be overemphasized that in the industrial world *only the United States and South Africa* lack national health insurance. The determinately unfair and inadequate health care system in the US is compounded by official AIDS policy, which has thus far been directed toward the detection and penalizing of those affected, and to the "protection" of the white, middle- and upper-class heterosexual population, while the incidence of AIDS grows exponentially in minority communities.

"Freedom of the press" remains a sacred—and thus largely unexamined—concept in the US. Examination might begin with the relationship between our profit-motivated mass media and AIDS hysteria, which has led to increased violence against gays and others and, even more seriously, to the increased spread of the epidemic because of public confusion and ignorance. But our examination cannot be limited to such specific questions as health care systems and press ownership. As long as the United States remains a class-, race-, and gender-structured society, the inequities of these divisions will reproduce themselves at every opportunity in every domain of public and private life. The AIDS crisis has only brought this fact more clearly into focus.

It is a common American conceit to neutralize criticism of negative prevailing conditions by assuming that things must be worse elsewhere. Certainly Germany, with its fascist heritage, and more certainly Marxist East Germany, ruled by iron-fisted goons and doddering apparatchiks, must be a nightmare by comparison.

DOUGLAS CRIMP

—AIDS: Questions and Answers
—AIDS: Get the Facts
—AIDS: Don't Die of Ignorance

The sloganeering of AIDS education campaigns suggests that knowledge about AIDS is readily available, easily acquired, and undisputed. Anyone who has sought to learn the "facts," however, knows just how hard it is to get them. Since the beginning of the epidemic, one of the very few sources of up-to-date information on all aspects of AIDS has been the gay press, but *this* is a fact that no education campaign (except those emanating from gay organizations) will tell you. As Simon Watney has noted, the British government ban on gay materials coming from the US until late in 1986 meant, in effect, that people in the UK were legally prohibited from learning about AIDS during a crucial period. The ban also meant that the British Department of Health had to sneak American gay publications into the country in diplomatic pouches in order to prepare the Thatcher government's bullying "Don't Die of Ignorance" campaign.[1]

Among information sources, perhaps the most acclaimed is the *New York Native*, which has published news about AIDS virtually every week since 1982. But, although during the early years a number of leading medical reporters wrote for the newspaper and provided essential information, the *Native*'s overall record on AIDS is not so admirable. Like other tabloids, the *Native* exploits the conflation of sex, fear, disease, and death in order to sell millions of newspapers. Banner headlines with grim predictions, new theories of "cause" and "cure," and scandals of scientific infighting combine with soft-core shots of hot male bodies to insure that we will rush to plunk down our two dollars for this extremely thin publication. One curious aspect of these headlines over the past few years is that they nearly always refer not to a major news or feature story, but to a short editorial column by the newspaper's publisher Charles Ortleb. These

---

1.   See Simon Watney, *Policing Desire: Pornography, AIDS, and the Media*, Minneapolis, University of Minnesota Press, 1987, p. 13.

weekly diatribes against the likes of Robert Gallo of the National Cancer Institute and Anthony Fauci of the National Institute for Allergy and Infectious Diseases might appear to be manifestations of a healthy skepticism toward establishment science, but Ortleb's distrust takes an odd form. Rather than performing a political analysis of the ideology of science, Ortleb merely touts the crackpot theory of the week, championing whoever is the latest outcast from the world of academic and government research. Never wanting to concede that establishment science could be right about the "cause" of AIDS — which is now generally (if indeed skeptically) assumed to be the retrovirus designated HIV — Ortleb latches onto any alternative theory: African Swine Fever Virus, Epstein-Barr Virus, reactivated syphilis.[2] The genuine concern by informed people that a full acceptance of HIV as *the* cause of AIDS limits research options, especially regarding possible cofactors, is magnified and distorted by Ortleb into ad hominem vilification of anyone who assumes for the moment that HIV is the likely primary causal agent of AIDS and ARC. Among the *Native*'s maverick heroes in this controversy about origins is the Berkeley biochemist Peter Duesberg, who is so confident that HIV is harmless that he has claimed to be unafraid of injecting it into his veins. When asked by *Village Voice* reporter Ann Giudici Fettner what he *does* think is causing the epidemic, Duesberg replied, "We don't have a new disease. It's a collection of [old] diseases caused by a lifestyle that was criminal 20 years ago. Combined with bathhouses, all these infections go with lifestyles which enhance them."[3] As Fettner notes, this is "a stunning regression to 1982," when AIDS was presumed to be a consequence of "the gay life-style."

A scientist pushing "the gay life-style" as the cause of AIDS in 1987 might seem a strange sort of hero for a gay newspaper to be celebrating, but then anyone who has read the *Native* regularly will have noted that, for Ortleb too, sex has been the real culprit all along. And, in this, Ortleb is not alone among powerful gay journalists. He is joined in this belief not only by right-wing politicians and ideologues, but by Randy Shilts, AIDS reporter for the *San Francisco Chronicle* and author of *And the Band Played On*, the bestselling book on AIDS.[4] That this book is pernicious has already been noted by many people working in the struggle against AIDS. For anyone suspicious of "mainstream" American culture, it might seem enough simply to note that the book *is* a bestseller, that it has been highly praised throughout the dominant media, or, even more damning, that the book has been optioned for a TV miniseries by Esther Shapiro, writer and producer of *Dynasty*. For some, the fact that Larry

2.   For an overview of theories of the cause of AIDS, see Robert Lederer, "Origin and Spread of AIDS: Is the West Responsible?" *Covert Action*, no. 28 (Summer 1987), pp. 43–54; and no. 29 (Winter 1988), pp. 52–65.
3.   Quoted in Ann Giudici Fettner, "Bad Science Makes Strange Bedfellows," *Village Voice*, February 2, 1988, p. 25.
4.   Randy Shilts, *And the Band Played On: Politics, People, and the AIDS Epidemic*, New York, St. Martin's Press, 1987. Page numbers for all citations from the book appear in parentheses in the text.

Kramer is said to be vying for the job of scriptwriter of the series will add to these suspicions (whoever reads the book will note that, in any case, the adaptation will be an easy task, since it is already written, effectively, *as* a miniseries). The fact that Shilts places blame for the spread of AIDS equally on the Reagan Administration, various government agencies, the scientific and medical establishments, *and the gay community*, is reason enough for many of us to condemn the book.

And the Band Played On is predicated on a series of oppositions; it is, first and foremost, a story of heroes and villains, of common sense against prejudice, of rationality against irrationality; it is also an account of scientific advance versus political maneuvering, public health versus civil rights, a safe blood supply versus blood-banking industry profits, homosexuals versus heterosexuals, hard cold facts versus what Shilts calls AIDSpeak.

We might assume we know what is meant by this neologism: AIDSpeak would be, for example, "the AIDS test," "AIDS victims," "promiscuity." But no, Shilts employs these imprecise, callous, or moralizing terms just as do all his fellow mainstream journalists, without quotation marks, without apology. For Shilts, AIDSpeak is, instead, a language invented to cover up the truth. An early indication of what Shilts thinks this language is appears in his account of the June 5, 1981, article in the *Morbidity and Mortality Weekly Report* about cases of *Pneumocystis* pneumonia in gay men. Shilts writes:

> The report appeared . . . not on page one of the *MMWR* but in a more inconspicuous slot on page two. Any reference to homosexuality was dropped from the title, and the headline simply read: *Pneumocystis* pneumonia — Los Angeles.
>
> Don't offend the gays and don't inflame the homophobes. These were the twin horns on which the handling of this epidemic would be torn from the first day of the epidemic. Inspired by the best intentions, such arguments paved the road toward the destination good intentions inevitably lead (pp. 68–69).

It was a great shock to read this in 1987, after six years of headlines about "the gay plague" and the railing of moralists about God's punishment for sodomy, or, more recently, statements such as "AIDS is no longer just a gay disease." Language destined to offend gays and inflame homophobia has been, from the very beginning—in science, in the media, and in politics—the main language of AIDS discussion, although the language has been altered at times in order that it would, for example, offend Haitians and inflame racism, or offend women and inflame sexism. But to Shilts AIDSpeak is not this language guaranteed to offend and inflame. On the contrary, it is

> . . . a new language forged by public health officials, anxious gay politicians, and the burgeoning ranks of "AIDS activists." The linguistic roots of AIDSpeak sprouted not so much from the truth as

from what was politically facile and psychologically reassuring. Se-
mantics was the major denominator of AIDSpeak jargon, because the
language went to great lengths never to offend.

A new lexicon was evolving. Under the rules of AIDSpeak, for
example, AIDS victims could not be called victims. Instead, they were
to be called People With AIDS, or PWAs, as if contracting this
uniquely brutal disease was not a victimizing experience. "Promiscuous" became "sexually active," because gay politicians declared "promiscuous" to be "judgmental," a major cuss word in AIDSpeak. . . .

. . . The new syntax allowed gay political leaders to address and
largely determine public health policy in the coming years, because
public health officials quickly mastered AIDSpeak, and it was a fundamentally political tongue (p. 315).

Shilts's contempt for gay political leaders, AIDS activists, and people with
AIDS, and his delusions about their power to influence public health policy are
deeply revealing of his own politics. But to Shilts, politics is something alien,
something others have, and political speech is AIDSpeak. Shilts has no politics,
only common sense; he speaks only the "truth," even if the truth is "brutal," like
being "victimized" by AIDS.

As an immediate response to this view, I will state my own political position:
*Anything said or done about AIDS that does not give precedence to the knowledge, the
needs, and the demands of people living with AIDS must be condemned.* The passage
from *And the Band Played On* quoted above—and indeed the entire book—is
written in flagrant disregard for these people. Their first principle, that they not
be called victims, is flaunted by Shilts. I will concede that people living with AIDS
are victims in one sense: they have been and continue to be victimized by all those
who will not listen to them, including Randy Shilts. But we cannot stop at
condemnation. Shilts's book is too full of useful information, amassed in part
with the help of the Freedom of Information Act, simply to dismiss it. But while
it may be extremely useful, it is also extremely dangerous—and thus has to be
read very critically.

In piecing together his tale of heroes and villains—which intersperses
vignettes about scientists from the Centers for Disease Control in Atlanta, the
National Institutes of Health in Bethesda, and the Pasteur Institute in Paris;
doctors with AIDS patients in New York, San Francisco, and Los Angeles;
blood-banking industry executives; various people with AIDS (always white,
usually gay men living in San Francisco); officials in the Department of Health
and Human Services and the Food and Drug Administration; gay activists and
AIDS service organization volunteers—Shilts always returns to a single complaint. With all the people getting sick and dying, and with all the scandals of
inaction, stonewalling, and infighting that are arguably the primary cause of
their illness and death, journalists never bothered to investigate. They always

bought the government's lies, never looked behind those lies to get the "truth." There was, of course, one exception, the lonely journalist for the *San Francisco Chronicle* assigned full-time to the AIDS beat. He is never named, but we know his name is Randy Shilts, the book's one unqualified hero, who appears discreetly in several of its episodes. Of course, that journalist knows the reason for the lack of investigative zeal on the part of his fellows: the people who were dying were gay men, and mainstream American journalists don't care what happens to gay men. Those journalists would rather print hysteria-producing, blame-the-victim stories than uncover the "truth."

So Shilts would print that truth in *And the Band Played On*, "investigative journalism at its best," as the flyleaf states. The book is an extremely detailed, virtually day-by-day account of the epidemic up to the revelation that Rock Hudson was dying of AIDS, the moment, in 1985, when the American media finally took notice.[5] But taking notice of Rock Hudson was, in itself, a scandal, because by the time the Rock Hudson story captured the attention of the media, Shilts notes, "the number of AIDS cases in the United States had surpassed 12,000 . . . of whom 6,079 had died" (p. 580). Moreover, what constituted a story for the media was only scandal itself: a famous movie star simultaneously revealed to be gay and to be dying of AIDS.

How surprised, then, could Shilts have been that, when his own book was published, the media once again avoided mention of the six years of political scandal that contributed so significantly to the scope of the AIDS epidemic? that they were instead intrigued by an altogether different story, the one they had been printing all along—the dirty little story of gay male promiscuity and irresponsibility?

In the press release issued by Shilts's publisher, St. Martin's, the media's attention was directed to the story that would ensure the book's success:

PATIENT ZERO: The Man Who Brought AIDS to North America

What remains a mystery for most people is where AIDS came from and how it spread so rapidly through America. In the most bizarre story of the epidemic, Shilts also found the man whom the CDC dubbed the "Patient Zero" of the epidemic. Patient Zero, a French-Canadian airline steward, was one of the first North Americans diagnosed with AIDS. Because he traveled through the gay communities of major urban areas, he spread the AIDS virus [*sic*] throughout the continent. Indeed, studies later revealed 40 of the first 200 AIDS cases in America were documented either to have had sex with Patient Zero or have had sex with someone who did.

5. The fact that Shilts chose this moment as the end point of his narrative suggests that the book's central purpose is indeed to prove the irresponsibility of all journalists but Shilts himself, making him the book's true hero.

The story of Gaetan Dugas, or "Patient Zero," is woven throughout the book in over twenty separate episodes, beginning on page 11 and ending only on page 439, where the young man's death is recounted. "At one time," Shilts writes in a typically portentous tone, "Gaetan had been what every man wanted from gay life; by the time he died, he had become what every man feared." It is interesting indeed that Shilts, a gay man who appears *not* to have wanted from gay life what Gaetan Dugas may or may not have been, should nevertheless assume that what all gay men want is identical.

The publisher's ploy worked, for which they appear to be proud. Included in the press kit sent to me were xeroxes of the following news stories and reviews:

—*New York Times:* Canadian Said to Have Had Key Role in Spread of AIDS

—*New York Post:* THE MAN WHO GAVE US AIDS

—*NY Daily News:* The man who flew too much

—*Time:* The Appalling Saga of Patient Zero

—*McClean's:* "Patient Zero" and the AIDS virus

People magazine made "Patient Zero" one of its "25 most intriguing people of '87," together with Ronald Reagan, Mikhail Gorbachev, Oliver North, Fawn Hall, Princess Diana, Vincent van Gogh, and Baby Jessica. Shilts's success in giving the media the scandalous story that would overshadow his book's other "revelations"—and that would ensure that the blame for AIDS would remain focused on gay men—can be seen even in the way the story appeared in Germany's leading liberal weekly *Der Spiegel.* Underneath a photograph of cruising gay men at the end of Christopher Street in New York City, the story's sensational title reads "Ich werde sterben, und du auch" ("I'm going to die, and so are you"), a line the Canadian airline steward is supposed to have uttered to his bathhouse sex partners as he turned up the lights after an encounter and pointed to his KS lesions.

Shilts's painstaking efforts at telling the "true" story of the epidemic's early years thus resulted in two media stories: the story of the man who brought us AIDS, and the story of the man who brought us the story of the man who brought us AIDS. Gaetan Dugas and Randy Shilts became overnight media stars. Being fully of the media establishment, Shilts's criticism of that establishment is limited to pitting good journalists against bad. He is apparently oblivious to the economic and ideological mechanisms that largely determine how AIDS will be constructed in the media, and he thus contributes to that construction rather than to its critique.

The criticism most often leveled against Shilts's book by its gay critics is that

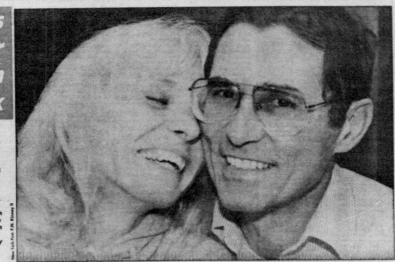

NEW YORK POST

FINAL

TONIGHT: Cloudy, mid 50s TOMORROW: Cloudy, mid 60s. Details: Page 2.

Stocks: P. 41

TV listings: P. 95

TUESDAY, OCT. 6, 1987   Founded by Alexander Hamilton in 1801   35 CENTS

Triggered 'gay cancer' epidemic in U.S.

THE MAN WHO GAVE US AIDS

— STORY ON PAGE THREE

His love's safe after ordeal on icy peak

Weekend hiker Millicent Moore Tomassetti nuzzles her husband, Louis, last night in Cherry Hill, N.J. She surprised him, and turned up safe and sound after being trapped in Sunday's freak snow storm atop Hunter Mountain in the Catskills. Mrs. Tomassetti and two companions made it down the slope to safety. Three more hikers walked down this morning on snow shoes dropped to them by helicopter.

SEE PAGE 5

it is a product of internalized homophobia. In this view, Shilts is seen to identify with the heterosexist society that loathes him for his homosexuality, and through that identification to project his loathing onto the gay community. Thus, "Patient Zero," the very figure of the homosexual as imagined by heterosexuals — sexually voracious, murderously irresponsible — is Shilts's homophobic nightmare of himself, a nightmare that he must constantly deny by making it true only of others. Shilts therefore offers up the scapegoat for his heterosexual colleagues in order to prove that he, like them, is horrified by such creatures.

It is true that Shilts's book reproduces virtually every cliché of homophobia. Like Queen Victoria's proverbial inability to fathom what lesbians do in bed, Shilts's disdain for the sexual habits of gay men extends even to finding certain of those habits "unimaginable." In one of his many fulminations against gay bathhouses, Shilts writes, "Just about every type of unsafe sex imaginable, and many variations that were unimaginable, were being practiced with carefree abandonment [*sic*] at the facilities" (p. 481).

Shilts's failure of imagination is in this case merely a trope, a way of saying that certain sexual acts are beyond the pale for most people. But in resorting to such a trope, Shilts unconsciously identifies with all those who would rather see gay men die than allow homosexuality to invade their consciousness.

And the Band Played On is written not only as a chronology of events, but also as a cleverly plotted series of episodes. Hundreds of narrative threads are woven around individual characters described in conventional novelistic fashion. Often Shilts uses peoples' regional accents and physiques metonymically to stand for their characters: "Everyone cheered enthusiastically when Paul Popham [president of the Gay Men's Health Crisis] addressed the crowd in his broad, plainspoken Oregon accent" (p. 139). A hundred pages earlier, Popham is introduced with the sentence, "At the Y, Larry [Kramer] had told Paul that he had such a naturally well-defined body that he didn't need to work out, and Paul responded with a shy aw-shucks ingenuousness that reminded Larry of Gary Cooper or Jimmy Stewart" (p. 26). Shilts's choice of novelistic form allows him these tricks of omniscient narration. Not only does he tell us what Paul said and Larry thought, he also reveals his characters' dreams and nightmares, and even, in a few cases, what people with AIDS were thinking and feeling at the moment of death. These aspects of bourgeois writing would seem to represent a strange choice indeed for the separation of fact from fiction,[6] but I want to argue that it is precisely this choice that determines Shilts's homophobia. For it is my contention not simply that Shilts has internalized homophobia, but that he has sought to

---

6.   Shilts writes in his "Notes on Sources," "This book is a work of journalism. There has been no fictionalization. For purposes of narrative flow, I reconstruct scenes, recount conversations and occasionally attribute observations to people with such phrases as 'he thought' or 'she felt.' Such references are drawn from either the research interviews I conducted for the book or from research conducted during my years covering the AIDS epidemic for the *San Francisco Chronicle*" (p. 607).

escape the effects of homophobia by employing a particular cultural form, one that is thoroughly outmoded but still very much with us in its vulgarized variants. In *Writing Degree Zero*, Roland Barthes writes:

> Until [the 1850s], it was bourgeois ideology itself which gave the measure of the universal by fulfilling it unchallenged. The bourgeois writer, sole judge of other people's woes and without anyone else to gaze on him, was not torn between his social condition and his intellectual vocation.[7]

"Sole judge of other people's woes and without anyone else to gaze on him," Shilts adopted a no-longer-possible universal point of view—which is, among other things, the *heterosexual* point of view—and thus erased his own social condition, that of being a gay man in a homophobic society. Shilts wrote the story of Gaetan Dugas not because it needed telling—because, in the journalist's mind it was true and factual—but because it was required by the bourgeois novelistic form that Shilts used as his shield. The book's arch-villain has a special function, that of securing the identity of his polar opposite, the book's true hero. Shilts created the character of "Patient Zero" to embody everything that the book purports to expose: irresponsibility, delay, denial—ultimately murder.[8] "Patient Zero" stands for all the evil that is "really" the cause of the epidemic, and Shilts's portrait of "Patient Zero" stands for Shilts's own heroic act of "exposing" that evil.

If I have dwelt for so long on *And the Band Played On*, it is not only because its enthusiastic reception demands a response. It is also because the book demonstrates so clearly that cultural conventions rigidly dictate what can and will be said about AIDS. And these cultural conventions exist everywhere the epidemic is constructed: in newspaper stories and magazine articles, in television documentaries and fiction films, in political debate and health-care policy, in scientific research, in art, in activism, and in sexuality. The way AIDS is understood is in large measure predetermined by the forms these discourses take. Randy Shilts

---

7.   Roland Barthes, *Writing Degree Zero*, trans. Annette Lavers and Colin Smith, Boston, Beacon Press, 1967, p. 60.
8.   I say *created* because, though Gaetan Dugas was a real person, his character—in both senses of the word—was invented by Shilts. Moreover, contrary to the St. Martin's press release, Shilts did not "discover" "Patient Zero." The story about how various early AIDS researchers were able to link a number of early cases of the syndrome—which was done not to locate the "source" of the epidemic and place blame, but simply to verify the transmissibility of a causal agent—was told earlier by Ann Giudici Fettner and William A. Check. Dugas is called "Eric" in their account, and his character is described significantly differently: " 'He felt terrible about having made other people sick,' says [Dr. William] Darrow [a CDC sociologist]. 'He had come down with Kaposi's but no one ever told him it might be infectious. Even at CDC we didn't know then that it was contagious. It is a general dogma that cancer is not transmissible. Of course, we now know that the underlying immune-system deficiency that allows the cancer to grow is most likely transmissible.' " (*The Truth about AIDS*, New York, Henry Holt, revised edition, 1985, p. 86). Thanks to Paula Treichler for calling this passage to my attention.

provided the viciously homophobic portrait of "Patient Zero" because his thriller narrative demanded it, and the news media reported that story and none of the rest because what is news and what is not is dictated by the form the news takes in our society. In a recent op-ed piece about his recognition that AIDS is now newsworthy, A. M. Rosenthal, executive editor of the *New York Times* during the entire five-year period when the epidemic was a *nonstory* for the *Times*, offered the following reflection on the news-story form: "Journalists call events, trivial or historic, 'stories' because we really are tellers of tales and to us there is no point in knowing or learning if we can't run out and tell somebody. That's just the way we are; go ask a psychiatrist why." [9]

"Patient Zero" is a news story while the criminal inaction of the Reagan Administration is not — "go ask a psychiatrist why." Rock Hudson is a story, but the thousands of other people with AIDS are not — "go ask a psychiatrist why." Heterosexuals with AIDS is a story; homosexuals with AIDS is not — "go ask a psychiatrist why." Shilts laments this situation. His book contributes nothing to understanding and changing it.

Among the heroes of *And the Band Played On* is Larry Kramer, who shares Shilts's negative view of gay politics and sexuality. Here is how Shilts describes the reception of Kramer's play about AIDS, *The Normal Heart*:

> April 21 [1985]
> PUBLIC THEATER
> *New York City*
> A thunderous ovation echoed through the theater. The people rose to their feet, applauding the cast returning to the stage to take their bows. Larry Kramer looked to his eighty-five-year-old mother. She had always wanted him to write for the stage, and Kramer had done that now. True, *The Normal Heart* was not your respectable Neil Simon fare, but a virtually unanimous chorus of reviewers had already proclaimed the play to be a masterpiece of political drama. Even before the previews were over, critics from every major news organization in New York City had scoured their thesauruses for superlatives to describe the play. NBC said it "beats with passion"; *Time* magazine said it was "deeply affecting, tense and touching"; the *New York Daily News* called it "an angry, unremitting and gripping piece of political theater." One critic said *Heart* was to the AIDS epidemic what Arthur Miller's *The Crucible* had been to the McCarthy era. *New York Magazine*'s critic John Simon, who had recently been overheard saying that he looked forward to when AIDS had killed all the homosexuals in New York theater, conceded in an interview that he left the play weeping (p. 556).

9.   A. M. Rosenthal, "AIDS: Everyone's Business," *New York Times*, December 29, 1987, p. A19.

How is it that for four years the deaths of thousands of gay men could leave the dominant media entirely unmoved, but Larry Kramer's play could make them weep? Shilts offers no explanation, nor is he suspicious of this momentary change of heart. *The Normal Heart* is a *pièce à clef* about the Gay Men's Health Crisis, the AIDS service organization Kramer helped found and which later expelled him—because, as the play tells it, he, like Shilts, insisted on speaking the truth.[10] In one of his many fights with his fellow organizers, Ned Weeks, the character that represents Kramer, explodes, "Why is anything I'm saying compared to anything but common sense?" (p. 100). Common sense, in Kramer's view, is that gay men should stop having so much sex, that promiscuity kills. But this common sense is, of course, conventional moral wisdom: it is not safe sex, but monogamy that is the solution. The play's message is therefore not only reactionary, it is lethal, since monogamy per se provides no protection whatsoever against a virus that might already have infected one partner in a relationship.

"I am sick of guys who can only think with their cocks" (p. 57), says Ned Weeks, and later, "Being defined by our cocks is literally killing us" (p. 115). For Kramer, being defined by sex is the legacy of gay politics; promiscuity and gay politics are one and the same:

> Ned [to Emma, the doctor who urges him to tell gay men to stop having sex]: Do you realize that you are talking about millions of men who have singled out promiscuity to be their principal political agenda, the one they'd die before abandoning? (pp. 37–38).

> Bruce [the president of GMHC]: . . . the entire gay political platform is fucking (p. 57).

> Ned: . . . the gay leaders who created this sexual liberation philosophy in the first place have been the death of us. Mickey, why didn't you guys fight for the right to get married instead of the right to legitimize promiscuity? (p. 85).

This is the view of someone who did not participate in the gay movement, and who has no sense of its history, its complexities, its theory and practice (was he too busy taking advantage of its gains?). Kramer's ignorance of and contempt for the gay movement are demonstrated throughout the play:

> Ned: Nobody with a brain gets involved in gay politics. It's filled with the great unwashed radicals of any counterculture (p. 37).

> Mickey: You know, the battle against the police at Stonewall was won

---

10.   Larry Kramer, *The Normal Heart*, New York and Scarborough, Ontario, New American Library, 1985. Page numbers for citations are given in the text.

by transvestites. We all fought like hell. It's you Brooks Brothers guys
who—
Bruce: That's why I wasn't at Stonewall. I don't have anything in
common with those guys, girls, whatever you call them.
Mickey: . . . and . . . how do you feel about Lesbians?
Bruce: Not very much. I mean, they're . . . something else.
Mickey: I wonder what they're going to think about all this? If past
history is any guide, there's never been much support by either half of
us for the other. Tommy, are you a Lesbian? (pp. 54–55).

I want to return to gay politics, and specifically to the role lesbians have
played in the struggle against AIDS, but first it is necessary to explain why I have
been quoting Kramer's play as if it were not fictional, as if it could be unprob-
lematically taken to represent Kramer's own political views. As I've already said,
The Normal Heart is a *pièce à clef*, a form adopted for the very purpose of
presenting the author's experience and views in dramatic form. But my criticism
of the play is not merely that Kramer's political views, as voiced by his characters,
are reactionary—though they certainly are—but that the genre employed by
Kramer will dictate a reactionary content of a different kind: because the play is
written within the most traditional conventions of bourgeois theater, its politics
are the politics of bourgeois individualism. Like *And the Band Played On, The
Normal Heart* is the story of a lonely voice of reason smothered by the deafening
chorus of unreason. It is a play with a hero, Kramer himself, for whom the play is
an act of vengeance for all the wrong done him by his ungrateful colleagues at
the Gay Men's Health Crisis. *The Normal Heart* is a purely personal—*not* a
political—drama, a drama of a few heroic individuals in the AIDS movement.
From time to time, some of these characters talk "politics":

> Emma: Health is a political issue. Everybody's entitled to good medical
> care. If you're not getting it, you've got to fight for it. Do you know
> this is the only industrialized country in the world besides South
> Africa that doesn't guarantee health care for everyone? (p. 36).

But this is, of course, politics in the most restricted sense of the word. Such
a view refuses to see that power relations invade and shape all discourse. It
ignores the fact that the choice of the bourgeois form of drama, for example, is a
political choice that will have necessary political consequences. Among these is
the fact that the play's "politics" sound very didactic, don't "work" with the
drama. Thus in *The Normal Heart*, even these "politics" are mostly pushed to the
periphery; they become décor. In the New York Shakespeare Festival production
of the play, "the walls of the set, made of construction-site plywood, were
whitewashed. Everywhere possible, on this set and upon the theater walls too,
facts and figures and names were painted, in black, simple lettering" (p. 19).
These were such facts as

—MAYOR   KOCH: $75,000—MAYOR   FEINSTEIN: $16,000,000. (For public education and community services.)

—During the first nineteen months of the epidemic, *The New York Times* wrote about it a total of seven times.

—During the first three months of the Tylenol scare in 1982, *The New York Times* wrote about it a total of 54 times (pp. 20–21).

No one would dispute that these facts and figures have political significance, that they are part of the political picture of AIDS. But in the context of *The Normal Heart*, they are absorbed by the personal drama taking place on the stage, where they have no other function than to prove Ned Weeks right, to vindicate Ned Weeks's—Larry Kramer's—rage. And that rage, the play itself, is very largely directed against other gay men.

Shilts's book and Kramer's play share a curious contradiction: they blame the lack of response to the epidemic on the misrepresentation of AIDS as a gay disease even as they themselves treat AIDS almost exclusively as a gay problem. Both display indifference to the other groups drastically affected by the epidemic, primarily, in the US, IV drug users, who remain statistics for the two writers, just as gay men do for the people the two authors rail against.

The resolution of this contradiction, which is pervasive in AIDS discourse, would appear to be simple enough. AIDS is not a gay disease, but in the US it affected gay men first and, thus far, has affected us in greater proportion. But AIDS probably did *not* affect gay men first, even in the US. What is now called AIDS was first *seen* in middle-class gay men in America, in part because of our access to medical care. Retrospectively, however, it appears that IV drug users —whether gay or straight—were dying of AIDS in New York City throughout the '70s and early '80s, but a class-based and racist health care system failed to notice, and an epidemiology equally skewed by class and racial bias failed to begin to look *until 1987*.[11] Moreover, AIDS has never been restricted to gay men

11.   In October 1987, the *New York Times* reported that the New York City Department of Health conducted a study of drug-related deaths from 1982 to 1986, which found an estimated 2,520 AIDS-related deaths that had not been reported as such. As a result, "AIDS-related deaths, involving intravenous drug users accounted for 53 percent of all AIDS-related deaths in New York City since the epidemic began, while deaths involving sexually active homosexual and bisexual men accounted for 38 percent." Even these statistics are based on CDC epidemiology that continues to see the beginning of the epidemic as 1981, following the early reports of illnesses in gay men, in spite of widespread anecdotal reporting of a high rate of deaths throughout the 1970s from what was known as "junkie pneumonia" and was likely *Pneumocystis* pneumonia. Moreover, the study was undertaken not through any recognition of the seriousness of the problem posed to poor and minority communities, but, as New York City Health Commissioner Stephen Joseph was reported as saying, because "the higher numbers . . . showed that the heterosexual 'window' through which AIDS presumably could jump to people who were not at high risk was 'much wider that we believed'" (Ronald Sullivan, "AIDS in New York City Killing More Drug Users," *New York Times*, October 22, 1987, p. B1).

in Central Africa, where the syndrome is a problem of apocalyptic dimensions, but to this day receives almost no attention in the US.

What is far more significant than the real *facts* of HIV transmission in various populations throughout the world, however, is the initial conceptualization of AIDS as a syndrome affecting gay men. No insistence on the facts will render that discursive construction obsolete, and not only because of the intractability of homophobia. The idea of AIDS as a gay disease occasioned two *interconnected* conditions in the US: that AIDS would be an epidemic of stigmatization rooted in homophobia, and that the response to AIDS would depend in very large measure on the very gay movement Shilts and Kramer decry.

The organization Larry Kramer helped found, the Gay Men's Health Crisis, is as much a part of the early construction of AIDS as were the first reports of the effects of the syndrome in the *Morbidity and Mortality Weekly Report.* Though it may be true that few, if any, of the founders of GMHC were centrally involved in gay politics, everything they were able to accomplish — from fundraising and recruiting volunteers to consulting with openly gay health care professionals and getting education out to the gay community — depended on what had already been achieved by the gay movement. Moreover, the continued life of GMHC as the largest AIDS service organization in the US has necessarily aligned it with other, considerably more radical grass-roots AIDS organizations both in the gay community and in other communities affected by the epidemic. The Gay Men's Health Crisis, whose workforce comprises lesbians and heterosexual women as well as gay men (heterosexual men are notably absent from the AIDS movement), is now an organization that provides services for infants with AIDS, IV drug users with AIDS, women with AIDS. It is an organization that every day puts the words *gay men* in the mouths of people who would otherwise never speak them. More importantly, it is an organization that has put the words *gay men* in the mouths of nongay people living with the stigma attached to AIDS by those very words. The Gay Men's Health Crisis is thus a symbol, in its very name, of the fact that the gay movement is at the center of the fight against AIDS. The limitations of this movement — especially insofar as it is riven by race and class differences — are therefore in urgent need of examination.

In doing this, we must never lose sight of the fact that the gay movement is responsible for virtually every positive achievement in the struggle against AIDS during the epidemic's early years. These achievements are not only those of politically organized response — of fighting repressive measures; of demanding government funding, scientific research, and media coverage; of creating service organizations to care for the sick and to educate the well. They are also the achievements of a sexual community whose theory and practice of sex made it possible to meet the epidemic's most urgent requirement: the development of safe sex practices. But who counts as a member of this community? Who will be protected by the knowledge of safe sex? Kramer's character Mickey was right in saying that it was transvestites who fought back at Stonewall. What he did not say was that those "guys in Brooks Brothers suits" very soon hounded transvestites out of the movement initiated by Stonewall, because the "gay good citizens"[12] didn't want to be associated with "those guys, girls, whatever you call them." Now, in 1988, what AIDS service organizations are providing transvestites with safe sex information? Who is educating hustlers? Who is getting safe sex instructions, printed in Spanish, into gay bars in Queens that cater to working-class Colombian immigrants?[13] It is these questions that cannot be satisfactorily answered by a gay community that is far from inclusive of the vast majority of people whose homosexual practices place them at risk. It is also these questions that we must ask even more insistently of AIDS education programs that are now being taken out of the hands of gay people — AIDS education programs devised by the state, outside of any existing community, whatever its limitations.

Kramer's summary dismissal of transvestites in *The Normal Heart* is followed by his assumption that lesbians will show no interest in the AIDS crisis. Not only has Kramer been proven dead wrong, but his assumption is grounded in a failure to recognize the importance of a gay *political* community that has always included both sexes. In spite of the very real tensions and differences between lesbians and gay men, our common oppression has taught us the vital necessity of forming a coalition. And having negotiated and renegotiated this coalition over a period of two decades has provided much of the groundwork for the coalition politics necessitated by the shared oppression of all the radically different groups affected by AIDS. But the question Larry Kramer and other gay men should be asking in any case is not "What are lesbians doing to help us?" but rather "What are we doing to help lesbians?" Although it is consistently claimed that lesbians, as a group, are the least vulnerable to HIV transmission, this would appear to be predicated, once again, on the failure to understand what lesbians do in bed. As Lee Chiaramonte wrote in an article entitled "The Very Last Fairy Tale,"

> In order to believe that lesbians are not at risk for AIDS, or that those who have already been infected are merely incidental victims, I would have to know and agree with the standards by which we are judged to be safe. Meaning I would have to believe we are either sexless or olympically monogamous; that we are not intravenous drug users; that we do not sleep with men; that we do not engage in sexual activities that could prove as dangerous as they are titillating. I would also have to believe that lesbians, unlike straight women, can get seven years'

12. I borrow the phrase from Guy Hocquenghem, who used it to describe a gay movement increasingly devoted to civil rights rather than to the more radical agenda issuing from the New Left of the 1960s.
13. I do not want to suggest that there are no gay community organizations for or including transvestites, sex workers, or Latino immigrants, but rather that no organization representing highly marginalized groups has the funding or the power to reach large numbers of people with sensitive and specific AIDS information.

worth of honest answers from their lovers about forgotten past lives.[14]

Chiaramonte goes on to cite a 1983 *Journal of Sex Research* study in which it was determined that lesbians have almost twice as much sex as straight women and that their numbers of partners are greater than straight women's by nearly fifteen to one. In a survey conducted by Pat Califia for the *Journal of Homosexuality*, over half the lesbians questioned preferred nonmonogamous relationships.[15] And, in addition to the risks of HIV infection, which only compound women's problems with a sexist health care system, lesbians have, along with gay men, borne the intensified homophobia that has resulted from AIDS.

Not surprisingly it was a lesbian — Cindy Patton — who wrote one of the first serious political analyses of the AIDS epidemic and who has more recently coauthored a safe sex manual for women.[16] "It is critical," says Patton, "that the experience of the gay community in AIDS organizing be understood: the strategies employed before 1985 or so grew out of gay liberation and feminist theory."[17] The most significant of these strategies was — again — the development of safe sex guidelines, which, though clearly the achievement of the organized gay community, are now being reinvented by "experts."

> At the 1987 lesbian and gay health conference in Los Angeles, many longtime AIDS activists were surprised by the extent to which safe sex education had become the province of high level professionals. The fact that safe sex organizing began and is highly successful as a grassroots, community effort seemed to be forgotten. . . . Heterosexuals — and even gay people only beginning to confront AIDS — express panic about how to make appropriate and satisfying changes in their sex lives, as if no one had done this before them. It is a mark of the intransigence of homophobia that few look to the urban gay communities for advice, communities which have an infrastructure and a track record of highly successful behavior change.[18]

As Patton insists, gay people invented safe sex. We knew that the alternatives — monogamy and abstinence — were *unsafe*, unsafe in the latter case because people do not abstain from sex, and if you only tell them "just say no,"

14.   Lee Chiaramonte, "Lesbian Safety and AIDS: The Very Last Fairy Tale," *Visibilities*, vol. 1, no. 1 (January–February 1988), p. 5.
15.   *Ibid.*, p. 7.
16.   Cindy Patton, *Sex and Germs: The Politics of AIDS*, Boston, South End Press, 1985; and Cindy Patton and Janis Kelly, *Making It: A Woman's Guide to Sex in the Age of AIDS*, Ithaca, New York, Firebrand Books, 1987.
17.   Cindy Patton, "Resistance and the Erotic: Reclaiming History, Setting Strategy as We Face AIDS," *Radical America*, vol. 20, no. 6 (Facing AIDS: A Special Issue), p. 68.
18.   *Ibid.*, p. 69.

they will have unsafe sex. We were able to invent safe sex because we have always known that sex is not, in an epidemic or not, limited to penetrative sex. Our promiscuity taught us many things, not only about the pleasures of sex, but about the great multiplicity of those pleasures. It is that psychic preparation, that experimentation, that conscious work on our own sexualities that has allowed many of us to change our sexual behaviors—something that brutal "behavioral therapies" tried unsuccessfully for over a century to force us to do—very quickly and very dramatically. It is for this reason that Shilts's and Kramer's attitudes about the formulation of gay politics on the basis of our sexuality is so perversely distorted, why they insist that our promiscuity will destroy us when in fact *it is our promiscuity that will save us.*

> The elaborateness of gay male sexual culture which may have once contributed to the spread of AIDS has been rapidly transformed into one that inhibits spread of the disease, still promotes sexual liberation (albeit differently defined), and is as marvelously fringe and offensive to middle America as ever.[19]

All those who contend that gay male promiscuity is merely sexual *compulsion* resulting from fear of intimacy are now faced with very strong evidence against their prejudices. For if compulsion were so easily overcome or redirected, it would hardly deserve the name. Gay male promiscuity should be seen instead as a positive model of how sexual pleasures might be pursued by and granted to everyone if those pleasures were not confined within the narrow limits of institutionalized sexuality.

Indeed, it is the lack of promiscuity and its lessons that suggests that many straight people will have a much harder time learning "how to have sex in an epidemic" than we did.[20] This assumption follows from the fact that risk reduction information directed at heterosexuals, even when not clearly antisex or based on false morality, is still predicated upon the prevailing myths about sexuality in our society. First among these, of course, is the myth that monogamous relationships are not only the norm but ultimately everyone's deepest desire. Thus, the message is often not about safe sex at all, but about how to find *a* safe partner.

As Art Ulene, "family physician" to the *Today Show* put it:

> I think it's time to stop talking about "safe sex." I believe we should be talking about safe partners instead. A safe partner is one who has never been infected with the AIDS virus [*sic*]. With a safe partner, you don't have to worry about getting AIDS yourself—no matter what

19.   *Ibid.*, p. 72.
20.   *How to Have Sex in an Epidemic* is the title of a 40-page pamphlet produced by gay men, including PWAs, as early as 1983. See Patton, *ibid.*, p. 69.

you do sexually, and no matter how much protection you use while you do it.[21]

The agenda here is one of maintaining the us/them dichotomy that was initially performed by the CDC's "risk group" classifications — "Only gay men and IV drug users get AIDS." But now that neat classifications of otherness no longer "protect" the "general population,"[22] how does one go about finding a safe partner? One obvious way of answering this question is to urge HIV antibody testing. If you and your sex partner both test negative, you can still have unbridled fun.[23] But Dr. Ulene has an additional solution:

> One way to find safer partners — though a bit impractical for most — is to move to a place where the incidence of AIDS is low. There are two states that have reported only four cases of AIDS since the disease was discovered, while others are crowded with AIDS patients. Although this near-freedom from AIDS cannot be expected to last forever, the relative differences between states like Nebraska and New York are likely to last.[24]

Dr. Ulene then graciously provides a breakdown of AIDS cases by state.

Most safe sex education materials for heterosexuals, however, presume that their audience consists of people who feel themselves to be at some risk, perhaps because they do not limit themselves to a single sex partner, perhaps because they are unable to move to Nebraska. Still, in most cases, these safe sex instructions focus almost exclusively on penetrative sex and always make it a woman's job to

---

21   Art Ulene, M.D., *Safe Sex in a Dangerous World*, New York, Vintage Books, 1987, p. 31.
22.   In fact there continue to be concerted efforts to deny that everyone is at risk of HIV infection. The *New York Times* periodically prints updated epidemiological information editorially presented so as to reassure its readers — clearly presumed to be middle class, white, and heterosexual — that they have little to worry about. Two recent articles that resurrect old myths to keep AIDS away from heterosexuals are Michael A. Fumento, "AIDS: Are Heterosexuals at Risk?" *Commentary*, November 1987; and Robert E. Gould, "Reassuring News About AIDS: A Doctor Tells Why *You* May Not Be at Risk," *Cosmopolitan*, January 1988. That such articles are based on racist and homophobic assumptions goes without saying. The "fragile anus/rugged vagina" thesis is generally trotted out to explain not only the differences between rates of infection in gays and straights, but also between blacks and whites, Africans and Americans (blacks are said to resort to anal sex as a primitive form of birth control). But Gould's racism takes him a step further. Claiming that only "rough" sex can result in transmission through the vagina, Gould writes, "Many men in Africa take their women in a brutal way, so that some heterosexual activity regarded as normal by them would be closer to rape by our standards and therefore be likely to cause vaginal lacerations through which the AIDS virus [*sic*] could gain entry into the bloodstream."
23.   Cindy Patton tells of similar advice given to gay men by a CDC official at the 1985 International AIDS Conference in Atlanta: "He suggested that gay men only have sex with men of the same antibody status, as if gay male culture is little more than a giant dating service. This advice was quickly seen as dehumanizing and not useful because it did not promote safe sex, but renewed advice of this type is seen as reasonable within the heterosexual community of late" ("Resistance and the Erotic," p. 69).
24.   Ulene, p. 49.

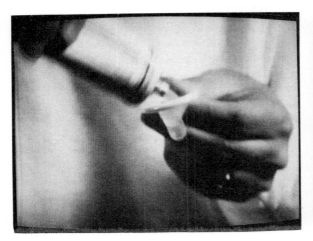
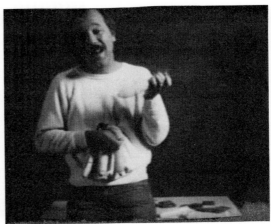

AIDSfilms. AIDS: Changing the Rules. *1987.*

get the condom on the cock. It appears to be a foregone conclusion that there is no use even trying to get straight men to take this responsibility themselves (the title of a recent book is *How to Persuade Your Lover to Use a Condom . . . And Why You Should*). The one exception is a segment of the video aired on PBS entitled *AIDS: Changing the Rules,* in which Rubén Blades talks to men directly, though very coyly, about condoms, but shows them only how to put one on a banana. Evidently condoms have now become too closely associated with gay men for straight men to talk straight about them. In addition, they have become too closely associated with AIDS for the banana companies to approve of *Changing the Rules*'s choice of props. The following letter was sent by the president of the International Banana Association to the president of PBS; I cite it to give some idea of how hilarious—if it weren't so deadly—the condom debate can be.

Dear Mr. Christiansen,

In this program, a banana is used as a substitute for a human penis in a demonstration of how condoms should be used.

I must tell you, Mr. Christiansen, as I have told representatives of WETA, that our industry finds such usage of our product to be totally unacceptable. The choice of a banana rather than some other inanimate prop constitutes arbitrary and reckless disregard for the unsavory association that will be drawn by the public and the damage to our industry that will result therefrom.

The banana is an important product and deserves to be treated with respect and consideration. It is the most extensively consumed fruit in the United States, being purchased by over 98 percent of

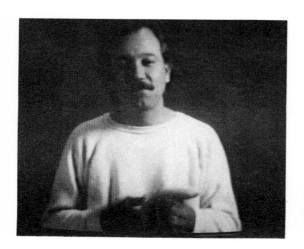 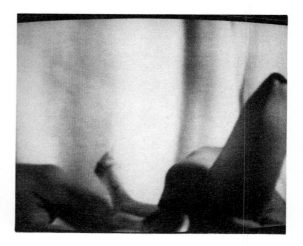

households. It is important to the economies of many developing Latin American nations. The banana's continued image in the minds of consumers as a healthful and nutritious product is critically important to the industry's continued ability to be held in such high regard by the public and to discharge its responsibilities to its Latin American hosts. . . .

Mr. Christiansen, I have no alternative but to advise you that we intend to hold PBS fully responsible for any and all damages sustained by our industry as a result of the showing of this AIDS program depicting the banana in the associational context planned. Further, we reserve all legal rights to protect the industry's interests from this arbitrary, unnecessary, and insensitive action.

Yours very truly,
Robert M. Moore

The debate about condoms, and safe sex education generally, is one of the most alarming in the history of the AIDS epidemic thus far, because it will certainly result in many more thousands of deaths that could be avoided. It demonstrates how practices devised at the grass-roots level to meet the needs of people at risk can be demeaned, distorted, and ultimately destroyed when those practices are coopted by state power. Perhaps no portion of this controversy is as revealing as the October 14, 1987, debate over the Helms amendment.[25]

In presenting his amendment to the Senate, Helms made the off-hand remark, "Now we had all this mob over here this weekend, which was itself a

25.   Unless otherwise indicated, all quotations of this debate are taken from the *Congressional Record*, October 14, 1987, pp. S14202–S14220.

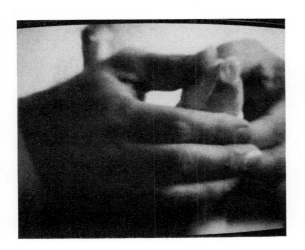
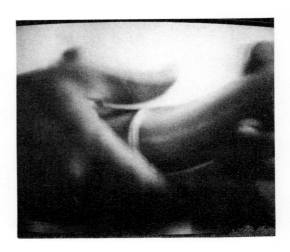

disheartening spectacle." He was referring to the largest civil rights demonstration in US history, in which over half a million people, led by PWAs and their friends, marched on Washington for lesbian and gay rights. Early in the morning before the march, the Names Project inaugurated its memorial quilt, whose panels with the names of people who had died of AIDS occupied a space on the Mall equivalent to two football fields. As the three-by-six-foot cloth panels made by friends, family, and admirers of the dead were carefully unfurled, 1,920 names were solemnly read to a crowd of weeping spectators. Though representing only a small percentage of the people who have died in the epidemic, the seemingly endless litany of names, together with the astonishing size of the quilt, brought home the enormity of our loss so dramatically as to leave everyone stunned.

But to Helms and his ilk this was just a "mob" enacting a "disheartening spectacle." In the following month's issue of the right-wing *Campus Review*, a front-page article by Gary Bauer, assistant to President Reagan and spokesperson for the Administration's AIDS policy, was accompanied by a political cartoon entitled "The AIDS Quilt." It depicts a faggot and a junkie sewing panels bearing the words *sodomy* and *IV Drugs*. Bauer's article explains:

> "Safe sex" campaigns are not giving students the full story about AIDS. Indeed many students are arguably being denied the information that is most likely to assist them in avoiding the AIDS virus [*sic*]. . . . Many of today's education efforts are what could be called "sexually egalitarian." That is, they refuse to distinguish or even appear to prefer one type of sexual practice over another. Yet medical research shows that sodomy is probably the most efficient method to transfer the AIDS virus [*sic*] as well as other diseases—for obvious

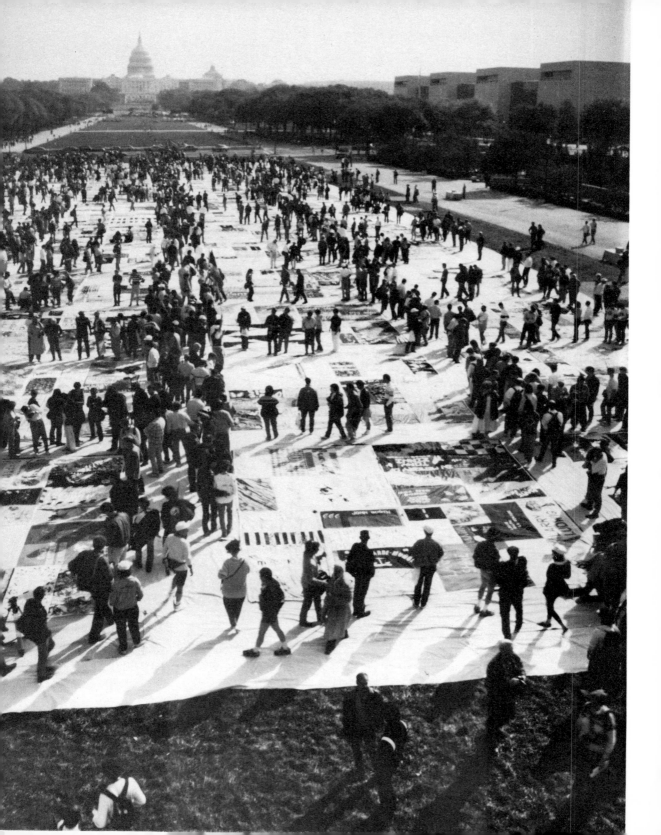

Campus Review

Volume 3 Number 8   The right side of the story   November 1987

AIDS and the College Student

Editor's note: Earlier this month an AIDS awareness class was sponsored by the rhetoric department at the University of Iowa. Rhetoric classes are required of nearly all U.I. students, and some instructors made the AIDS class mandatory. A university official told Campus Review that the program was rammed through by pressure from the university's gay community.

Thus we offer this article from a White House official as a balance to the often one-sided presentation that so many students were subjected to.

by Gary Bauer,
Assistant to the President

On hundreds of college and university campuses this year, students have returned not only to be greeted by the usual panoply of activities and issues, but also by a new crusade — safe sex. Reacting to the growing national

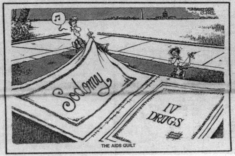

THE AIDS QUILT

to be aimed at promoting the most obvious and effective measure to slow down the AIDS epidemic.— abstinence. Yet, as Surgeon General C. Everett Koop has indicated time and time again, abstinence is the only foolproof way to avoid this disease. Are we to assume that highly educated young Americans are so enslaved by their passions that they are unable to limit their number of partners or sexual activities — even if failing to do so risks death? Actually, much research shows that many students do abstain or establish a mutual faithful relationship, with marriage as the long-term goal. Why the hesitancy to build on these healthy tendencies, particularly when the issue is life or death?

Second, many of today's educational efforts are what could be called "sexually egalitarian." That is, they refuse to distinguish or even appear to prefer one type of sexual practice over another. Yet medical research shows that sodomy is

reasons. Why is this information censored on so many campuses? Does it illustrate the growing power of gay rights activists who not only want to be tolerated, but want the culture at large to affirm and support the legitimacy of the gay life-style?[26]

Three days after the historic march on Washington and the inauguration of the Names Project, Jesse Helms would seek to ensure that such affirmation and support would never occur — at least in the context of AIDS. The senator from North Carolina introduced his amendment to a Labor, Health and Human Services, and Education bill allocating nearly a billion dollars for AIDS research and education in fiscal 1988. Amendment no. 956 began:

> Purpose: To prohibit the use of any funds provided under this Act to the Centers for Disease Control from being used to provide AIDS education, information, or prevention materials and activities that promote, encourage, or condone homosexual sexual activities or the intravenous use of illegal drugs.

26.   Gary Bauer, "AIDS and the College Student," *Campus Review*, November 1987, pp. 1, 12.

Inauguration of the Names Project Quilt, 1987. (Photo: Jane Rosett.)

GMHC. Safer Sex Comix #4. *Artwork by Donelan.*
Story by Greg.

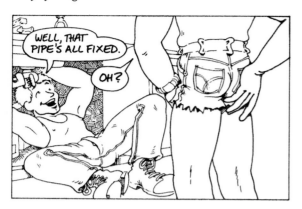 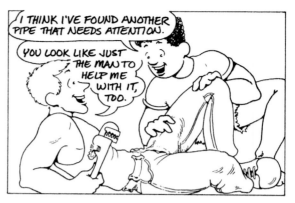

The "need" for the amendment and the terms of the ensuing debate (involving only two other senators) were established by Helms in his opening remarks:

> About 2 months ago, I received a copy of some AIDS comic books that are being distributed by the Gay Men's Health Crisis, Inc., of New York City, an organization which has received $674,679 in Federal dollars for so-called AIDS education and information. These comic books told the story, in graphic detail, of the sexual encounter of two homosexual men.
>
> The comic books do not encourage and change [*sic*] any of the perverted behavior. In fact, the comic book promotes sodomy and the homosexual lifestyle as an acceptable alternative in American society. . . . I believe that if the American people saw these books, they would be on the verge of revolt.
>
> I obtained one copy of this book and I had photostats made for about 15 or 20 Senators. I sent each of the Senators a copy—if you will forgive the expression—in a brown envelope marked "Personal and Confidential, for Senator's Eyes Only." Without exception, the Senators were revolted, and they suggested to me that President Reagan ought to know what is being done under the pretense of AIDS education.
>
> So, about 10 days ago, I went down to the White House and I visited with the President.
>
> I said, "Mr. President, I don't want to ruin your day, but I feel obliged to hand you this and let you look at what is being distributed under the pretense of AIDS educational material. . . ."
>
> The President opened the book, looked at a couple of pages, and shook his head, and hit his desk with his fist.

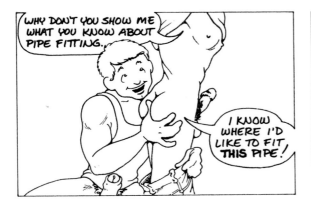

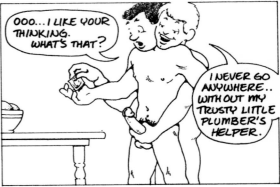

Helms goes on to describe, with even greater disdain, the grant application with which GMHC sought federal funds (none of which were, in any case, spent on the production of the safe-sex comics). GMHC's proposal involved what any college-level psychology student would understand as prerequisite to the very difficult task of helping people change their sexual habits. Helms read GMHC's statement of the problem:

> As gay men have reaffirmed their gay identity through sexual expression, recommendations to change sexual behavior may be seen as oppressive. For many, safe sex has been equated with boring, unsatisfying sex. Meaningful alternatives are often not realized. These perceived barriers must be considered and alternatives to high-risk practices promoted in the implementation of AIDS risk-reduction education.

After reading this thoroughly *un*extraordinary statement, Helms fumes:

> This Senator is not a goody-goody two-shoes. I have lived a long time. I have seen a lot of things. I have served 4 years in the Navy. I have been around the track. But every Christian, religious, moral ethic within me cries out to do something. It is embarrassing to stand on the Senate floor and talk about the details of this travesty.

Throughout the floor debate, Helms continued in this vein:

> —We have got to call a spade a spade and a perverted human being a perverted human being.

> —Every AIDS case can be traced back to a homosexual act.

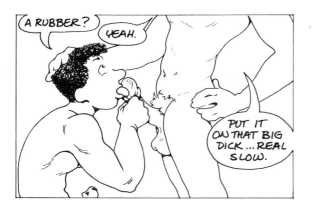
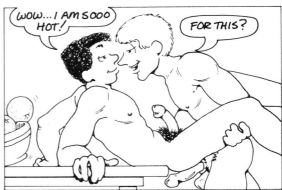

—It [the amendment] will force this country to slam the door on the wayward, warped sexual revolution which has ravaged this Nation for the past quarter of a century.[27]

—I think we need to do some AIDS testing on a broad level and unless we get around to that and stop talking about all of this business of civil rights, and so forth, we will not stop the spread of AIDS. We used to quarantine for typhoid fever and scarlet fever, and it did not ruin the civil liberties of anybody to do that.

There were, all told, two responses on the Senate floor to Helms's amendment. The first came from Senator Chiles of Florida, who worried about the amendment's inclusion of IV drug users among those to whom education would effectively be prevented by the legislation — worried because this group includes heterosexuals:

I like to talk about heterosexuals. That is getting into my neighborhood. That is getting into where it can be involved with people that I know and love and care about, and that is where it is getting to children. And again, these children, when you think about a child as an AIDS victim, there is just no reason in the world that should happen. And so we have to try to do what we can to prevent it.

The ritual hand-wringing sentiments about innocent children with AIDS pervade the debate, as they pervade the discussion of AIDS everywhere. This

27.   Compare Larry Kramer's character Ned Weeks's statement: "You don't know what it's been like since the sexual revolution hit this country. It's been crazy, gay or straight" (p. 36).

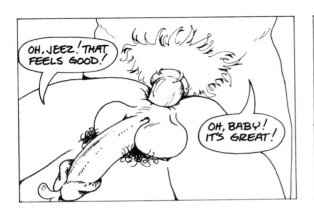

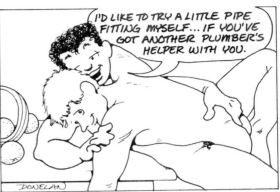

unquestioned sentiment must be seen for what it is: *a vicious apportioning of degrees of guilt and innocence to people with AIDS*. It reflects, in addition, our society's extreme devaluation of life and experience. (The hypocrisy of this distorted set of values does not, however, translate into funding for such necessities for the welfare of children as prenatal care, child care, education, and so forth.)

Because Chiles only liked to talk about heterosexuals, it was left to Senator Weicker of Connecticut to defend safe sex education for gay people. "It is not easy to stand up in the face of language such as this and oppose it," said Weicker, "but I do." Weicker's defense was not made any easier by the fact that he knew what he was talking about: "I know exactly the material that the Senator from North Carolina is referring to. I have seen it. I think it is demeaning in every way." And later, ". . . this is as repugnant to me as it is to anybody else." Because Weicker finds innocuous little drawings of gay male sex as demeaning and repugnant as the North Carolina senator does, he must resort to "science" to oppose Helms's " philosophy":[28] "We better do exactly what we have been told to do by those of science and medicine, which is, No. 1, put our money into research and, No. 2, put our money into education." "The comic book," says Weicker, "has nothing to do with the issue at hand."

28.   In the Senate debate, positions such as Helms's are referred to as philosophical. Thus Senator Weicker: "This education process has been monkeyed around with long enough by this administration. This subcommittee over 6 months ago allocated $20 million requested by the Centers for Disease Control for an educational mailer to be mailed to every household in the United States. . . . That is yet to be done. It is yet to be done not because of anybody in the Centers for Disease Control, or not anybody in Secretary [of Health and Human Services] Bowen's office, but because the philosophers in the White House decided they did not want a mailer to go to every household in the United States. So the education effort is set back" (*Congressional Record*, October 14, 1987, p. S14206).

But of course the comic book has everything to do with the issue at hand—because it is precisely the sort of safe sex education material that has been proven to work, developed by the organization that has produced the greatest amount of safe sex education material of any in the country, including, of course, the federal government.[29]

Given the degree of Senate agreement that gay men's safe sex education material was "garbage," in Helms's word, it seemed possible to compromise enough on the amendment's language to please all three participants in the debate. The amendment was thus reworded to eliminate any reference to IV drug users, thereby assuaging Senator Chiles's fears that someone he knows and cares about—or someone in his neighborhood, or at least someone he doesn't mind talking about—could be affected. Helms very reluctantly agreed to strike the word *condone*, but managed to add *directly or indirectly* after *promote or encourage* and before *homosexual sexual activity*. Thus the amendment now reads:

> . . . none of the funds made available under this Act to the Centers for Disease Control shall be used to provide AIDS education, information, or prevention materials and activities that promote or encourage, directly or indirectly, homosexual sexual activities.

After further, very brief debate, during which Weicker continued to oppose the amendment, a roll-call vote was taken. Two senators—Weicker and Moynihan—voted against; *ninety-four senators voted for the Helms amendment*, including all other Senate sponsors of the federal gay and lesbian civil rights bill. Senator Kennedy perhaps voiced the opinion of his fellow liberal senators when he said, "The current version [the reworded amendment] is toothless and it can in good conscience be supported by the Senate. It may not do any good, but it will not do any harm." Under the amendment, as passed, most AIDS organizations providing education and services to gay men, the group most affected and, thus far, at

---

29. "George Rutherford of the San Francisco Department of Public Health last year told a US Congressional Committee investigating AIDS that the spread of the virus dramatically slowed in 1983, when public health education programmes directed at gay men began. The year before, 21 percent of the unexposed gay population had developed antibodies to HIV, indicating that they had been exposed to the virus over the previous three months. But in 1983, that figure plummeted to 2 percent. In 1986 it was 0.8 percent, and researchers expect that it will continue to fall. . . . The campaigns to promote safe sex among gay men, and educate them about AIDS have been almost totally successful in less than four years. Such rapid changes in behaviour contrast sharply with the poor response over the past 25 years from smokers to warnings about the risks to their health from cigarettes" ("'Safe Sex' Stops the Spread of AIDS," *New Science*, January 7, 1988, p. 36).

In a study of the efficacy of various forms of safe sex education materials, commissioned by GMHC and conducted by Dr. Michael Quadland, professor of psychiatry at Mount Sinai School of Medicine, it was determined that explicit, erotic films are more effective than other techniques. Dr. Quadland was quoted as saying, "We know that in trying to get people to change risky behavior, stopping smoking, for example, or wearing seat belts, that fear is effective. But sex is different. People cannot just give sex up" (Gina Kolata, "Erotic Films in AIDS Study Cut Risky Behavior," *New York Times*, November 3, 1987).

highest risk in the epidemic, would no longer qualify for federal funding.[30] Founded and directed by gay men, the Gay Men's Health Crisis is hardly likely to stop "promoting or encouraging, directly or indirectly, homosexual sexual activity." Despite the fact that GMHC is the oldest and largest AIDS service organization in the US; despite the fact that it provides direct services to thousands of people living with AIDS, whether gay men or not; despite the fact that GMHC's safe sex comics are nothing more scandalous than simple, schematically depicted scenarios of gay male safe sex; despite the fact that they have undoubtedly helped save thousands of lives — GMHC is considered unworthy of federal funding.

When we see how compromised any efforts at responding to AIDS will be when conducted by the state, we are forced to recognize that all productive practices concerning AIDS will remain at the grass-roots level. At stake is the cultural specificity and sensitivity of these practices, as well as their ability to take account of psychic resistance to behavioral changes, especially changes involving behaviors as psychically complex and charged as sexuality and drug use.[31] Government officials, school board members, public health officers, Catholic cardinals insist that AIDS education must be sensitive to "community values." But the values they have in mind are those of no existing community affected by AIDS. When "community values" are invoked, it is only for the purpose of *imposing* the purported values of those (thus far) unaffected by AIDS on the people (thus far) most affected. Instead of the specific, concrete languages of those whose behaviors put them at risk for AIDS, "community values" require a "universal" language that no one speaks and many do not understand. "Don't exchange bodily fluids" is nobody's spoken language. "Don't come in his ass" or "pull out before you come" is what *we* say. "If you have mainlined or skinpopped now or in the past you may be at risk of getting AIDS. If you have shared needles, cookers, syringes, eyedroppers, water, or cotton with anyone, you are at risk of getting AIDS."[32] This is not abstract "community values" talking. This is the language of members of the IV drug using community. It is therefore essential that the word *community* be reclaimed by those to whom it belongs, and that abstract

30.   After the House of Representatives passed the amendment by a vote of 368–47, a full-scale lobbying effort was undertaken by AIDS organizations and gay activists to defeat it in House-Senate Conference Committee. Ultimately, the amendment was retained as written, although *indirectly* was stricken and the following rider added: "The language in the bill should not be construed to prohibit descriptions of methods to reduce the risk of HIV transmission, to limit eligibility for federal funds of a grantee or potential grantee because of its nonfederally funded activities, nor shall it be construed to limit counseling or referrals to agencies that are not federally funded."
31.   Richard Goldstein has written about the necessity to take account of the social and psychic dimensions of IV drug use in trying to bring about behavior changes: "Rescuing the IV-user may involve some of the same techniques that have worked in the gay community. The sharing of needles must be understood in the same context as anal sex — as an ecstatic act that enhances social solidarity" ("AIDS and the Social Contract," *Village Voice*, December 29, 1987, p. 19).
32.   Quoted from a pamphlet issued by ADAPT (Association for Drug Abuse Prevention and Treatment), Brooklyn, New York.

usages of such terms be vigorously contested. "Community values" are, in fact, just what we need, but they must be the values of our actual communities, not those of some abstract, universalized community that does not and cannot exist.

One curious aspect of AIDS education campaigns devised by advertising agencies contracted by governments is their failure to take into account any aspect of the psychic but fear. An industry that has used sexual desire to sell everything from cars to detergents suddenly finds itself at a loss for how to sell a condom. This paralysis in the face of sex itself on the part of our most sophisticated producers of propaganda is perhaps partially explained by the strictures placed on the industry by the contracting governments—by their notion of "community values"—but it is also to be explained by advertising's construction of its audience only as a group of largely undifferentiated consumers.

In *Policing Desire*, Watney writes of the British government's AIDS propaganda campaign, produced for them by the world's largest advertising firm, Saatchi and Saatchi:

> Advertisements spelled out the word "AIDS" in seasonal gift wrapping paper, together with the accompanying question: "How many people will get it for Christmas?" Another advert conveys the message that "Your next sexual partner could be that very special person"—framed inside a heart like a Valentine—with a supplement beneath which tersely adds, "The one that gives you AIDS." The official line is clearly anti-sex, and draws on an assumed rhetoric from previous AIDS commentary concerning "promiscuity" as the supposed "cause" of AIDS.[33]

Similar ploys were used for ads paid for by the Metropolitan Life Insurance Company and posted throughout the New York City subway system by the city health department. One is a blow-up of a newspaper personals section with an appealing notice circled (intended to be appealing, that is, to a heterosexual woman) and the statement "I got AIDS through the personals." The other is a cartoon of a man and woman in bed, each with a thought bubble saying "I hope he [she] doesn't have AIDS!" And below: "You can't live on hope."

"What's the big secret?" asked the poster that was pasted over the city's worse-than-useless warnings, "You can protect yourself from AIDS." And, below, carefully designed and worded safe sex and clean works information. This was a guerrilla action by an AIDS activist group calling itself the Metropolitan Health Association (MHA), whose members also pasted strips printed with the words *government inaction* over *the personals* or *hope* to work the changes "I got AIDS from government inaction" or "You can't live on government inaction." But saving lives is clearly less important to the city than protecting the

33.   Watney, p. 136.

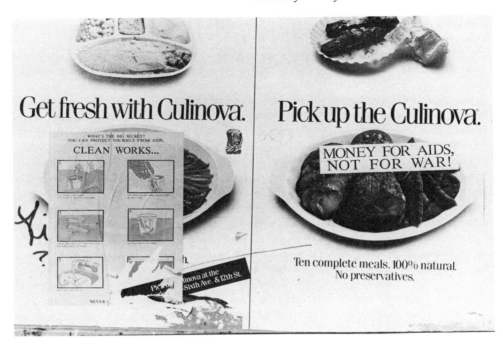

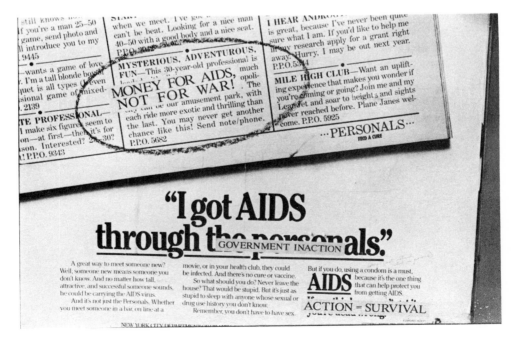

transit authority's advertising space, so MHA's "reinformation" was quickly removed.[34]

The city health department's scare tactics were next directed at teenagers —and specifically teenagers of color—in a series of public service announcements made for television. Using a strategy of enticement followed by blunt and brutal admonishment, one of these shows scenes of heavy petting in cars and alleys over a sound track of the pop song "Boom Boom": "Let's go back to my room so we can do it all night and you can make me feel right." Suddenly the music cuts out and the scene changes to a shot of a boy wrapped in a blanket, looking frightened, miserable, and ill. A voice-over warns, "If you have sex with someone who has the AIDS virus [sic], you can get it, too. So before you do it, ask yourself how bad you really want it. Don't ask for AIDS, don't get it." The final phrase serves as a title for the series—"AIDS: Don't get it." The confusion of antecedents for *it*—both sex and AIDS—is, of course, deliberate. With a clever linguistic maneuver, the health department tells kids that sex and AIDS are the same thing. But the ability of these PSAs to shock their intended audience is based not only on this manipulative language and quick edit from scenes of sexual pleasure to the close-up of a face with KS lesions on it—the media's standard "face of AIDS." The real shock comes because images of sexy teenagers and sounds of a disco beat are usually followed on TV by Pepsi Cola and a voice telling you to get it. One can only wonder about the degree of psychic damage that might result from the PSAs' substitution. But AIDS will not be prevented by psychic damage to teenagers caused by ads on TV. It will only be stopped by respecting and celebrating their pleasure in sex and by telling them exactly what they need and want to know in order to maintain that pleasure.

> The ADS epidemic
> Is sweeping the nation
> Acquired dread of sex
>
> Fear and panic
> In the whole population
> Acquired dread of sex
>
> This is not a Death in Venice
> It's a cheap, unholy menace
> Please ignore the moral message
> This is not a Death in Venice

---

34.   I borrow the term *reinformation* from Michael Eisenmenger and Diane Neumaier, who coined it to describe cultural practices whose goal is to counter the disinformation to which we are all constantly subject.

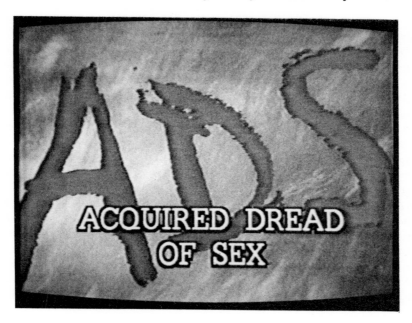

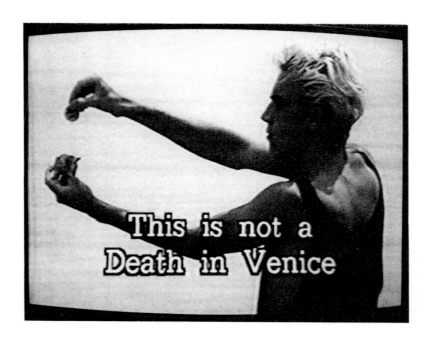

This is the refrain of John Greyson's music-video parody of *Death in Venice*. The plague in Greyson's version of the tale is ADS, acquired dread of sex — something you can get from, among other things, watching TV. Tadzio is a pleasure-loving blonde who discovers that condoms are "his very favorite thing to wear," and Aschenbach is a middle-class bigot who, observing the sexy shenanigans of Tadzio and his boyfriend, succumbs to acquired dread of sex. Made for a thirty-six-monitor video wall in the Square One shopping mall in Mississauga, a suburb of Toronto, *The ADS Epidemic*, like the PSAs just described, is directed at adolescents and appropriates a format they're used to, but in this case the message is both pro-sex and made for the kids most seriously at risk — sexually active gay boys. The playfulness of Greyson's tape should not obscure this immensely important fact: not a single piece of government-sponsored education about AIDS for young people, in Canada or the US, has been targeted at a gay audience, even though governments never tire of emphasizing the statistics showing that the overwhelming numbers of reported cases of AIDS occur in gay and bisexual men.

The impulse to counteract the sex-negative messages of the advertising industry's PSAs also informs British filmmaker Isaac Julien's *This Is Not an AIDS Advertisement*.[35] There is no hint of a didactic message here, but rather an attempt to give voice to the complexities of gay subjectivity and experience at a critical historical moment. In Julien's case, the specific experience is that of a black gay man living in the increasingly racist and homophobic atmosphere of Thatcher's Britain.[36] Using footage shot in Venice and London, *This Is Not an AIDS Advertisement* is divided into two parts, the first elegiac, lyrical; the second, building upon and repeating images from the first, paced to a Bronski Beat rock song. Images of gay male sexual desire are coupled with the song's refrain, "This is not an AIDS advertisement. Feel no guilt in your desire."

Greyson's and Julien's videos signal a new phase in gay men's responses to the epidemic. Having learned to support and grieve for our lovers and friends; having joined the fight against fear, hatred, repression, and inaction; having adjusted our sex lives so as to protect ourselves and one another — we are now reclaiming our subjectivities, our communities, our culture . . . and our promiscuous love of sex.

---

35.   Available through Third World Newsreel, New York City.
36.   In late 1987, a Helms-style anti-gay clause was inserted in Britain's Local Government Bill. Clause 28 says, "A local authority shall not (a) promote homosexuality or publish material for the promotion of homosexuality; (b) promote the teaching in any maintained school of the acceptability of homosexuality as a pretended family relationship by the publication of such material or otherwise; and (c) give financial assistance to any person for either of the purposes referred to in paragraphs (a) and (b) above." Unlike the Helms Amendment, however, the British bill, though a more sweeping prohibition of pro-gay materials, specifically forbids the use of the bill "to prohibit the doing of anything for the purpose of treating or preventing the spread of disease."

Isaac Julien. This Is Not an AIDS Advertisement.
1987.

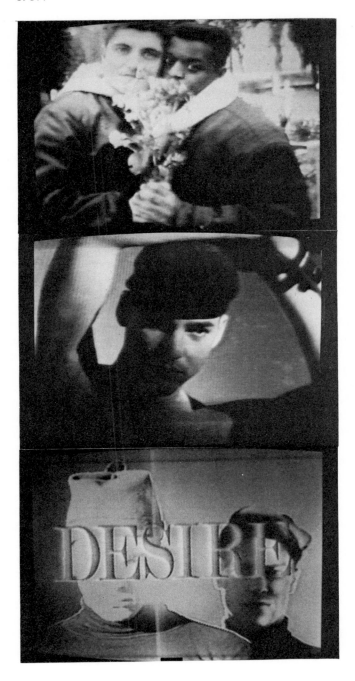

Contributors

LEO BERSANI is Professor of French at the University of California, Berkeley. His most recent books are *The Forms of Violence* (with Ulysse Dutoit) and *The Freudian Body*.

GREGG BORDOWITZ is a member of the Testing the Limits collective and of ACT UP (AIDS Coalition to Unleash Power). His video *Some Aspects of a Shared Lifestyle* was shown at the 1987 American Film Institute Video Festival.

JOHN BORNEMAN, a doctoral candidate in social anthropology at Harvard, is currently conducting research in West Berlin.

MARTHA GEVER is editor of *The Independent*, a film and video monthly, and has published widely on issues of the media.

SANDER L. GILMAN is Goldwin Smith Professor of Humane Studies at Cornell University and, for the spring semester of 1988, Mellon Visiting Professor of Humanities at Tulane University. His most recent books are *Oscar Wilde's London* and *Disease and Representation*.

JAN ZITA GROVER teaches a course entitled Media(ted) AIDS at the California Institute of the Arts. She spent a year as an AIDS volunteer in San Francisco and currently works as medical editor of an AIDS textbook at San Francisco General Hospital/University of California, San Francisco.

AMBER HOLLIBAUGH is Video Producer/Educator in the AIDS Discrimination Unit of the New York City Commission on Human Rights. A founding member of the San Francisco Lesbian and Gay History Project, her writing has appeared in *Pleasure and Danger, The Politics of Desire, Socialist Visions,* and *All-American Women*.

MITCHELL KARP is Supervising Attorney in the AIDS Discrimination Unit of the New York City Commission on Human Rights and a member of the board of directors of Men of All Colors Together, New York.

CAROL LEIGH, a member of COYOTE, is a contributor to the anthology *Sex Work: Writings by Women in the Sex Industry.* As a performance artist, her current work is devoted to AIDS organizing and safe sex education for prostitutes.

MAX NAVARRE, a founding member of the PWA Coalition, is the editor of their monthly *Newsline*. He was the first publicly identified person with AIDS to serve on the Gay Men's Health Crisis executive board.

SUKI PORTS, a longtime community activist, was Executive Director of the New York City Minority Task Force on AIDS from its inception in November 1985 until November 1987.

KATY TAYLOR is Deputy Director of the AIDS Discrimination Unit of the New York City Commission on Human Rights. Formerly with the Working Women's Institute, she was a member of the editorial collective of the *Heresies* issue on women and violence and is currently on the board of the Lesbian and Gay Anti-Violence Project.

PAULA A. TREICHLER teaches in the medical school and in communications at the University of Illinois, Urbana. The coauthor of *A Feminist Dictionary* and coeditor of *For Alma Mater: Theory and Practice of Feminist Scholarship*, she is currently at work on a study of AIDS and language.

SIMON WATNEY serves on the board of the Health Education Committee of the Terrence Higgens Trust, a London-based AIDS service organization. He is the author of *Policing Desire: AIDS, Pornography, and the Media*, recently published by the University of Minnesota Press.

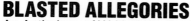

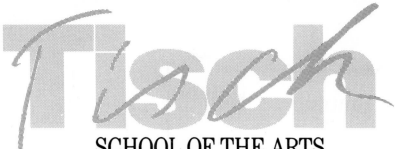

SCHOOL OF THE ARTS

Film scholarship demands the finest resources.

We provide them.

The Department of Cinema Studies at the Tisch School of the Arts, New York University, offers graduate students the resources essential to the scholarly study of film. Our M.A. and Ph.D. programs in cinema studies provide:

■ Rigorous study of history, criticism, and aesthetics

■ Exposure to new methodologies— semiotics, psychoanalysis, structuralism, and post-structuralism

■ Personal viewing/study facilities— flatbeds, analytic projector, and video equipment

■ Access to materials—the department's own holdings; rare material from the William Everson Collection, the Museum of Modern Art, and New York City's many cinemas, libraries, and archives.

Our faculty includes Jay Leyda, Annette Michelson, William K. Everson, Robert Sklar, William Simon, and Robert Stam.

For information, call (212) 998-1600.

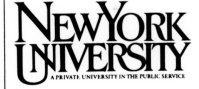

NEW YORK UNIVERSITY
A PRIVATE UNIVERSITY IN THE PUBLIC SERVICE

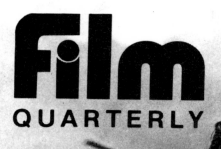